Technology in Physical Activity and Health Promotion

As technology becomes an ever more prevalent part of everyday life and population-based physical activity programmes seek new ways to increase lifelong engagement with physical activity, so the two have become increasingly linked. This book offers a thorough, critical examination of emerging technologies in physical activity and health, considering technological interventions within the dominant theoretical frameworks, exploring the challenges of integrating technology into physical activity promotion and offering solutions for its implementation.

Technology in Physical Activity and Health Promotion occupies a broadly positive stance toward interactive technology initiatives and, while discussing some negative implications of an increased use of technology, offers practical recommendations for promoting physical activity through a range of media, including:

- social media
- mobile apps
- global positioning and geographic information systems
- wearables
- active video games (exergaming)
- virtual reality settings.

Offering a logical and clear critique of technology in physical activity and health promotion, this book will serve as an essential reference for upper-level undergraduates, postgraduate students and scholars working in public health, physical activity and health and kinesiology, and healthcare professionals.

Zan Gao is a faculty member at the School of Kinesiology in the University of Minnesota-Twin Cities, USA, specializing in physical activity and health. His research has primarily focused on promoting health through population-based physical activity interventions with emerging technologies, such as active video games, online social media and mobile device apps.

Routledge Research in Physical Activity and Health

The *Routledge Research in Physical Activity and Health* series offers a multidisciplinary forum for cutting-edge research in the broad area of physical activity, exercise and health. Showcasing the work of emerging and established scholars working in areas ranging from physiology and chronic disease, psychology and mental health to physical activity and health promotion and socio-economic and cultural aspects of physical activity participation, the series is an important channel for ground-breaking research in physical activity and health.

Physical Activity and the Gastro-Intestinal Tract
Responses in Health and Disease
Roy J. Shephard

Technology in Physical Activity and Health Promotion
Edited by Zan Gao

Technology in Physical Activity and Health Promotion

Edited by Zan Gao

Routledge
Taylor & Francis Group
LONDON AND NEW YORK

First published 2017 by Routledge

2 Park Square, Milton Park, Abingdon, Oxfordshire OX14 4RN
52 Vanderbilt Avenue, New York, NY 10017

Routledge is an imprint of the Taylor & Francis Group, an informa business

First issued in paperback 2019

British Library Cataloguing in Publication Data
A catalogue record for this book is available from the British Library

Library of Congress Cataloging in Publication Data
A catalog record for this book has been requested

ISBN: 978-1-138-69576-4 (hbk)
ISBN: 978-0-367-37449-5 (pbk)

Typeset in Times New Roman
by Wearset Ltd, Boldon, Tyne and Wear

Contents

Illustrations

Figures

Table

Contributors

Zan Gao is a faculty member at the School of Kinesiology in the University of Minnesota-Twin Cities, USA, specializing in physical activity and health. His research has primarily focused on promoting health through population-based physical activity interventions with emerging technologies such as active video games, online social media and mobile device apps. Gao has been the principal investigator of National Institute of Health research grants, and of the Robert Wood Johnson Foundation Grant. He has published more than 100 research articles in peer-reviewed journals, and book chapters.

Jung Eun Lee is an Assistant Professor at the University of Minnesota at Duluth, USA. Her research interests are the psychological correlates of physical activity, technology-based physical activity promotion, and motor skill enhancement.

Zachary Pope is a researcher focused on the use of smartphone applications, wearable tech, GPS/GIS, and active video games in health promotion across diverse populations. Other interests include epidemiological studies of the antecedents/correlates of physical activity participation.

Haichun Sun is an Associate Professor at the University of South Florida, USA. Her research focuses on children and adolescent physical activity program design and evaluation as related to the physical, cognitive, and motivational domains.

Nan Zeng is a researcher focused on the behavior aspects of physical activity, such as physical activity intervention and health promotion in a diverse array of populations using modern technology, including but not limited to active video games, fitness wristband, and smartphone applications.

Preface

In the past decades, research has documented the numerous benefits of regular physical activity participation, such as preventing obesity and diabetes, treating mental problems, preventing falls among the elderly, and decreasing chronic heart diseases. However, nowadays, most young people and adults are not active regularly, and in many countries they tend to discontinue structured physical activity programs, especially those underserved populations with limited resources in the developed countries. Given the fact that many physical activity interventions were not as effective as expected in the past, population-based physical activity programs (i.e., working site, after-school programs) have taken an approach more aligned with public health in recent years. With this public health emphasis has come the search for activity modalities which can impact individuals' lifelong physical activity participation and physical activity determinants, such as self-efficacy and social support. As technology continues to become ever more pervasive in our daily lives, and is of great interest to this generation, professionals have begun to integrate emerging technology not only into population-based physical activity programs to promote health, but also into assessment methods of individuals' physical activity, fitness, and health.

Early integration of technology within the population-based physical activity programs involved video cameras and audio players, but the advent of new interactive technology including new generations of active video gaming (a.k.a., exergaming; e.g., Wii, Xbox), smartphone/tablet-based applications (a.k.a., apps), global positioning systems (GPS), among others, has offered new opportunities for studying and applying this technology to the field of physical activity and health. For example, new generations of active video games have seen a rapid rate of growth in physical activity settings over the past decade. We currently live in a digital world—encompassed by technology in a diverse array of settings. In fact, the current youth generation's leisure time is increasingly spent on mobile devices, using apps, playing video games, texting, and perusing social media. It is almost as if the majority of our leisure time is consumed interacting with screen-based technology. Therefore, it is only logical to ask how the omnipresence of screen-based technology impacts our lifestyles, health, and fitness. Further, what does this technology-laden environment mean with regard to exercising in a digital world?

In response, this book has been written to help the audience exercise regularly with the use of emerging technologies, in addition to exploring the challenges of integrating new interactive and emerging technology in promoting physical activity and health—addressing core problems and offering practical and meaningful implications for health professionals. Developing emerging technology to promote physical activity participation, while also studying human-technology interaction in physical activity and health, has the potential to have a clear and important impact on improving the effectiveness of physical activity and healthcare programs—ultimately improving the health status and quality of life among various populations.

In summary, *Technology in Physical Activity and Health Promotion* offers novel contributions in the following ways:

1 This book will critically scrutinize the latest development of emerging technologies in the past decade, and will demonstrate the important role that emerging technologies play in a grand societal challenge toward improved health and wellbeing.
2 Instead of concentrating on the potentially negative health impact and risks a digital world poses, this book will counter with information on how to integrate apps, active video games, social media, and other technologies in a manner capable of promoting physical activity and health. This book will provide individualized physical activity prescriptions capable of being adopted in and integrated with a digital world—steering away from prescribing a blanket solution to the integration of emerging technology in promoting health and physically active lifestyles.
3 This book features a unique assemblage of several widely used theoretical frameworks in promoting physical activity and behavioral changes relevant to technology interventions, including the Self-efficacy Theory, the Self-determination Theory, the Transtheoretical Model, Social Cognitive Theory, and the Social Ecologic Model.
4 Although academic in nature, this book will still be written in an inclusive manner for use by scholars, graduate/undergraduate students, and healthcare professionals.

Part I

Introduction to emerging technology and physical activity health

1 Foundations of technology and health effects of physical activity

Zan Gao, Zachary Pope, and Nan Zeng

Take a look around the room in which you are currently sitting. What do you see? Most likely, you see a smartphone, maybe a tablet and/or laptop, and a television. Maybe you are a fan of video games and have a gaming console in the room as well. Regardless of the presence of one or more of these items in your room, however, all of these technologies serve various purposes in your life. Your smartphone and tablet/laptop allow you to connect with friends and do work. Conversely, your television and gaming console allow for entertainment and relaxation. Indeed, these technologies, together with hundreds of thousands of other technological innovations, provide you with unprecedented access to the world around you and make life easier in innumerable ways. Notably, the aforementioned technologies, as well as several others, are currently being used to promote physical activity (PA) participation and improved health outcomes in numerous populations and settings.

Throughout this book, readers will be treated to a comprehensive discussion of emerging technologies currently being used in PA and health promotion. Some of these technologies one might have guessed would be used for health promotion (e.g., a health wearable like a Fitbit) while other technologies might be novel to the reader in their use as public health tools (e.g., using virtual technology to create an artificial world in which the player can be more active). Whether you are a student, health professional, or scholar, it is hoped that the content of this book will inform your future career direction, current practice, or future research, respectively. That said, it is important for readers to understand the foundations of technology and how some of the most frequently used emerging technologies in the promotion of PA and health were developed. As such, the first section of this chapter will devote itself to a brief review of the history of these technologies. Following the preceding discussion, the remainder of this chapter will concentrate on the physiological and psychological effects of PA before ending with an overview of the importance of mastering the effective implementation of these technologies in the community health and medical fields (Figure 1.1). Therefore, sit back and watch as technology meets health!

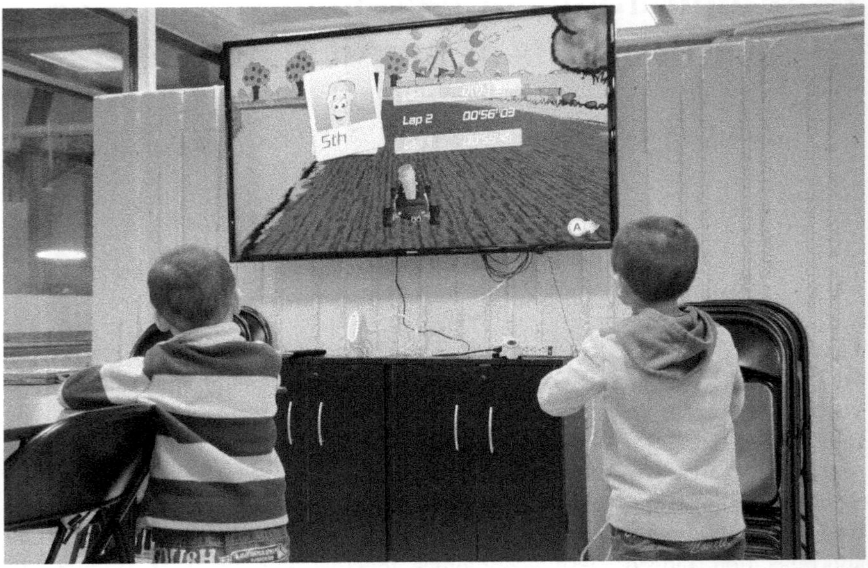

Figure 1.1 Two kids playing active video games.
Source: Photo by Zan Gao.

Understanding the foundations of technology

A remarkable evolution in twenty-first-century technology is currently being observed. Notably, however, the eighteenth through the twentieth centuries also experienced rapid technological advances. Indeed, the Industrial Revolution from the mid-eighteenth century to the start of the twentieth century necessitated advances in technology as business and commerce were beginning to increase within and between more developed countries—resulting in the need for better communication, transportation, and power sources, among other technologies (Buchanan, 2016). Yet, as Buchanan (2016) highlights, it was nearer 1900 when technology started to become fully realized as a crucial part of civilized life in developed countries. As a result of this realization, the 20th century up to the present day has been filled with technological milestones—fueled in large part by the increasing globalization of our world (i.e., the need to do business and connect with individuals around the globe) and the desire to improve the health and well-being of the world's population. While many technological milestones during the twentieth century could be highlighted, for the purposes of this book, only a select group will be concentrated on below given these technologies' current use in PA and health promotion.

The computer, the Internet, social media and pertinent products

Given the great integration of computers in our daily life, it is easy to forget just how recent an innovation computers are. From traditional personal computers/laptops to computers' placement within our smartphones and even many household appliances, computers have revolutionized the way we interact and obtain information in addition to how we carry out our daily tasks. In the mid- to late-1940s, Alan Turing was the first to develop the concept of the modern digital computer, later joining the National Physical Laboratory where he began to develop the prototype for this computer (Turing, 1937, 1946). It was not until several years later in 1952, however, with the first description of the integrated circuit by Geoffrey Dummer (Dummer, 1978), that the age of the digital computer really began to progress. Briefly, the integrated circuit Dummer proposed and developed made the microchips in present-day computers and other electronic devices (e.g., smartphones, video game consoles) possible. By the 1980s, computers as we know them today were becoming more common with companies like Microsoft and Apple developing and selling progressively smaller computers to the general consumer (Computer History Museum, 2016). However, the computers of the 1980s were used mainly for text and data-processing purposes. It was not until nearly 1990 with advent of the World Wide Web, which allowed individuals to connect on what is more commonly known as the Internet, that computers began to gain capabilities which have forever changed our world (Pew Research Center, 2014).

In the early 1990s, the Internet was used mainly for communication, with companies like AOL creating the first forms of email and messenger services. It was not until the mid- to late-1990s that large search engines such as Yahoo and Google became available—adding another dimension to the Internet as users could now search and find any information they desired with a few keystrokes (Pew Research Center, 2014). Towards the turn of the century, however, computer and Internet technology were becoming advanced enough to allow for the streaming of music and videos, offering users more than just text-based mediums by which to gather information and interact with one another. Indeed, in 2003, MySpace, the first widely used social media site launched. By 2005, Facebook and Twitter had launched as well (Terrel, 2015). Each of these sites had features which allowed users to post text, audio forms, and video-based forms of media, read national and world news, and interact with friends via embedded groups and messaging services. Notably, Facebook is currently the largest site of this type with 1.71 billion users as of mid-2016 (Statista, 2016b).

Other interactive platforms also emerged with the advent of the Internet. For example, blogs, akin to online diaries, have become one of the most popular technologies among users, allowing for the sharing of personal reflections on specific topics such as barriers to participation in PA and the enjoyment of sports events. Further, the development of Wikis, a type of server software, allows users to freely create and edit web content simultaneously online. Wikis are interactive in nature in that they allow users to contribute to certain content while communicating with other users who share common interests. Using a similar platform, Google has developed Google Drive (formerly known as Google Docs). This platform acts as a file storage and synchronization service provided by Google, allowing users to store files in the cloud and share and edit files simultaneously with other collaborators (Mossberg, 2012). In addition, Google has also developed Google Hangouts—a communication platform which includes instant messaging, video chat, Short Message Service and Voice over Internet Protocol features. Collectively, these are interactive means of communicating via the Internet.

Indeed, computers, the Internet, and social media have become nearly inseparable aspects of our daily lives. With computing technology continuing to advance at an exponential pace, researchers/health professionals have been increasingly examining the effectiveness of the Internet and social media in the delivery of PA and health interventions over the past decade (Nigg, 2003). Specifically, researchers/health professionals can tailor websites to impart health-related knowledge or develop social media groups which allow the intervention of participants to support one another as they each try to improve their health through greater participation in exercise and healthy eating behaviors. In detail, the Internet and social media have advantages over traditional face-to-face interventions as interventionists can reach a large and more diverse sample of individuals while also reducing the burdens that might arise during typical face-to-face interventions (e.g., the need for transportation). These advantages and the relevant literature will be highlighted in Chapters 4 and 5. Nonetheless, it is safe to say that computers, the Internet, and social media will play a part in PA intervention delivery for many years to come.

Mobile devices

Alexander Bell is credited with inventing and patenting the first modern-day telephone in 1876 (Borth, 2015). Bell's phone was far from portable, however. In fact, it was not until just over 100 years after Bell's patent in 1983 that the first commercial, mobile phone became available (Borth, 2016). This phone was large and bulky with the ability to make calls only. Yet, as time went on, mobile phones began to gain new capabilities, such as the ability to send and receive text messages and, later, to send pictures, videos, and access the Internet via 4G and WiFi connectivity—resulting in terming these mobile phones "smartphones." Today, there are very few individuals without a smartphone. The most recent Pew Research Group report states that 64% of adults now own a smartphone, with this number continuing to increase steadily (Pew Research Center, 2014). Notably, however, smartphones represent just one type of popular mobile device. Tablet computers (a.k.a., tablets) are also popular mobile devices seen nowadays.

Tablets offer capabilities akin to that of a laptop computer, but are smaller and typically bigger than smartphones. In 1987, the modern-day tablet was introduced to the market in the form of Cambridge Researcher's Z88 and Linus Technologies'

Write top (Gregersen, 2016). Although, as Gregersen (2016) notes, while the aforementioned tablets sparked a number of other companies' endeavors to break into the tablet market, the popularity of the tablet was low until the introduction of Apple's iPad in 2010. Indeed, the introduction of the iPad to the market has resulted in a booming present-day tablet industry, with most of the major technology companies marketing tablets to consumers. Since 2012, the number of tablet shipments has consistently been between 40 and 80 million (Statista, 2016c)—indicating the popularity of these powerful mobile devices among consumers. Nonetheless, whether a user prefers to use a smartphone or tablet, these mobile devices offer researchers/health professionals the capability to use mobile device applications (a.k.a., apps) to promote health and wellness.

As of 2015, Google Play and the Apple Store offered 1.6 and 1.5 million apps, respectively, for users to download to their mobile device (Statista, 2016a). Moreover, 165,000 of these apps were considered mobile health (a.k.a., mHealth) apps—providing the user with the ability to track or manage their PA routines, healthy eating habits, and stress levels, among other health behaviors (Intercontinental Marketing Services [IMS] Institute of Health Informatics, 2015). As such, researchers/health professionals have recently capitalized on the use of mHealth apps in the promotion of health and wellness in numerous general and clinical populations using researcher-developed or commercially available mHealth apps. Given the fact that intervention participants may find the need to carry around a laptop computer to participate in an intervention to be burdensome, the small and portable nature of smartphones and tablets in the promotion of PA and health is a promising field of research in a generation in which individuals are increasingly using mobile device apps to assist in daily activities. That said, the use of mHealth apps in the promotion of PA and health will be reviewed in Chapter 6.

Global positioning systems (GPS) and geographic information systems (GIS)

While researchers and health professionals appreciate the provision of PA intensity data through accelerometers and other devices equipped with accelerometry (e.g., Fitbit), these devices cannot provide health professionals with information regarding the location of PA in one's environment. This inability to track PA location is unfortunate, as researchers over the past 15 years have made clear the negative impact that the built environment (e.g., sidewalk construction, land use, trail systems) can have on PA (Handy, Boarnet, Ewing, & Killingsworth, 2002; Krenn et al., 2011). Global positioning systems (GPS) or geographic information systems (GIS), however, have shown great promise in providing researchers/health professionals information regarding PA location, after which detailed analyses of the relationship of PA and the built environment can be explored.

The technology behind GPS was developed approximately 40 years ago for exclusive use by the military (Maddison & Mhurchu, 2009). In 2000, however,

President Clinton made GPS technology available for civilian use—citing the incredible potential of this technology to provide highly accurate positioning data for everyone (U.S. Government Information, 2000). High-tech GIS software was then marketed, allowing for the upload, storage, and analysis of the GPS data (National Geographic Society, 2016). In brief, GIS software gives researchers the power to construct highly specific maps which allow these investigators to correlate individuals' GPS-measured PA data with different locations to assess where changes in the built environment might be needed to facilitate greater PA participation.

As a result of the commercialization of GPS, GPS units have become widely available over the last 15 years in the form of GPS watches and other units which can be attached around the waist or carried like a backpack (Maddison & Mhurchu, 2009) (Figure 1.2). Researchers/health professionals can provide individuals with these small GPS devices which serve to assist these professionals in conducting PA environment audits which, again, through later analysis via GIS, can allow these professionals to advocate for changes in the built environment (e.g., increased sidewalk connectivity, greater access to trails and parks) that facilitate PA. Furthermore, recent research using minimalistic GPS devices (e.g., the Spi Elite™) has been conducted to investigate athlete velocity, changes in direction,

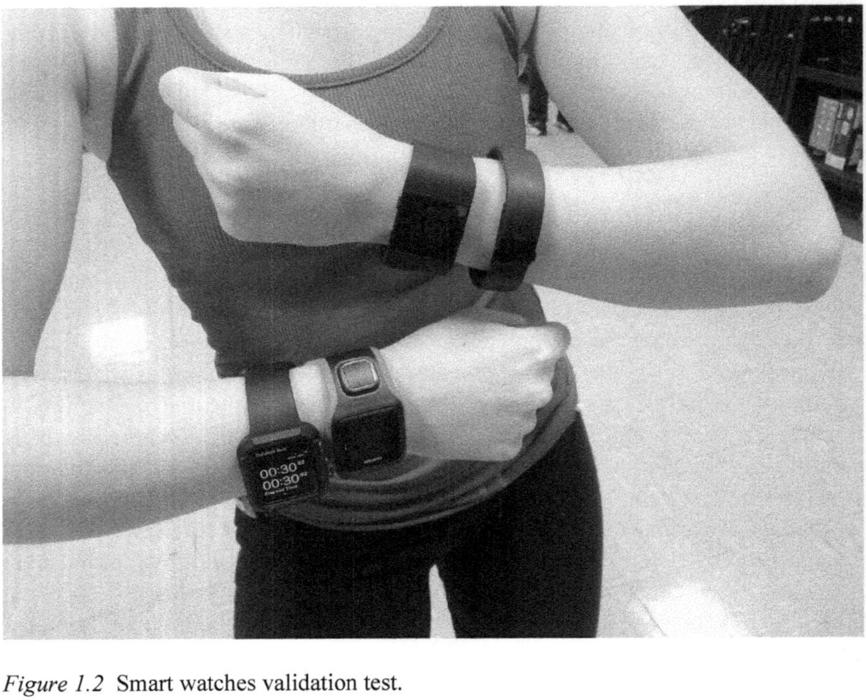

Figure 1.2 Smart watches validation test.

Source: Photo by Zan Gao.

and training load—all with the aim of reducing injury and improving performance (MacLeod, Morris, Nevill, & Sunderland, 2009; Malone et al., 2015). Therefore, it should be clear that GPS/GIS technology offers a unique and needed solution regarding how to evaluate and assess PA location and intensity in order to promote health and wellness among the general population and safety/performance in athletes. The aforementioned benefits and more will be discussed in Chapter 7.

Health wearables

Activity trackers (a.k.a., health wearables) are likely the newest type of emerging technology used by researchers and health professionals to promote PA and health in various populations. Although pedometers and accelerometers have been available for some time, these technologies were either limited in their ability to track multiple types of PA (e.g., pedometers are poor at assessing activities other than walking or running) or, like accelerometers, were expensive and primarily only used in research settings. In 2007, however, the company Fitbit was founded—selling the first of its kind health wearable devices to consumers in order to give health-conscience individuals the ability to track and self-regulate health behaviors (e.g., steps taken per day) (Fitbit, 2016). While the first Fitbit was attached to the waist and had limited capabilities other than tracking PA, subsequent iterations of this device have been wrist-mounted and equipped to track a number of health metrics (Figure 1.3). Regardless of the limited functionality of the first Fitbit, at the time of

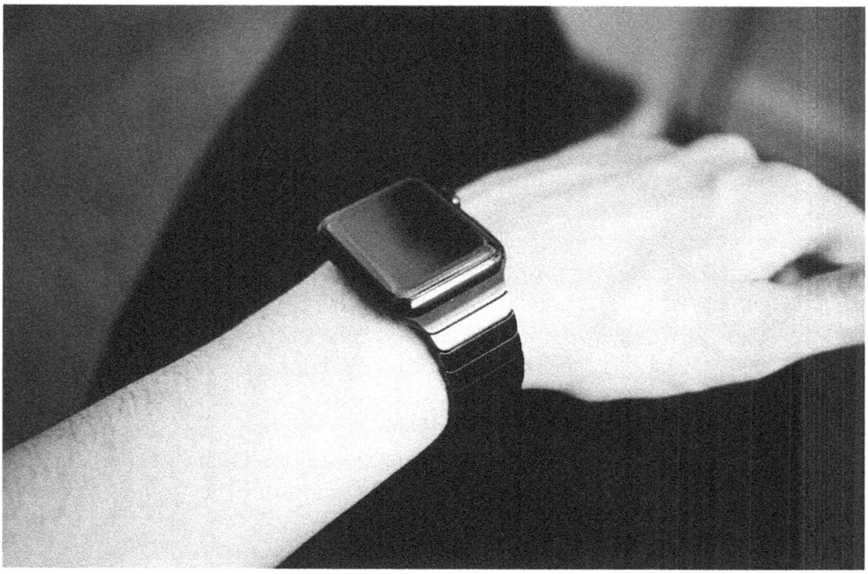

Figure 1.3 Use of a smart watch in health promotion.

Source: pixabay.com.

its release the Fitbit inspired a whole market of health wearables (e.g., the Jawbone) and pushed these devices from relative obscurity into the mainstream. Although the style and placement (e.g., wrist, belt, ankle) may differ for various health wearables, the majority of these devices sync wirelessly with mobile devices via associated mHealth apps and are now equipped to evaluate a number of different health metrics such as steps per day, sleep duration/quality, steps climbed, and heart rate, among other indices. Yet, while the popularity of health wearables like the Fitbit continues to be high, the introduction of The Pebble smartwatch in 2012 changed the landscape of health wearables once again.

Indeed, smart watches are poised to be the next generation of common health wearable technology—with major technology companies such as Apple capitalizing on the current popularity of smart watches with devices like the Apple Watch. While functions vary, depending on the smart watch in question, these devices offer a number of advantages over other, more traditional health wearable technologies. As Rawassizadeh and colleagues (2015) state, the two biggest advantages to smart watches is these devices' consistent wear location at the wrist and the continual contact these devices have with the user's skin. Specifically, the consistent wear location is notable, given the fact it can be assumed the user is wearing the device in the same location over multiple days—increasing the validity of the health data collected—while the continual contact that smart watches have with users' skin allows for the measurement of a number of health indices including, but not limited to: heart rate, galvanic skin response, blood oxygen levels, and heart rate variability (Rawassizadeh, Price, & Petre, 2015). Aside from the aforementioned advantages, smart watches also allow the user to engage in tasks such as reading texts/emails, playing music, and checking the weather—functions that most traditional health wearables have not yet gained the ability to complete. It should also be noted, however, that some research-grade accelerometry companies have noted the trends in health wearables and have begun developing their own "smart" products. For example, ActiGraph Co. recently released a smart watch-like wearable device called the ActiGraph GT9X Link, which provides data via a sleek and high resolution liquid crystal display screen for optional real-time feedback. The GT9X Link also offers a variety of wireless features, including proximity detection, heart rate monitoring, and communication with its mobile app through Bluetooth®Smart technology.

Regardless of whether researchers and/or health professionals use a more traditional health wearable, such as a Fitbit or Jawbone or ActiGraph Link, or a smart watch, such as The Pebble or Apple Watch, it is clear these devices hold promise in the tracking and self-regulation of PA and other health behaviors. In Chapter 8, readers will be treated to a discussion of the extant literature on the use of health wearables in the promotion of PA and health.

Active video gaming and virtual reality

Home video games are a relatively recent innovation which certainly have benefited from the technological advances made in the personal computer industry over the last half of the twentieth century up to the present day. In 1972, an engineer by the name of Ralph Baer patented what was then termed the "television gaming apparatus" for a video game console called the Magnavox Odyssey which allowed users to play a game called *Fox and Hounds* (Lowood, 2016). Not long after the release of the Magnavox Odyssey Atari released their first video gaming consoles—most notably, the Atari 2600 Video Computer System. The first active video game, however, was not released until 1988 with Atari's *Foot Craz*, requiring players to run in place on a track displayed on a television screen while trying to beat a virtual opponent (Montfort & Bogost, 2009). However, *Foot Craz* and other early active video games achieved only limited success. It was not until 1998, with the release of *Dance Revolution* on the PlayStation, that active video gaming really started to attract consumer interest (Chamberlin & Maloney, 2013). Moreover, as technology advanced, so did the active video gaming consoles. During the mid- to late-2000s PlayStation's EyeToy, Nintendo's Wii, and Microsoft's Kinect were all released, with the Wii experiencing enormous success. As Chamberlin and Maloney (2013) state, it did not take long for the Wii and other similar consoles to gain the interest of researchers/health professionals regarding their use in PA and health promotion. Notably, active video games are also considered a form of virtual reality. Specifically, active video games are considered a form of non-immersive virtual reality as these games typically do not fully immerse players in a virtual environment—using only television screens and associated gamepads or motion-sensing cameras during user gameplay (Pasco, 2013). Virtual reality, as most have come to know it, is immersive, often employing headset displays, body motion sensors worn by the user, and/or helmets to completely simulate an environment (Figure 1.4).

Virtual reality has a similar timeline to active video gaming, given this technology's similar dependence on advances in the computer industry. Modern-day virtual reality was first conceived in the 1960s and was used almost exclusively in the job training of individuals such as pilots in a controlled and low-risk manner (Lowood, 2015). However, as Lowood (2015) states, it was not until the 1990s that virtual reality companies began to aggressively develop virtual reality systems for the general consumer for entertainment purposes. Today, personal virtual reality systems such as the Ocular Rift, Samsung Gear VR, PlayStation VR, HTC Vive dominate the market—providing relatively inexpensive virtual reality experiences (Lamkin, 2016). Indeed, researchers/health professionals can use these virtual reality systems to create virtual worlds of PA for intervention participants wherein the movements required to participate in certain activities can be mimicked (e.g., a golf swing or free throw in basketball), which will hopefully lead to increased confidence in participating in these sports in the real world.

Finally, augmented reality, a technology format combining the physical and virtual worlds—most commonly using a smartphone app—has also become popular in recent years with games like Zombies, Run! and the recently released Pokémon Go among the most popular (Figure 1.5). Of interest to researchers/health professionals is the health benefits which might arise from playing these

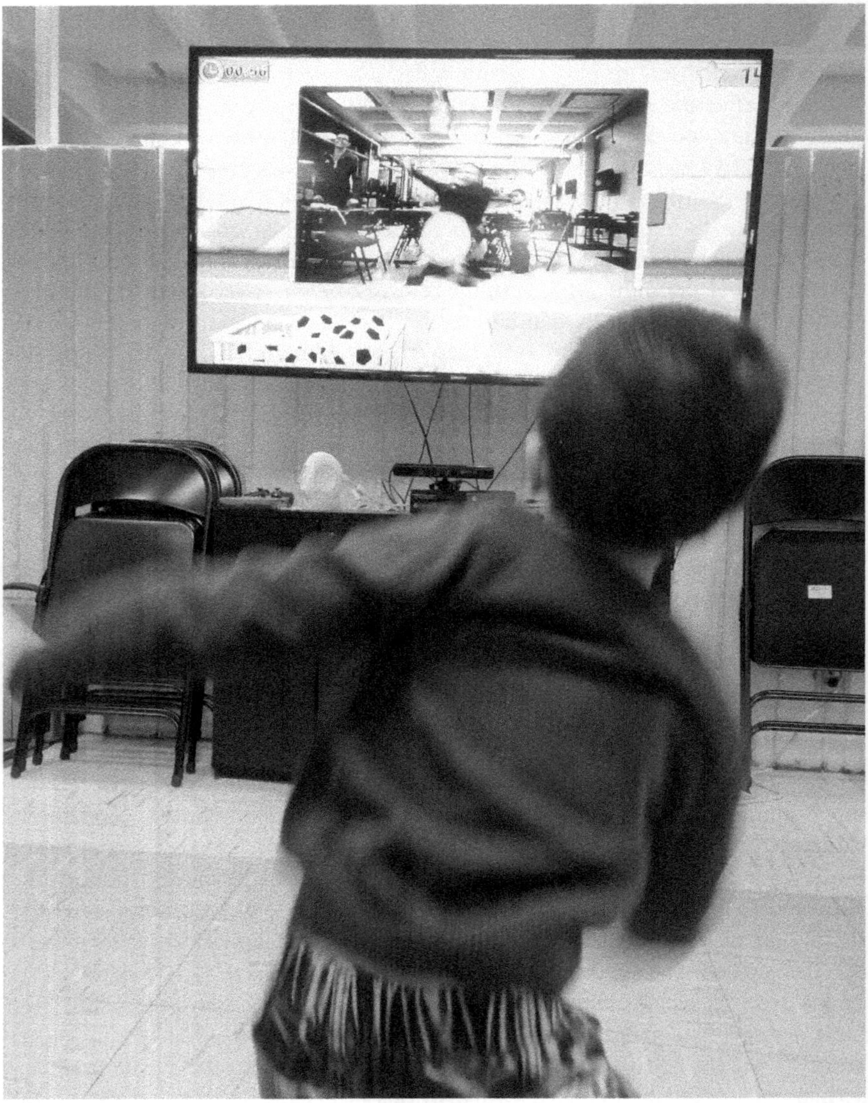

Figure 1.4 A kid playing soccer video games.
Source: Photo by Zan Gao.

augmented reality games as the games require players to move to different locations in the environment to engage in gameplay (Baranowski, 2016). Chapters 9 and 10 will cover the extant literature to date regarding active video gaming and various types of virtual reality, respectively.

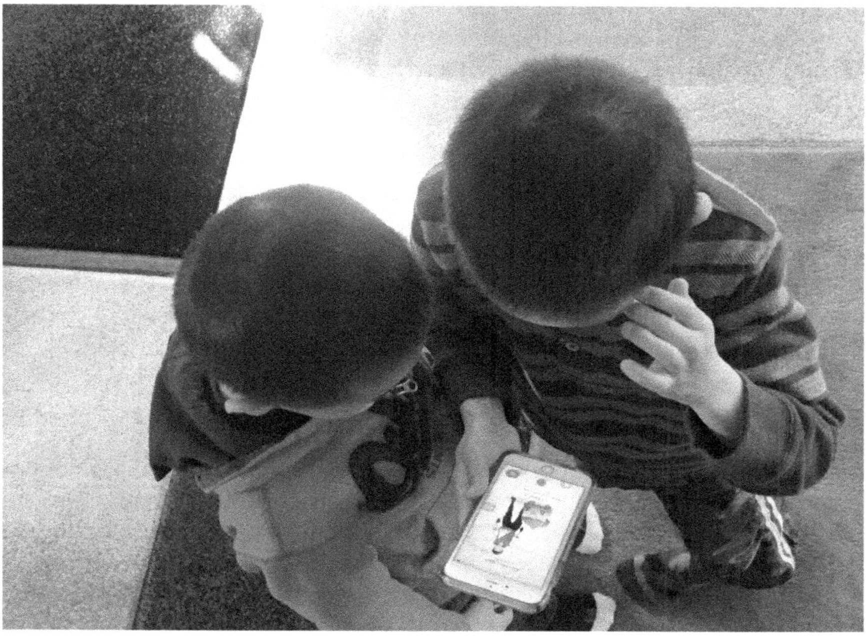

Figure 1.5 Kids playing Pokémon Go.
Source: Photo by Zan Gao.

Throughout the remainder of this chapter, the readers will be treated to a review of the physiological and psychological benefits related to PA—providing the basis for why the preceding technologies might prove vital to public health initiatives.

Understanding the underlying science behind the health benefits of PA

Physical activity (PA) refers to any bodily movement produced by the skeletal muscles that results in a substantial increase in energy expenditure above resting levels (Claude, Steven, & William, 2012). Regular PA promotes health and fitness. More specifically, moderate-to-vigorous-intensity aerobic PA helps build and maintain healthy bones and muscles; reduces the risk of developing obesity and chronic diseases, such as diabetes and cardiovascular disease; and reduces symptoms of depression and anxiety, thereby promoting cardiorespiratory fitness (CRF) and psychological well-being (U.S. Department of Health and Human Services [USDHHS], 2008). However, only 21% American adults meet the 2008 PA Guidelines, and less than three in ten (29%) high school students get at least

60 minutes of PA every day (Centers for Disease Control and Prevention [CDC], 2014). Even more unfortunate is that nearly half of preschool children do not meet the recommended 60 daily minutes of PA for this age group (Tucker, 2008) (Figure 1.6). Indeed, globally, 81% of adolescents aged 11–17 years and approximately 23% of adults aged 18 and over were insufficiently physically active in 2010 (World Health Organization [WHO], 2016). In fact, physical inactivity is one of the ten leading risk factors for global mortality, which is on the rise in many countries, adding to the burden of non-communicable diseases (e.g., cardiovascular diseases, cancer and diabetes) and affecting general health worldwide (WHO, 2016). As global inactivity has rapidly increased due to individuals spending less time performing PA, this section provides an overview of the scientific evidence linking PA to physiological and psychological health—furthering the rationale behind the use of emerging technology in PA promotion.

Cardiorespiratory health

Since the late 1950s, numerous scientific studies have examined the relationships between PA and cardiovascular health. Expert panels, convened by national organizations and other international organizations, along with the 1996 U.S. Surgeon General's Report on PA and Health, have reinforced scientific evidence regarding the ability of regular PA to positively impact various measures of cardiovascular health. Based upon more than five decades of epidemiological studies, it is now widely accepted that physically active individuals tend to develop less coronary heart disease (CHD) than their sedentary peers, with higher PA patterns and CRF levels associated with better health outcomes (Myers et al., 2015).

The human body responds to PA through a series of integrated changes in function that involve most, if not all, of its physiological systems. For example, movement requires activation and control of the musculoskeletal system, with the cardiovascular and respiratory systems providing the ability to sustain this movement over extended periods of time. If an individual engages in PA several times a week, each of the aforementioned physiological systems undergoes specific adaptations that increase the body's efficiency and capacity. Generally,

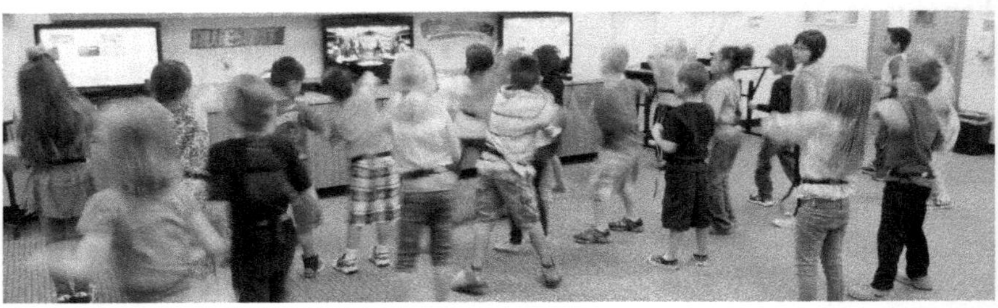

Figure 1.6 A group of kids playing active video games.

Source: Photo by Zan Gao.

regular PA participation improves cardiovascular function by lowering resting heart rate and increasing stroke volume at submaximal workloads (Vella & Robergs, 2005). Additionally, the muscles used during aerobic activities show improvements in strength and endurance while the muscles used for breathing (i.e., the intercostals and abdominals) become more resistant to fatigue. Finally, individuals who regularly participate in endurance exercises develop the ability to sustain a higher fractional utilization of their maximal oxygen uptake—becoming more physiologically efficient during various aerobic activities (Ghosh, 2004). The preceding result is almost entirely a result of increased maximal cardiorespiratory endurance (VO_2 max) increases along with the ability of the muscle to extract oxygen to power PA. Given the preceding physiological adaptations, fitter individuals can more easily participate in PA at a given workload as compared to less fit individuals.

Regular participation in PA is also associated with an improved atherogenic dyslipidemia profile, resulting in increased high-density lipoprotein (HDL) cholesterol, lower total cholesterol, and lower triglyceride levels. Additionally, improvements in autonomic nerve function, increases in aerobic and anaerobic enzymes, increased lactate threshold (max), improved glucose homeostasis, improved endothelial function, and reduced inflammation related to oxidative stress are also common physiological adaptations observed regular PA participation (Kohl & Murray, 2012). Notably, high-intensity PA results in increases of both glycolytic and oxidative enzymes (Bogdanis, 2012). Last but not least, increased total energy expenditure and reduced body fat percentage and waist circumference have been seen over time among various populations when regularly performing PA at a moderate- or vigorous-intensity level.

Metabolic health

The Physical Activity Guidelines Advisory Committee (PAGAC, 2008) reported clear and strong scientific evidence indicating regular PA improves the metabolic health of individuals who are at least moderately active by 30–40% compared to sedentary populations. The benefits of PA on metabolic health apply equally for a variety of populations. Generally, PA-related adaptations that positively influence metabolic health are the same as those seen in conjunction with cardiorespiratory adaptations to PA. Explicitly, regular PA participation results in increased HDL levels and reduced low-density lipoprotein (LDL) levels (Kokkinos & Fernhall, 1999), as well as reduced triglyceride levels (LeBlanc & Janssen, 2010). Further, both aerobic and resistance exercises increase glucose transporter type 4 (GLUT4) abundance and blood glucose (BG) uptake (Colberg et al., 2010). As GLUT4 levels increase with PA, insulin resistance is prevented (Ross, 2003) while improvements in insulin sensitivity are observed (Duncan et al., 2003)—a key factor in diabetes prevention and treatment. Existing evidence also indicates regular PA to be highly related to improved glucose tolerance (Aller & van Baak, 2013) in addition to an improved protein synthesis rate and amino acid uptake into skeletal muscle (van Loon, 2014). Overall, significant metabolic adaptations occur in response to PA and exercise. Indeed, by improving metabolic health, individuals decrease the likelihood of chronic disease and improve their quality of life.

Musculoskeletal health

Participating in activities such as strength and resistance training has been proven effective in improving musculoskeletal function (Baechle & Earle, 2008). Even with moderate-intensity PA (e.g., carrying heavy loads, climbing stairs, etc.), improvements in muscular strength and endurance are observed in most healthy individuals.

Increases in VO_2 max (5% change) have been observed in those who participated in interval training combining resistance training and aerobic exercise, while sedentary individuals have demonstrated VO_2 max improvements of 3% with resistance training alone (Gettman & Pollock, 1981). Increases in strength and power have also been observed over time when PA regimens incorporate resistance training (Bogdanis, 2012; Hong, Hong, & Shin, 2014). The preceding musculoskeletal strengthening is facilitated by the body's ability to recruit more motor units (i.e., the motor neuron and the muscle fibers it innervates), the increased size of individual muscle fibers, the increased numbers of anaerobic enzymes, and the higher amounts of anaerobic energy store such a phosphocreatine and glycogen (Kohl & Murray, 2012). Notably, all of the aforementioned health benefits are critical for performing short-duration and high-intensity musculoskeletal activity.

Of clinical importance, increased ligament and tendon strength and increased collagen content are the results of connective tissues changes caused by the stress placed on specific muscles during musculoskeletal strengthening activities—which may reduce the risk of injury for those of all ages. Further, resistance training activities can trigger positive hormonal changes that allow for the remodeling of bone, which can improve bone mineral density (BMD) in some people, while delaying bone mass loss for individuals at risk of osteoporosis—particularly females. Finally, exercise physiology research has clearly demonstrated that regular PA and musculoskeletal strengthening exercise participation increase lean muscle mass by way of improved muscle quality and quantity while also reducing body fat and aiding in maintenance or loss of weight (Chaput et al., 2011). Of note, the amount of physiological adaptation associated with each of the benefits of PA and exercise reviewed to this point are dose-dependent—indicating that lower doses of PA have smaller physiological effects and changes than performing higher doses (Kohl & Murray, 2012). This dose-response relationship must be kept in mind when critiquing literature regarding PA interventions or developing an intervention of your own.

Mental health

Mental disorders are of major public health significance. Specifically, mental disorders have a long-lasting impact on an individual's mood or affect, personality, cognition, and perception (USDHHS, 1996). The Physical Activity Guidelines Advisory Committee (PAGAC; 2008) listed common mental disorders or problems that have been investigated in relation to PA, which included mood disorders, anxiety disorders, psychological distress, low self-esteem, age-related decline in cognitive function, and eating or exercise-related disorders. Of the most frequently examined outcomes of mental health examined in relation to PA, investigations have included mood (e.g., anxiety, depression, positive affect, and negative affect), self-efficacy, self-esteem, and cognitive functioning. Among these outcomes, affective (mood) and anxiety disorders are the most frequently reported.

Current scientific evidence supports the assertion that regular PA and exercise lower the risk/symptoms of depression (Mammen & Faulkner, 2013), anxiety (Stonerock, Hoffman, Smith, & Blumenthal, 2015), psychological distress (Matzka et al., 2016), and age-related decline in cognitive function (Chang et al., 2010). Furthermore, improvements in positive affect, general psychological well-being (Brown et al., 2013), and self-esteem (Awick et al., 2016) were also observed. Overall, physically inactive populations are twice as likely to have symptoms of depression and anxiety compared to those who are more active. The general consensus is that people who are physically active or have higher levels of cardiorespiratory fitness trend to have enhanced mood (greater positive affect and less negative affect), higher self-esteem, greater confidence in their ability to perform tasks requiring PA (i.e., greater self-efficacy), and better cognitive functioning than those who are physically inactive or live a sedentary lifestyle. Notably, it has been claimed that light PA (e.g., performing activities of daily living, for example) is likely not intense enough to elicit significant physiological responses. As such, it is still recommended that PA must be at a moderate or vigorous intensity to generate the physiological stimulus necessary to promote mental health (Kohl & Murray, 2012).

Despite substantial research in the area, however, PA has not been shown to be effective in the treatment of mental health disorders. That said, only a paucity of research has been conducted on the role that PA might play in the prevention of mental health disorders. Indeed, the extant literature studying individuals with mental health disorders, such as depression and anxiety, represents the best current evidence available regarding attempts to promote PA in the prevention of mental health disorders. Unfortunately, the literature is less clear regarding the psychological effects of regular PA for individuals who have relatively good health status, or those with other mental disorders, including sleep and eating disorders, schizophrenia, dementia, personality disorders, and substance-related disorders. Therefore, more studies are warranted to further explore the effects of PA on mental health.

In summary, PA has numerous beneficial and well-documented physiological effects. Most widely appreciated are its effects on the cardiorespiratory and musculoskeletal systems, but benefits for the functioning of the metabolic systems of the body are also considerable. These beneficial physiological effects have been observed in individuals of all race/ethnicity, gender, and ages. Moreover, emerging positive effects of PA on relieving symptoms of anxiety and depression, and improving mood, self-esteem, cognitive functioning, and general psychological well-being are promising. Nevertheless, most physiological and psychological health benefits from PA are dose-dependent. That is, regular PA must be performed at moderate-to-vigorous intensity and in episodes of at least 10 minutes in duration to generate the necessary physiological stimulus to promote overall health.

Application of emerging technologies in promoting PA and health

The physiological and psychological benefits of regular PA participation have been well documented and include improved cardiorespiratory fitness, enhanced self-efficacy, and reduced risk of non-communicable chronic diseases such as obesity, type 2 diabetes, and cardiovascular diseases, among numerous other positive outcomes. Despite the recognized benefits, the majority of Americans do not meet the recommended levels of PA on a daily basis. As known, technology is embedded in our society and is changing our lives in positive and negative ways. Traditionally, technology-based media such as television, video games, and computer games have been blamed for their negative effects on individuals' health, as these media usually result in increased screen time and reduced PA levels in various populations, contributing to public health concerns such as obesity and type 2 diabetes. Fortunately, just like the famous Chinese saying "fight fire with fire," the present-day health professionals are intentionally using emerging technology to promote PA participation through the provision of technologies such as health wearable devices and active video games that are now available on the market. In fact, these emerging technologies have entered into homes, schools, communities, and other places, and have been very popular among various populations. For example, nowadays smartphones not only allow us to regularly communicate with others through phone calls and text messages, but also let us monitor our health status and monitor PA behaviors via multiple health-oriented apps.

Health professionals can play a valuable role in the selection and integration of emerging technology. This section will equip the reader with the requisite knowledge base regarding the use of emerging technology for PA assessment and promotion. It is hoped that such knowledge will promote further integration of emerging technology into PA and health by researchers and health professionals alike.

Emerging technology for PA assessment

Technology is constantly changing our living environment and lifestyles. Approximately a decade ago, electronic devices that monitor PA by detecting and processing human movement made an impact with regard to assessing habitual PA levels due to their accuracy and ease of use—replacing the widely used

PA questionnaires. Particularly, the most popular electronic devices, such as pedometers, accelerometers, and heart rate monitors, provide details of PA measures, including but not limited to: steps, estimated distance, energy expenditure, time in different intensity levels of PA, and heart rate. Beyond their measurement attributes, these devices also play an important role in providing feedback to clients which can act to motivate these individuals to participate in more PA.

With the rapid development of technology, accelerometers capable of assessing sedentary behavior, light PA, and moderate-to-vigorous PA are now appearing in smartphones and GPS devices. While technology advancement offers opportunities for the public to engage in sedentary behavior, the integration of accelerometers into a greater number of electronic devices is providing opportunities for health professionals to objectively assess PA and sedentary behavior to address various health issues. In fact, the extant electronic devices are attractive for health professional in that they have achieved greater ease of use, greater precision, and greater scope (i.e., data from various sources in one device) by integrating innovative emerging technologies such as mobile device apps, GPS units, and health wearables. This is imperative for health professionals implementing PA interventions, because more precise assessments allow for a better understanding of when, where, and how PA participation occurs—improving subsequent behavioral change strategies.

Currently many mobile devices (smartphones and tablets) and fashion accessories (belt, necklace, bracelet, and rings) have embedded GPS and accelerometer technologies which are being used to identify and promote PA participation as well as understand naturalistically occurring activities (Graham & Hipp, 2014). Some smart devices are even taking advantage of the camera function of mobile devices. For example, SenseCam, a wearable digital camera that takes photos automatically without user intervention, along with mobile apps and other visual devices can provide details of PA contexts and an individual's lifestyle.

Furthermore, technology advancement has included the development of multiple sensor systems, enabling better identification of previously non-identifiable physical activities (e.g., bench press, stair climbing) through pedometers or accelerometers alone. Presently, the vast majority of monitors (i.e., Actigraph), devices (i.e., Polar M400 Sports Watch), or apps (i.e., MapMyFitness) are able to send data to an individual's account and relevant communities via remote servers. This invites the further embrace of online technology (e.g., adopting online social-networks like MapMyFitness Friends as a source of extrinsic motivation to achieve predetermined personal health goals), and PA promotion websites such as Stickk.com that let individuals make public contracts visible to other users and also use monetary incentives to promote PA behavioral changes. Additionally, technological advances like crowdsourcing (i.e., applies to the masses, or crowds, of individuals using the Internet, social media, and smartphone apps) allows for input from a large base of diverse users that can help to identify and improve the infrastructure for PA. For example, professionals can identify environmental features that are inhibiting or facilitating PA behavior on a regional or even national scale, based upon the input from large groups.

Overall, although validity testing is warranted when applying emerging technologies in assessing and evaluating PA behavior, it is critical and noteworthy that researchers and practitioners should embrace new technologies give the fact that: (1) emerging technologies can greatly increase our capability to analyze PA behavior patterns; (2) the ease of use and transferability can significantly impact large populations from a longitudinal perspective; (3) emerging technologies can improve the ongoing, systematic process evaluation of any intervention program, given their real-time data sharing capabilities; (4) researchers are calling for new strategies to deal with big data through data mining or data texting (PA data, posts on social media, GPS and/or GIS data, etc.). With the improvements in mathematical models and computer algorithms, researchers will empower themselves to allow greater capacity for assessing and evaluating PA data; and (5) increasingly blurred boundaries between PA assessment and intervention (e.g., self-tracking PA) may require a re-evaluation of the traditional scientific model to design and evaluate these types of studies (Graham & Hipp, 2014).

Emerging technology in PA promotion

As previously stated, researchers and health professionals have taken advantage of the emerging technology that is available in PA promotion. However, it should be noted that some emerging technologies such as GPS/GIS have only been used to measure and track PA behavior, with few interventions of this type having the aim of changing an individual's PA behaviors—the core element of PA promotion. Fortunately, the introduction of persuasive technology shows great potential for emerging technology application in PA promotion. More specifically, persuasive technology refers to a technology that is designed to change individuals' attitudes or behaviors through persuasion and social influence but not through coercion (Fogg, 2003). Research involving persuasive technology focuses primarily on interactive and computational technologies such as video games, desktop computers, the Internet, and mobile devices, yet it also incorporates behavioral theories and human-computer interactions (Dominic, Hounkponou, Doh, Ansong, & Brighter, 2013) (Figure 1.7). Indeed, persuasive technology is designed with the goal of changing a particular aspect of human behavior, including PA behavior, in a predefined way in non-commercial domains.

Some emerging technologies play key roles in persuading individuals to engage in greater PA participation in that: (1) they serve as the tool (e.g., recording heart rates and calories with the Apple watch); (2) they are linked to social media (e.g., synchronize exercise app data to Facebook or Twitter); and (3) they offer social interaction (e.g., Kinect Just Dance 5 allow for dancing with another person from the online community). The applications of such technology have been increasingly seen in our daily life. For example, MapMyFitness, a popular smartphone exercise app, is a good intervention strategy in PA promotion, as it integrates with the music on the smartphone and provides instant feedback from a bout of exercise to users. Users can also share their accomplishments with their

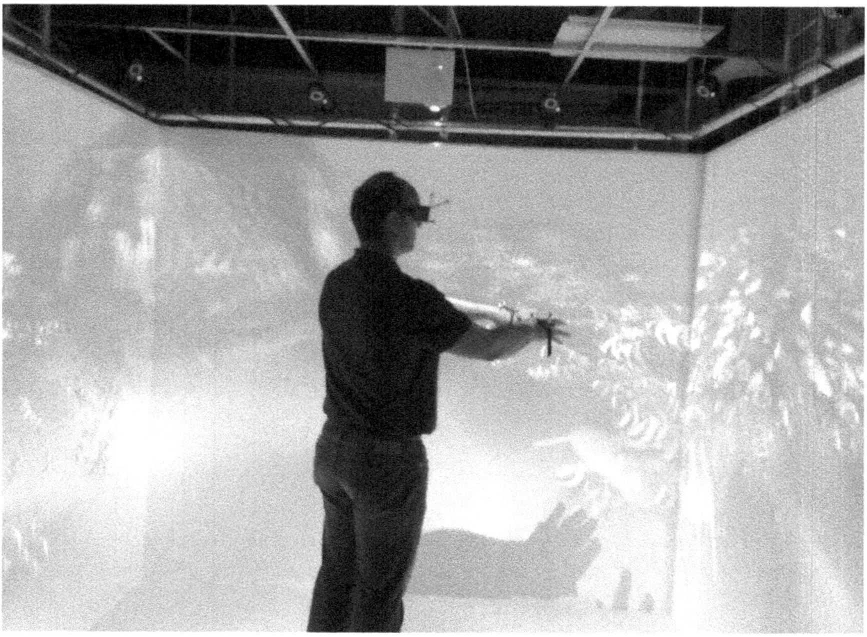

Figure 1.7 Application of virtual reality CAVE.
Source: Photo by Zan Gao.

friends using this app or can synchronize data to Facebook. Further, this app once even partnered with Sears soon after the app's release to offer monetary incentives to users who engaged in exercise. Another example is Just Dance, a type of active video game with dance movement. Just Dance provides scores and instant feedback to users for each of their movements while allowing users to compete with others simultaneously on site or online. Most importantly, this technology's interactive feature captures users' attention so that they play the dance game without knowing that they are actually exercising.

According to Dominic et al. (2013), emerging technology is generally deemed as a tool thus far, and the technology use alone may not lead to ideal persuasion and expected intervention outcomes. Changing behavior is never an easy task. Therefore, it is critical to integrate emerging technology and behavioral theories to promote PA among various target populations. In fact, a number of behavioral theories have been widely used in some PA interventions involving emerging technology. The reader will be treated to details concerning theory application in PA interventions using emerging technology in Chapter 3.

Finally, health professionals should keep in mind several technologies have been integrated into singular applications over the past several years. By embracing the strengths of each technology, an integrated technology application may be very powerful and convenient for users. In fact, a number of products are now available on the market to combine PA assessment and intervention delivery in a single application. Presently, the aforementioned MapMyFitness, XBox Kinect, and the Apple watch are such applications. Thus, more research will be warranted on using these multi-technologies devices.

Overall, technology is continuously evolving and constantly changing our lives. On the horizon are novel and exciting cutting-edge technologies that have great potential for PA promotion. Indeed, human beings have applied technology in promoting PA for some time. Yet, in this day and age, emerging technologies and relevant behavioral theories are providing us with needed and exciting opportunities to assess and promote PA on a larger scale—particularly when discussing novel technologies and methodologies such as augmented reality games, crowdsourcing, and online active gaming. Undoubtedly, the technology era appears to be a prime time for researchers and health professionals in PA and health.

References

Aller, E. E., & van Baak, M. A. (2013). Physical activity improves glucose tolerance independent of weight loss in severe obesity. *Journal of Diabetes & Metabolism*, *4*(3), 254.

Awick, E. A., Ehlers, D., Fanning, J., Phillips, S. M., Wójcicki, T., Mackenzie, M. J., … & McAuley, E. (2016). Effects of a home-based DVD delivered physical activity program on self-esteem in older adults: Results from a randomized controlled trial. *Psychosomatic Medicine* (In Press).

Baechle, T. R., & Earle, R. W. (2008). National strength and conditioning association. In *Essentials of strength training and conditioning*. (3rd ed.). Champaign, IL: Human Kinetics.

Baranowski, T. (2016). Pokémon Go, go, go, gone? *Games for Health Journal*, *5*(5), 1–2.

Bogdanis, G. C. (2012). Effects of physical activity and inactivity on muscle fatigue. *Frontiers in Physiology*, *3*, 142.

Borth, D. (2015). Telephone. In *Encyclopedia Britannica*. Retrieved from www.britannica.com/technology/telephone.

Borth, D. (2016). Mobile telephone. In *Encyclopedia Britannica*. Retrieved from www.britannica.com/technology/mobile-telephone.

Brown, H. E., Pearson, N., Braithwaite, R. E., Brown, W. J., & Biddle, S. J. (2013). Physical activity interventions and depression in children and adolescents. *Sports Medicine*, *43*(3), 195–206.

Buchanan, R. (2016). History of technology. In *Encyclopedia Britannica*. Retrieved from www.britannica.com/technology/history-of-technology.

Centers for Disease Control and Prevention (CDC) (2014, May 20). Facts about physical activity. Retrieved from www.cdc.gov/physicalactivity/data/facts.htm.

Chamberlin, B., & Maloney, A. (2013). *Active video games: Impacts and research*. Oxford Handbooks Online. Retrieved from www.oxfordhandbooks.com/view/10.1093/oxfordhb/9780195398809.001.0001/oxfordhb-9780195398809-e-18.

Chang, M., Jonsson, P. V., Snaedal, J., Bjornsson, S., Saczynski, J. S., Aspelund, T., … & Gudnason, V. (2010). The effect of midlife physical activity on cognitive function among older adults: AGES—Reykjavik Study. *The Journals of Gerontology Series A: Biological Sciences and Medical Sciences*, *65*(12), 1369–1374.

Chaput, J.-P., Klingenberg, L., Rosenkilde, M., Gilbert, J.-A., Tremblay, A., & Sjödin, A. (2011). Physical activity plays an important role in body weight regulation. *Journal of Obesity*, *2011*, 360257. http://doi.org/10.1155/2011/360257.

Claude, B., Steven, N. B., & and William, H. (2012). *Physical activity and health* (2nd ed.). Champaign, IL: Human Kinetics.

Colberg, S. R., Sigal, R. J., Fernhall, B., Regensteiner, J. G., Blissmer, B. J., Rubin, R. R., … & Braun, B. (2010). Exercise and type 2 diabetes: The American College of Sports Medicine and the American Diabetes Association: Joint position statement. *Diabetes Care*, *33*(12), e147–e167.

Computer History Museum. (2016). Timeline of computers. Retrieved from www.computerhistory.org/timeline/computers.

Dominic, D., Hounkponou, F., Doh, R., Ansong, E., & Brighter, A. (2013). Promoting Physical Activity through Persuasive Technology, *CiteSeerX*, *2*(1), 16–22.

Dummer, G. (1978). *Electronic inventions and discoveries (applied electricy and electronics)* (2nd ed.). Oxford: Pergamon Press.

Duncan, G. E., Perri, M. G., Theriaque, D. W., Hutson, A. D., Eckel, R. H., & Stacpoole, P. W. (2003). Exercise training, without weight loss, increases insulin sensitivity and postheparin plasma lipase activity in previously sedentary adults. *Diabetes Care*, *26*(3), 557–562.

Fitbit. (2016). Who we are. Retrieved from www.fitbit.com/about.

Fogg, B. J. (2003). *Persuasive technology: Using computers to change what we think and do*. New York: Morgan Kaufmann Publishers.

Gettman, L. R., & Pollock, M. L. (1981). Circuit weight training: A critical review of its physiological benefits. *The Physician and Sports Medicine*, *9*(1), 44–60.

Ghosh, A. K. (2004). Anaerobic threshold: Its concept and role in endurance sport. *The Malaysian Journal of Medical Sciences*, *11*(1), 24–36.

Graham, D. J., & Hipp, J. A. (2014). Emerging technologies to promote and evaluate physical activity: Cutting-edge research and future directions. *Frontiers in Public Health*, *2*(June), 66.

Gregersen, E. (2016). Tablet computer. In *Encyclopedia Britannica*. Retrieved from www.britannica.com/technology/tablet-computer.

Handy, S., Boarnet, M., Ewing, R., & Killingsworth, R. (2002). How the built environment affects physical activity: Views from urban planning. *American Journal of Preventive Medicine*, *23*(2S), 64–73.

Heyward, V. H., & Gibson, A. L. (2014). *Advanced fitness assessment and exercise prescription* (7th ed.). Champion, IL: Human Kinetics.

Hong, A.-R., Hong, S.-M., & Shin, Y.-A. (2014). Effects of resistance training on muscle strength, endurance, and motor unit according to ciliary neurotrophic factor polymorphism in male college students. *Journal of Sports Science & Medicine*, *13*(3), 680–688.

IMS Institute of Health Informatics. (2015). *Patient adoption of mHealth*. Retrieved from www.imshealth.com/en/thought-leadership/ims-institute/reports/patient-adoption-of-mhealth.

Kohl III, H., & Murray, T. (2012). *Foundations of physical activity and public health*. Champaign, IL: Human Kinetics.

Kokkinos, P. F., & Fernhall, B. (1999). Physical activity and high density lipoprotein cholesterol levels. *Sports Medicine*, *28*(5), 307–314.

Krenn, P., Mag, D., Titze, S., Oja, P., Jones, A., & Ogilvie, D. (2011). Use of global positioning systems to study physical activity and the environment. *American Journal of Preventive Medicine, 41*(5), 508–515.

Lamkin, P. (2016). The best VR headsets: The virtual reality race is on. Retrieved from www.wareable.com/headgear/the-best-ar-and-vr-headsets.

LeBlanc, A. G., & Janssen, I. (2010). Dose-response relationship between physical activity and dyslipidemia in youth. *Canadian Journal of Cardiology, 26*(6), e201–e205.

Lowood, H. (2015). Virtual reality (VR). In *Encyclopedia Britannica.* Retrieved from www.britannica.com/technology/virtual-reality.

Lowood, H. (2016). Electronic game. In *Encyclopedia Britannica.* Retrieved from www.britannica.com/topic/electronic-game.

MacLeod, H., Morris, J., Nevill, A., & Sunderland, C. (2009). The validity of a non-differential global positioning system for assessing player movement patterns in field hockey. *Journal of Sports Sciences, 27*(2), 121–128.

Maddison, R., & Mhurchu, C. (2009). Global positioning system: A new opportunity in physical activity measurement. *International Journal of Behavioral Nutrition and Physical Activity, 6*(73).

Malone, J., Michele, R., Morgans, R., Burgess, D., Morton, J., & Drust, B. (2015). Seasonal training-load quantification in elite English Premier League soccer players. *International Journal of Sports Physiology and Performance, 10*, 489–497.

Mammen, G., & Faulkner, G. (2013). Physical activity and the prevention of depression: A systematic review of prospective studies. *American Journal of Preventive Medicine, 45*(5), 649–657.

Matzka, M., Mayer, H., Köck-Hódi, S., Moses-Passini, C., Dubey, C., Jahn, P., … & Eicher, M. (2016). Relationship between resilience, psychological distress and physical activity in cancer patients: A cross-sectional observation study. *PloS one, 11*(4), e0154496.

Montfort, N., & Bogost, I. (2009). *Racing the beam: The Atari video computer system.* Cambridge, MA: The MIT Press.

Mossberg, W. S. (2012, April 25). Google stores, syncs, edits in the Cloud. *The Wall Street Journal.* Retrieved from www.wsj.com/articles/SB10001424052702303459004577362111867730108.

Myers, J., McAuley, P., Lavie, C. J., Despres, J. P., Arena, R., & Kokkinos, P. (2015). Physical activity and cardiorespiratory fitness as major markers of cardiovascular risk: Their independent and interwoven importance to health status. *Progress in Cardiovascular Diseases, 57*(4), 306–314.

National Geographic Society. (2016). *Encyclopedic entry: GIS (geographic information system).* Retrieved from http://nationalgeographic.org/encyclopedia/geographic-information-system-gis/.

Nigg, C. (2003). Technology's influence on physical activity and exercise science: the present and the future. *Psychology of Sport and Exercise, 4*, 57–65.

Pasco, D. (2013). The potential of using virtual reality technology in physical activity settings. *Quest, 65*(4), 429–441.

Pew Research Center. (2014). *World Wide Web timeline.* Retrieved from www.pewinternet.org/2014/03/11/world-wide-web-timeline/.

Rawassizadeh, R., Price, B., & Petre, M. (2015). Wearables: Has the age of smartwatches finally arrived? *Communications of the ACM, 58*(1), 45–47.

Ross, R. (2003). Does exercise without weight loss improve insulin sensitivity? *Diabetes Care, 26*(3), 944–945.

Statista. (2016a). Number of apps available in leading apps stores as of July 2015. Retrieved from www.statista.com/statistics/276623/number-of-apps-available-in-leading-app-stores/.

Statista. (2016b). Number of monthly active Facebook users worldwide as of 2nd quarter 2016 (in millions). Retrieved from www.statista.com/statistics/264810/number-of-monthly-active-facebook-users-worldwide/.

Statista. (2016c). Worldwide tablet shipments from 2nd quarter 2010 to 2nd quarter 2016 (in million units). Retrieved from www.statista.com/statistics/272070/global-tablet-shipments-by-quarter/.

Stonerock, G. L., Hoffman, B. M., Smith, P. J., & Blumenthal, J. A. (2015). Exercise as treatment for anxiety: Systematic review and analysis. *Annals of Behavioral Medicine, 49*(4), 542–556.

Terrel, K. (2015). The history of social media. Retrieved from http://historycooperative.org/the-history-of-social-media.

Tucker, P. (2008). The physical activity levels of preschool-aged children: A systematic review. *Early Childhood Research Quarterly, 23*(4), 547–558.

Turing, A. (1937). On computable numbers, with an application to the entscheidungproblem. *Proceedings of the London Mathmatical Society, s2–42*(1), 230–265.

Turing, A. (1946). Proposed electronic calculator. In B. Carpenter & R. Doran (Eds.), *A. M. Turing's ACE Report of 1946 and Other Papers*. Cambridge, MA: MIT Press.

U.S. Department of Health and Human Services. (1996). *Physical activity and health: A report of the Surgeon General*. Washington, DC: diane Publishing.

U.S. Department of Health and Human Services (2008). *Physical Activity Guidelines Advisory Committee report.* Washington, DC: U.S. Department of Health and Human Services.

U.S. Government Information. (2000). Civilians can use military GPS data. Retrieved from http://usgovinfo.about.com/library/news/aa050300b.htm.

U.S. Public Health Service, Office of the Surgeon General. (1996). *Physical activity and health: A report of the Surgeon General*. Atlanta, GA: US Department of Health and Human Services, Centers for Disease Control and Prevention, National Center for Chronic Disease Prevention and Health Promotion.

van Loon, L. J. (2014). Is there a need for protein ingestion during exercise? *Sports Medicine, 44*(1), 105–111.

Vella, C. A., & Robergs, R. A. (2005). A review of the stroke volume response to upright exercise in healthy subjects. *British Journal of Sports Medicine, 39*(4), 190–195.

World Health Organization. (2016, June). Physical activity. Retrieved from www.who.int/mediacentre/factsheets/fs385/en/.

Zhu, W. (2008). Promoting physical activity using technology. *Research Digest, 9*(3).

2 Overview

Promoting physical activity and health through emerging technology

Haichun Sun, Nan Zeng, and Zan Gao

Physical inactivity has been identified as one of the main causes of premature death and many chronic diseases such as cancer, cardiovascular disease, stroke, type 2 diabetes, some cancers, and obesity. Technology plays a complicated role in physical inactivity—much like a double-edged sword. On one hand, some technologies, such as sedentary video games, TV and computers, have contributed to the epidemic of physical inactivity and sedentary leisure-time behavior (e.g., playing sedentary video games). Conversely, some newly emerged technologies have been increasingly used to assess and promote physical activity (PA) and health. For example, pedometers and accelerometers have been extensively used as tools in assessing and promoting PA among various populations. Within the past decade, emerging technology including online social media, mobile devices applications, health wearable devices, GPS, GIS, and AVGs have been used to promote PA participation. Therefore, although technology has potential negative effects on a healthy and active lifestyle, technology does also have great possibilities to facilitate PA promotion.

Notably, this chapter does not include an overarching review of all the technologies used in the PA and health field, such as the metabolic assessment devices used in highly advanced laboratory settings. Instead, this chapter begins by providing a broad picture of the traditional and current emerging technologies that have been employed in promoting PA and health on a large scale in population-based settings, including communities, schools (Figure 2.1), and homes, as well as findings regarding the application of each technology in PA contexts. The following section describes the opportunities and challenges concerning the emerging technology integration in the promotion of PA and health.

Traditional technology in PA promotion

Technology has long been used as a means for PA promotion. Traditionally, many technologies for PA promotion were categorized into four groups: (1) telephone; (2) mass media; (3) computer/Internet; and (4) electronic devices. We describe each of these groups in the following subsections.

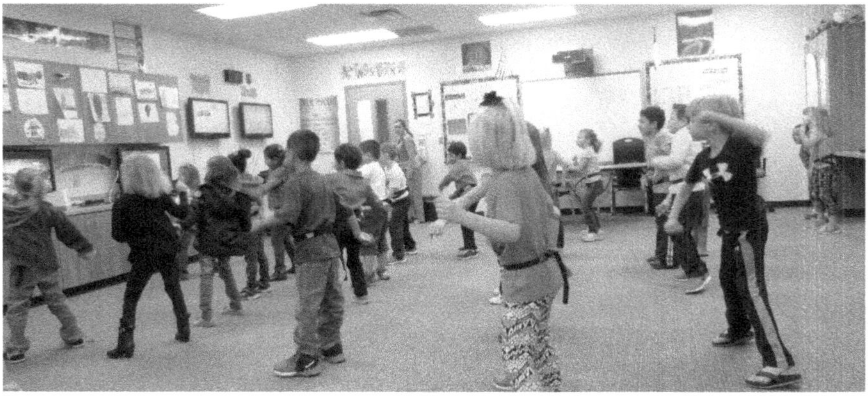

Figure 2.1 Young kids playing Kinect Just Dance.
Source: Photo by Zan Gao.

Telephone

Telephone-based intervention/program delivery is one of the most accessible approaches to PA promotion and has been used by major health agencies and organizations to conduct national surveillance studies which survey population-level rates of PA participation. As a result of telephone-based surveillance, previous research has provided strong evidence supporting telephone-based technologies as an effective method to promote PA behavior changes, with the ability to scale telephone-based interventions to the population level. This represents a major advantage of this technology (Goode, Reeves, & Eakin, 2012). Given the strength of evidence regarding telephone-based PA interventions, Goode et al. (2012) stated that the evaluation of the longer-term effects after cessation of this type of intervention as well as greater emphasis on the dissemination of the study methodology are warranted.

As mobile phones have become more ubiquitous over the last two decades, text messaging has also emerged as a telephone-based method to communicate with and promote individuals' participation in health-related behaviors. However, a recent systematic review identified that only a small group of researchers had conducted studies with regard to text message-based PA promotion (Buchholz et al., 2013). That said, these limited text message-based PA intervention studies did show promising results for increasing PA. Buchholz et al., therefore, argued that further research in this area is imperative.

Mass media

The mass media have diversified and continues to diversify communication methods, allowing for quick and efficient dissemination of information to large groups of people. Traditional mass media include radio, television, and print media (e.g., newspapers and magazines). A meta-analysis regarding the use of mass media for PA promotion indicated mixed results (Abioye, Hajifathalian, & Danaei, 2013). Nonetheless, Abioye et al. (2013) concluded that the mass media might promote greater walking participation, but may not be effective in reducing sedentary behavior or helping individuals participate in the recommended levels of PA. As such, the researchers stated that further research is needed to examine the effects of the mass media on outcomes such as objectively assessed PA and the necessary intensity and frequency of health messages delivered during mass media PA interventions. Further, more studies are warranted in low- and middle-income countries and in a sample of more diverse race/ethnicity. Studies addressing the aforementioned limitations are vital, given the mass media's ability to deliver content to large populations at low cost.

Computer and Internet use

The Internet and the World Wide Web represent information technology inventions and applications that have remarkably altered our lifestyles. Hundreds of thousands of websites have been developed to promote PA via information dissemination or direct PA intervention purposes. Research on Internet-based PA interventions, however, is still a relatively new area of inquiry. Previous Internet-based PA intervention studies have focused on developing programs tailored to participants' specific characteristics using interactive self-monitoring and feedback tools. As a result of the Internet-based PA interventions that use complex computer algorithms to offer tailored feedback to participants, it is not surprising that a meta-analysis recently reported that the delivery of Internet-based interventions is effective in producing positive PA behavioral changes (Davies, Spence, Vandelanotte, Caperchione, & Mummery, 2012). However, the authors indicated that the effect sizes of Internet-based interventions were relatively small. Similarly, Hamel, Robbins, and Wilbur (2011) reviewed 14 randomized controlled trials or quasi-experimental studies, concluding that while most Internet-based PA interventions have promoted significantly increased PA or positive PA-related behavioral changes, these findings were small and, notably, short-lived. Future research will be required to discover how to more effectively increase PA participation, as well as how to ensure the sustainability of PA behavioral change in the long term. With the preceding limitations of past research in mind, researchers have stated that future Internet-based PA interventions should include the use of objective PA measures, more programs tailored toward males, the involvement of greater social support, the integration into school curricula, the implementation of sound theoretical frameworks for intervention development, and individually tailored interventions (Hamel et al., 2011).

Electronic devices for PA assessment

Electronic devices have also been used to detect and process human body movement—subsequently providing quantifiable data on PA levels. The most popular electronic devices for this purpose are pedometers, accelerometers, and heart rate monitors. We discuss each of these devices in the following paragraphs.

A pedometer is a device that counts and monitors the number of steps taken during PA. Specifically, pedometers count the number of steps an individual takes by lifting an internal lever arm mechanically, electrically, or using a piezoelectric strain gauge (e.g., New Lifestyles NL-1000). Pedometers can be attached to a firm waistband, carried in a shirt/pants pocket, in a bag held close to the body, or worn on the ankle or in a shoe (Tudor-Locke et al., 2011)—with research indicating the positioning of the pedometer in a pants pocket or backpack might decrease accuracy (Hasson, Haller, Pober, Staudenmayer, & Freedson, 2009). Nevertheless, research has shown pedometers to be effective as both motivational tools and PA measurement devices. Bravata and colleagues (2007) reported that pedometer users increased their PA by 27% over baseline, which significantly decreased their body mass index, body weight, and systolic blood pressure. Importantly, researchers have developed health benefit thresholds for walking using pedometers (Tudor-Locke et al., 2011). Further, using criterion-referenced approaches, researchers can identify youth-specific walking thresholds for good health with these devices as well. In the future, it will also be critical to establish health risk thresholds for steps per day related to cardiovascular diseases (CVD), obesity, and osteoporosis—a task in which pedometers may play a major role.

Similar to pedometers, accelerometers are small portable electronic devices that record minute-by-minute information about the frequency, duration, intensity, and patterns of body movement. In detail, accelerometers are designed to assess total ambulatory activity levels via measurement of tri-axial accelerations and are, therefore, capable of providing an estimate of energy expenditure. Accelerometers have shown acceptable validity and good reliability and have been acknowledged as an accurate objective field measure for PA (Freedson & Miller, 2000). Accelerometers have also been used in national surveillance studies to objectively measure and monitor PA levels among the U.S. population. However, large-scale PA interventions using accelerometers are scarce due to the relatively high cost of accelerometers. Future development of lower-cost accelerometers are warranted in order to facilitate greater use of this device in national surveillance studies and smaller community-based interventions.

Motion sensors, such as pedometers and accelerometers, are considered practical, objective, and valid assessments of PA (Sirard & Pate, 2001). These instruments have advantages, such as minimal participant and experimenter burden, being unobtrusive to participants, and being comfortable and acceptable for the subjects to wear. Notably, pedometers are less expensive (approximately \$20–\$50) than accelerometers (e.g., approximately \$100–\$500), and are ideal for measuring the number of steps during a designated time period, recording distances, and providing estimated calories. However, accelerometers can provide very detailed information regarding the PA intensity (sedentary, light, moderate, and vigorous), the time spent at different PA intensity levels, and provide more accurate estimations of energy expenditure as compared to pedometers. Nonetheless, both types of motion sensors can accurately measure PA among children in real-world settings (e.g., physical education). That said, these devices are not yet equipped to adequately capture PA levels during such activities as stationary cycling and weightlifting (Freedson & Miller, 2000; Sirard & Pate, 2001).

Finally, heart rate monitors are devices that monitor individuals' PA intensity and can be used to estimate the individual's energy expenditure. Heart rate monitors have been widely used to estimate calories burned during PA due to the linear relationship between heart rate and energy expenditure during steady-state exercise. However, heart rate monitors are unable to accurately distinguish between light- and moderate-intensity activities or record the frequency of activity within a limited time frame (Hands, Parker, & Larkin, 2006). Moreover, the accuracy of heart rate monitors can also be affected by environmental factors, such as temperature, heat, and humidity. Therefore, future research is warranted to improve the measurement capabilities of this technology.

Emerging technology and its applications in PA promotion

The world is going through a cultural technological revolution. Over the course of the past several years, "Fourth screen" technology—smartphones, tablets, etc.—has occupied substantial amounts of personal time and changed the way we interact with one another. Indeed, smartphones and tablets have become broadly accessible and major channels for accessing social media or various types of apps. Wearable devices are also increasing in popularity and ubiquity (Figure 2.2). This section reviews these technologies and their application in PA interventions.

Online social media

Over the past two decades, the rapid rise of online social media such as Facebook, Twitter, and YouTube, among others, has resulted in these social media formats being investigated as intervention modalities, given their great potential to reach large groups of participants at a lower cost. A recent survey reported that in the U.S., 91% of young adults aged 18–29 years used online social media sites such as Facebook and Twitter. Different from traditional Web-based interventions, interventions using online social media allow participants to obtain health-related information, form social connections, and log health behaviors and activities any time without limited access (Zhang, Brackbill, Yang, & Centola, 2015).

As a global phenomenon—particularly among young adults—online social media have gained popularity among PA researchers. Research findings are promising, yet mixed. Some studies have suggested that online social media could be effective tools for both PA participation and weight loss. For example,

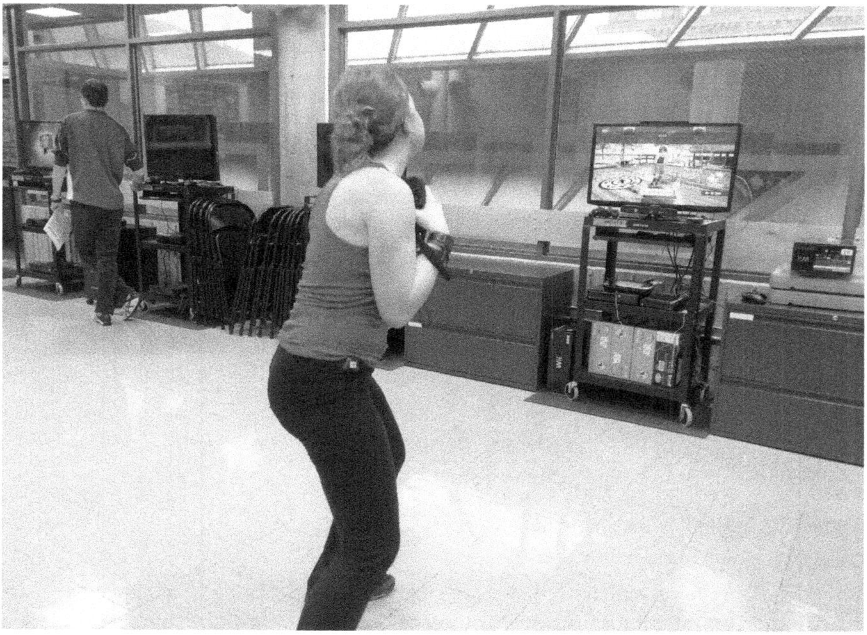

Figure 2.2 Testing smart watches.
Source: Photo by Zan Gao.

Hales, Davidson, and Turner-McGrievy (2014) found engagement in Facebook support groups was significantly associated with weight loss during the 4-month maintenance period of the intervention, even after adjusting for face-to-face meeting attendance. Other studies, however, did not suggest such positive results. Cavallo et al. (2012) conducted a randomized controlled trial among female undergraduate students to promote PA via a Facebook page. Researchers observed no differences between the online social media/Facebook PA page intervention group and the control group without access to a Facebook PA page. Taken together, more studies are needed to determine the effectiveness of online social media on PA and PA-related outcomes (Figure 2.3).

Recently, researchers have started to explore the effects of different types of posts on individuals' engagement with online social media. Strekalova and Krieger (2015) examined the impact of post type on audience engagement in association with the classification of a social media post as a photo, status update, video, or link. Findings indicated that photos have significantly greater impact on audience engagement than other media post types. Although this study was not completed within the context of PA, the findings certainly provide researchers with an idea of how to increase the effectiveness of their online social media-based PA interventions via experimentation with post type.

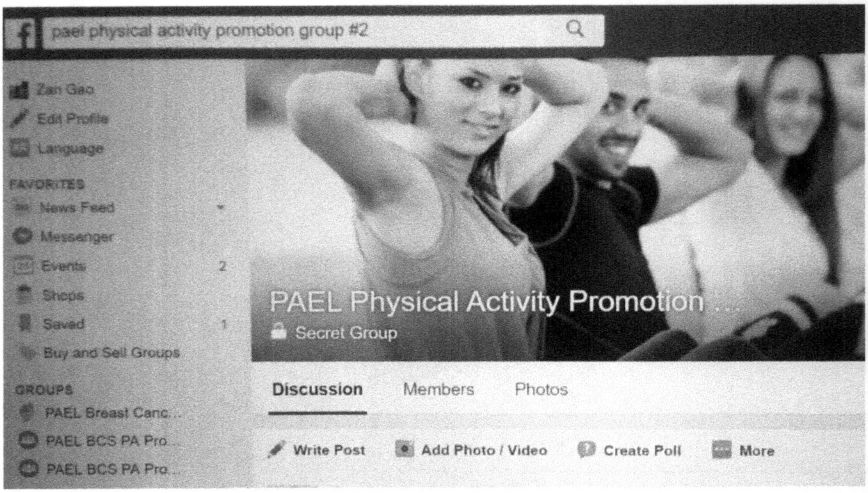

Figure 2.3 Facebook social media.

Source: Photo by Zan Gao.

Another popular function of the Internet is electronic publishing. Self-video publishing, in particular, may serve as a new dimension of Internet-based PA interventions. YouTube is the most popular video-sharing website—allowing users to upload, view, and share video clips. Like other online social media, self-video publishing sites, such as YouTube, can reach a large group of people rapidly. As such, these sites have a great potential to deliver health-related PA information and facilitate PA behavior changes. Clearly, there is a vital need to explore effective ways to use these new Internet opportunities to promote PA.

Mobile devices and apps

The mobile phone has also been widely acknowledged as a viable intervention delivery method that is easily accessible by a large number of individuals. Over the past several decades, mobile phones have developed dramatically in both design and function. Newly developed smartphones can be as sophisticated as tablets or a mini-personal computer, in addition to the capability to call and text. According to the Pew Research Center (Perrin, 2015), 64% of American adults own a smartphone, increasing the rationale for implementation of mobile phone-based PA interventions. Indeed, mobile phones and smartphones have unique features and components, including the ability to aid in self-monitoring and goal-setting, which can be utilized in PA interventions to promote behavior change (Duncan et al., 2014).

In recent years, mobile/smart phones have been implemented in PA interventions in addition to being integrated into existing online Internet-based programs.

For example, Kirwan et al. (2012) examined the effectiveness of a smartphone application, the iStepLog, on PA behaviors. Specifically, the application was designed to allow participants to record their daily PA levels on their smartphones. Through the built-in tracking software, researchers were able to monitor the time participants spent using the application, the frequency they logged their steps, and the most popular functions of the application. Their findings revealed that the application helped participants to maintain PA participation as compared to participants in the control group who showed a significant decline in the frequency and numbers of steps logged during the intervention period.

Although mobiles/smartphones have been observed to provide users more convenient access to the research-designed materials or information than print-based mediums, mobiles-/smartphone-based PA interventions might not be superior to print-based interventions in their effectiveness at promoting or changing PA behaviors. Duncan et al. (2014) compared the effectiveness of a 9-month Internet and mobile phone-based intervention to a print-based intervention on middle-aged males' PA, dietary behaviors, and health-related literacy. They found that participants in both groups had significant improvements in self-reported minutes and sessions of PA and overall dietary behaviors over time. However, there were no significant differences between the Internet/mobile phone-based group and the print-based group, suggesting that both methods could effectively deliver PA-related interventions. More importantly, Duncan et al. (2014) provided empirical evidence for future mobile phone/smart phone-based interventions. Specifically, these researchers revealed that participants are more likely to initiate PA challenges than the healthy eating challenges—further suggesting that light-strength PA challenges were the ones most frequently selected and completed by middle-aged males.

In general, mobile-/smartphone-based interventions allow participants to receive automated feedback, which provides these individuals with the additional ability to self-monitor their progress toward meeting their PA goals. Indeed, research has shown positive effects of mobile-/smartphone-based PA interventions. More studies are needed, however, exploring the long-term impact of mobile-/smartphone-based PA interventions on individuals' PA behavior.

Health wearable devices

In recent years, PA monitoring devices have gained popularity, with commercially available wearable activity monitors and trackers—health wearables (i.e., fitness bands and sports watches)—representing a rapidly growing health-focused industry. Health wearables use sensors to help users automatically track and set goals regarding PA (e.g., calories burned, step counts, distance traveled, etc.), sleep, diet, and other behaviors so as to optimize health behaviors (Almalki, Gray, & Sanchez, 2015). Over the last five years, health wearable technology has fast become a popular accessory. These health wearables can aid in the design and implementation of personal PA plans. Frequently, health wearables are used to motivate people to engage in more PA by viewing data and the results captured in real time, after which structured PA plans can be developed. Rapid developments in technology have encouraged the use of health wearable devices (e.g., Fitbit, Apple Watch, TomTom sports watch, Microsoft Band, etc.) in PA research and have generated new opportunities for promoting healthy lifestyles across diverse populations. Advances in the technology of health wearable devices also provide professionals and researchers a variety of PA measurement options to assess multiple health-related outcomes.

Thorndike and colleagues (2014) demonstrated that utilizing health wearable technology (Fitbit) may have potential for promoting healthier lifestyles among clinical populations. Further, Cadmus-Bertram et al. (2015) found that employing the Fitbit associated Internet-based app can promote postmenopausal women's moderate-to-vigorous PA (MVPA) and steps. Similarly, Wang and colleagues (2015) combined the Fitbit and short message service (SMS) text-messaging prompts to increase PA in overweight and obese adults. These researchers found the Fitbit One is capable of promoting a small increase in MVPA. Conversely, Melton and colleagues (2016) found that health wearables (Jawbone) are not effective in improving PA participation or sleep quality among African American college women. Moreover, while Jakicic and colleagues (2016) found individuals using health wearable devices that monitor and provide feedback on PA did have significant improvements in body composition, fitness, PA, and diet, these health wearable devices did not offer an advantage over standard behavioral weight loss approaches.

Although evidence regarding the effectiveness of health wearable devices in promoting PA and health is inconclusive, studies have demonstrated that these devices hold great promise for promoting healthier lifestyles among a diverse array of populations. Overall, the market for health wearable devices continues to grow in popularity, and the potential usefulness of using these devices to promote health is considerable.

GPS/GIS

As one of the most sophisticated modern technologies to be used in PA and health promotion, GPS and GIS—two related technologies, only recently popularized for health and fitness—show great promise in the public health field. Briefly, GPS calculates geographic locations and accurately tracks activity using 24 satellites and ground stations as reference points, which can be used in conjunction with accelerometers to assess and monitor PA parameters, such as activity time, distance, altitude, and average velocity (Rodriguez, Brown, & Troped, 2005; Troped et al., 2008). GIS is a computer system that caches information in relation to location and the surrounding environment (Heyward & Gibson, 2014). PA data captured by GPS can then be analyzed by GIS in relation to the locations where these activities took place—facilitating researchers' ability to discern associations between locations where the PA participation occurred and features of the built environment (e.g., sidewalk construction, land use, and trail systems) which may inhibit or facilitate PA participation.

As more sophisticated GPS technology has been developed within the past several years, research has shifted concentration from testing the reliability and validity of GPS and GIS to using these technologies to promote PA participation and health promotion. Indeed, the majority of the literature to date on the topic of GPS/GIS and PA and health focuses on the assessment of PA patterns instead of on PA promotion interventions. Furthermore, researchers using GPS/GIS are investigating how PA participation and promotion can be improved, implemented, and achieved by modifying the built environment to facilitate PA behavior change among youth and adults (Maddison et al., 2010; Wheeler, Cooper, Page, & Jago, 2010) (Figure 2.4). In addition to the built environment, GPS technology has also been employed in professional sports to assess PA patterns and examine position differences in intensity during the game such as: overall time in light, moderate, and vigorous exercise; distance traveled; and average/peak velocities (Kempton, Sullivan, Bilsborough, Cordy, & Coutts, 2015; Macutkiewicz & Sunderland, 2011).

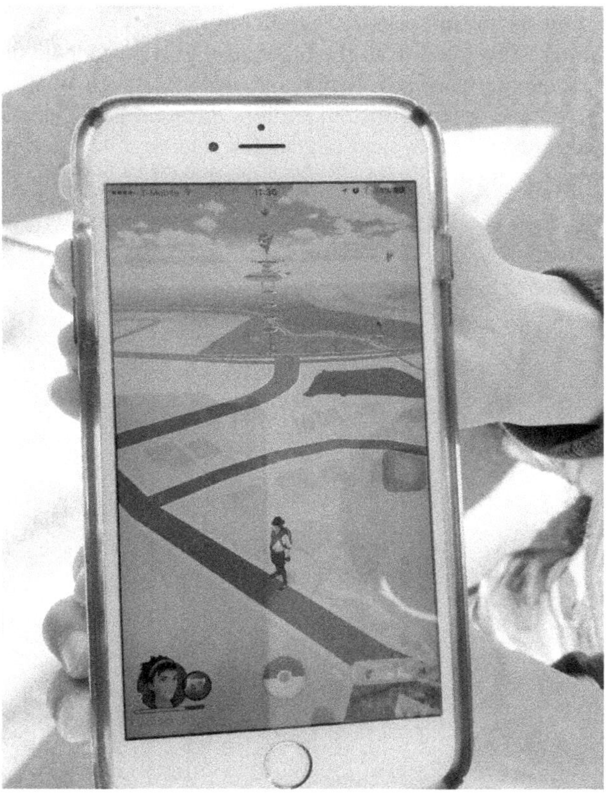

Figure 2.4 A kid playing Pokémon Go.

Source: Photo by Zan Gao.

Overall, GPS and GIS systems show promise as a way of improving our understanding of the relationship between environmental attributes and PA behavior at the population level, despite the relative paucity of literature using these technologies in the field of PA intervention and health promotion. That said, with the use of GPS/GIS for PA and health promotion among the general population continuing to increase, it is clear that the potential of GPS/GIS technology in PA and health promotion is considerable.

Active video games (AVGs)

AVGs are active video games that require players' bodily movement during gameplay. AVGs were originally designed to engage players in a more active mode of video game play, with research indicating AVGs have great potential to serve as a motivational source to initially engage players in PA (Sun, 2015). For example, Sun (2012) compared students' perceived situational interest between an AVG unit and a cardiovascular fitness-education unit. Findings indicated that students had significantly higher levels of situational interest in the AVG unit than they did in the fitness-education unit. Specifically, researchers found that increased situational interest resulted from the fact that AVGs provided a unique opportunity for players to experience new features, to use high levels of attention throughout gameplay, to have opportunities to explore different game situations, and be offered both cognitive and physical challenges, and be able to achieve a high level of instant enjoyment (Figure 2.5). Nonetheless, although AVGs

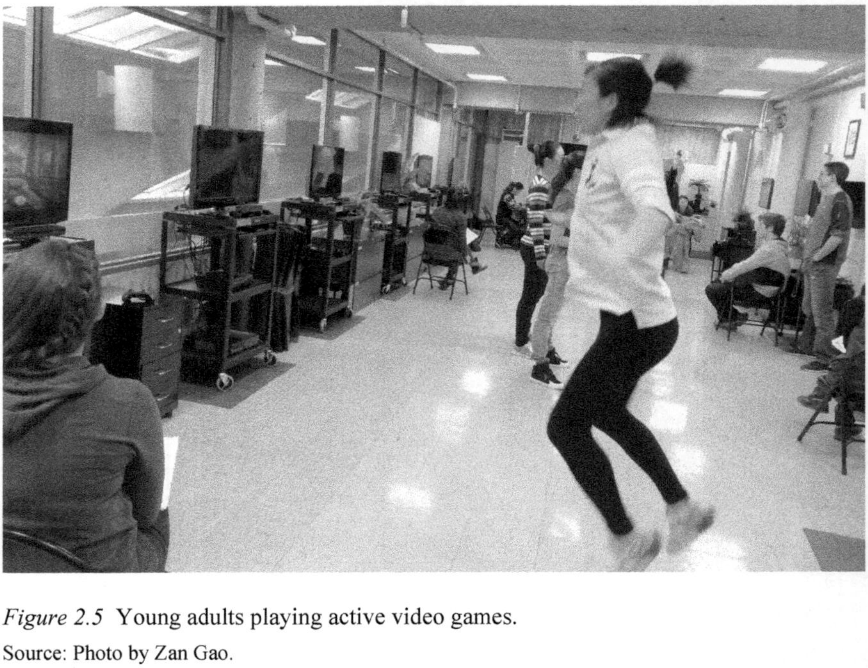

Figure 2.5 Young adults playing active video games.

Source: Photo by Zan Gao.

demonstrate an ability to motivate individuals during gameplay, the sustainability of this motivational function is questionable. How to achieve sustainable motivation as well as motivate sustainable PA behaviors outside of AVG play should be the focus of future AVG development and AVG-based interventions.

In addition to their motivational function, previous studies have demonstrated AVGs' ability to increase energy expenditure and produce positive health benefits while also examining the influence of gender, intensity, and active body mass on the overall energy cost of AVGs (Bailey & McInnis 2011) (Figure 2.6).

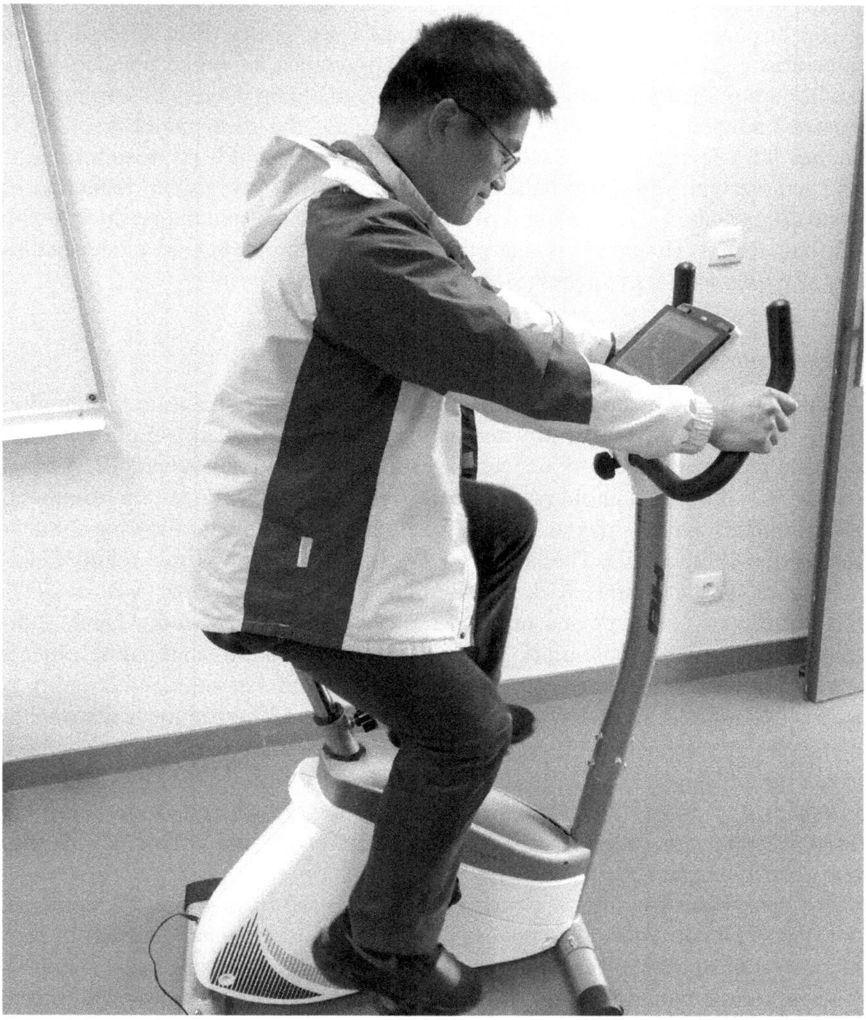

Figure 2.6 Active bike game.

Source: Photo by Denis Pasco.

Moreover, while participants generally enjoyed the AVGs, perceived enjoyment varied by gender and BMI classifications. Notably, children with higher BMIs enjoyed AVGs with greater social interaction offering intermittent high-intensity gameplay than children with lower BMIs. This finding is significant in that it provides empirical data for future AVG design and interventions that specifically target adolescents "at-risk" for overweight.

Recently, Sun (2015) further indicated the great potential of AVGs to facilitate players' cognitive development. For instance, Gao and colleagues (2013) examined the impact of Dance Revolution (DDR) on Latino children's physical fitness and academic achievement. They found that children in the intervention group displayed greater improvement on math test scores than children in the comparison group. The results are of great importance for future practice. More studies are needed to identify the role of AVGs in aiding players in learning PA-related knowledge, concepts, or strategies. While the great majority of AVG studies have focused on children, this technology also holds promise for adults and seniors with respect to balance improvement, fall prevention, reduction of premature disability, increasing functional independence, and maintaining health (deJong, 2010). The reader is referred to Chapter 9 to obtain a deep understanding of AVGs on PA and health.

Virtual reality

Among emerging technologies poised to aid in the assessment and promotion of PA and health, virtual reality and augmented reality (a.k.a., simulation technology) are arguably the most exciting and technologically advanced. Virtual reality is a digital technology that replicates a real or imagined environment, and simulates a user's physical presence in this environment, allowing for user interaction (Figure 2.7). The latest commercially available virtual reality headsets, such as the Oculus Rift, PlayStation VR, Samsung Gear VR, or HTC Vive artificially generate sensory experiences, which can include visual, auditory, touch, and scent stimuli, while allowing a user to manipulate objects within the virtual environment (Isaac, 2016). By contrast, augmented reality is a direct or indirect live view of a physical, real-world environment whose elements are supplemented by computer-generated sensory input such as sound, video, graphics or GPS data (Graham, Zook, & Boulton, 2013). Augmented virtual reality games, like Pokémon Go, Zombies, Run!, and Geocaching are unique in that they overlay aspects from the physical and virtual worlds into one cohesive experience.

To date, virtual reality has been extensively used in many health domains, with most virtual reality systems used for the purpose of rehabilitation. In fact, the potential of virtual reality in PA and health promotion has been explored, with improved motor function (McEwen, Taillon-Hobson, Bilodeau, Sveistrup, & Finestone, 2014; Saposnik et al., 2016), cognitive learning (Man, Chung, & Lee, 2012), and psychological well-being (Gaggioli et al., 2014) observed among various populations using this technology. Yet, while considered a cutting-edge

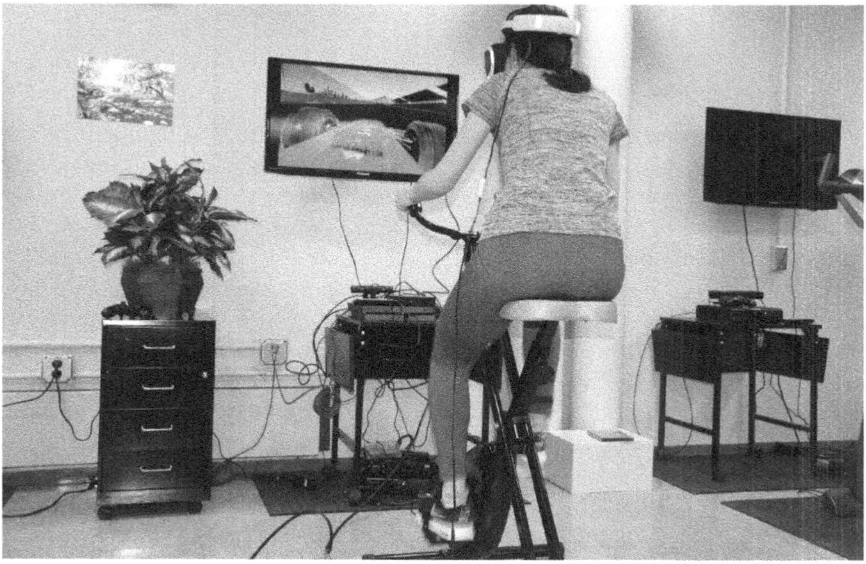

Figure 2.7 A young adult playing virtual reality games.

Source: Photo by Zan Gao.

technology possessing great potential in promoting PA, the use of virtual reality technology to promote PA is still in its infancy (Pasco, 2013). Nonetheless, the preceding literature review regarding the use of virtual reality in various PA settings indicates virtual reality technologies can have current applications in physical education and sports settings to promote PA and athletic performance. However, few large-scale, methodologically rigorous studies have been conducted in the literature, with no high-quality study completed in a physical education class. Therefore, researchers and practitioners should continue to explore the benefits of virtual reality and harness its potential in the promotion of PA and health among a variety of populations.

Opportunities and challenges

Technology has changed our lives tremendously over the past several decades and played a paramount role in shaping our lifestyles and health status. Emerging technologies bring exciting or even stunning opportunities for the promotion of PA and health. Yet, not all contributions from emerging technologies have been positive. The emerging field of PA and health, coupled with the rapid development of technology, has presented both challenges and opportunities that deserve further considerations for researchers. According to King and colleagues (2015), challenges and opportunities can be classified into four categories: (1) data collection and data expansion; (2) technical considerations; (3) areas for "bridging the gap"; and (4) privacy protection.

Data collection and data expansion

While processing data gathered from emerging technologies, a number of challenges have emerged. First, there has been a lack of Big Data analysis, despite the potential large amount of PA data that can be retrieved from multiple emerging technologies (e.g., PA data, posts on social media, GPS/GIS data, etc.) to improve the population's health. Thus, great opportunities exist to deal with Big Data via improved mathematical models and computer algorithms. Undoubtedly, researchers will find it vital to empower themselves to assess and analyze PA data through data and text mining within the next decade. Indeed, the ability to conduct Big Data analysis will be paramount in offering users constant personalized exercise prescriptions through mobile device apps in the future. Second, there has been little use of crowdsourcing data in the PA field. Further, many emerging technologies are not yet capable of capitalizing on the ubiquity and heterogeneity of potential environmental data sources or of employing crowdsourcing to evaluate and manage large datasets in an effort to improve public health. As such, crowdsourcing data in PA and health is an emerging field. For example, researchers have started to use crowdsourcing to complete PA evaluation and surveillance (Amazon Mechanic Turk; www.mturk.com). It appears promising to take advantage of crowdsourcing data in promoting PA in the future. Third, there is a lack of GIS infrastructure in many regional and local areas. Indeed, discrepancies exist for GIS infrastructure between major metropolitan areas and small towns. Thus, it is recommended that local municipalities and/or companies share GIS resources. Fourth, there is still a lack of sufficient PA data. Recruiting and training more researchers to study PA and emerging technologies are strongly encouraged. Finally, little understanding of person–environment interactions in studies using emerging technologies has been seen. It is, therefore, warranted to increase the number of studies that investigate different dimensions of an individual's personal attributes (e.g., self-esteem, attitudes, cognition, weight status) and environments (e.g., social environment, physical environment).

Technical considerations

Technology is rapidly developing at an amazing speed, thus offering numerous challenges and opportunities. First, a challenge exists in keeping up to date with the latest technological advances. Nowadays it is not uncommon for researchers to find that their recently purchased products have become outdated after a short period of time. King et al. (2015) suggested the centralization of technological resources for researchers with links, critiques, etc. It is also recommended to partner with companies in the public sector to begin developing and testing emerging technologies. Second, it is noteworthy that a virtual exercise advisor has now been applied in PA promotion. For example, a culturally and linguistically adapted virtual exercise advisor (i.e., Carmen) was used to provide tailor-based PA advice and support to the elderly. Given the major potential of this type of interactive technology, it is advisable for health professionals and researchers to solicit small business research grants to develop cutting-edge technologies for PA promotion. Third, augmented reality games (e.g., Pokémon Go) have successfully gained attention from users in recent years. These reality games are attractive as they integrate the physical and virtual worlds into one interface on mobile devices, particularly the apps of smartphone devices. Of note for health professionals, augmented reality games require users to walk around and explore their local surroundings; hence increasing PA participation. However, physical harm may occur, such as playing these games while walking or driving. Playing the games also increases the economic burden as a result of in-app purchasing and heavy data usage, and potentially leads the users to enter inappropriate or dangerous areas. In addition, the goe-locating feature embedded within some games can result in crime (e.g., criminals using the "lure" function of Pokémon Go). It is, therefore, imperative to offer safety guidelines for users of such games. Fourth, the cost of recent technology and relevant equipment and supplies can be a problem. In many cases, researchers provide subjects with the required equipment and supplies, assuming the investment will increase consistency in intervention across participants and decrease the potential barriers to participation and adherence. Yet, it can be quite expensive to offer lots of devices to a large population at one time. To deal with this issue, researchers can solicit research funds and industry donations for technology-based PA promotion programs. Researchers can also enroll participants in cohorts to decrease the number of devices needed. For some programs, it is possible to request participants cover the costs (e.g., when using smartphone and its apps as intervention strategies)—potentially providing a more contextually relevant evaluation of the intervention program. Additionally, it is challenging to secure funds for longitudinal data collection. Indeed, with longitudinal or prospective research studies, external funds may be necessary to fully integrate emerging technologies and examine their effectiveness. In these circumstances, researchers can again use established relationships with stakeholders to cover implementation costs. Finally, challenges exist due to the discrepancies in access to emerging technology among individuals from different socioeconomic status. It is suggested to locate and use publicly available technological resources or to employ widely used low-fee mobile devices, such as smartphones for PA promotion.

Areas for "bridging the gap"

To bridge the gap between research on the use of emerging technologies to promote PA and the real world, researchers face a number of challenges. First, technology is continuously becoming more sophisticated, and experts in various disciplines are needed to develop and implement technology applications to improve health in field-/clinic-based settings. Many times, some well-functioning applications are designed by computer scientists while neglecting the needs of clients, which leads to little or no intervention impact. Hence, to design and implement an effective technology application for PA promotion, it is critical to recruit researchers and practitioners from different disciplines, including PA specialists, computer scientists, and health practitioners as well as consulting the end users. Once more, forming institutional collaborations with initiatives and monetary incentives is encouraged. Notably, with the increasing application of the Social Ecological Model, the built environment inevitably becomes an indispensable component of PA promotion. As such, partnering with experts across disciplines (e.g., PA, planning, transportation, technology) is also encouraged. Second, with the integration of electronic devices, mobile devices, and apps, bridging the gap between PA assessment and intervention becomes a challenge for researchers. Thus, working with all stakeholders, including clients, to identify the leverage points for behavioral change and integrating everyday PA data seamlessly into the lives of participants to promote behavioral change strategies will be important in the years to come. Finally, to effectively implement technology-based PA promotion, it is imperative to understand the community and organizational systems, as well as all the other stakeholders' needs and interests. For example, in school-based PA programs, technology can offer more choice to students. Children may be able to choose from different active video games, such as Wii Fit, Kinect Just Dance, and Dance Revolution and other games. This increased autonomy acts as a motivational tool to make children be active and improve class participation. Yet, it is quite challenging to implement such programs in schools due to lack of support from the school administration, space limitations, curricular conflicts, and budget shortages. As a result, King et al. (2015) recommended teaming up with organizational personnel from different community sectors, engaging with supportive decision-makers, and collaborating with industry to assess technology applications in PA and health field.

Privacy protection

There are substantial concerns regarding how the digital world has compromised and is compromising anonymity. Briefly, emerging technologies that continuously collect data regarding PA behavior as well as other social and environmental aspects related to PA invite several important ethical considerations for researchers in the areas of anonymity, privacy, and participants' informed consent. Therefore, researchers should develop standardized protocols for privacy protection. More details will be discussed in Chapter 12.

References

Abioye, A. I., Hajifathalian, K., & Danaei, G. (2013). Do mass media campaigns improve physical activity? A systematic review and meta-analysis. *Archives of Public Health*, *71*(1), 20–30.

Almalki, M., Gray, K., & Sanchez, F. M. (2015). The use of self-quantification systems for personal health information: Big Data management activities and prospects. *Health Information Science and Systems, 3*(1), 1–11.

Bailey, B. W., & McInnis, K. (2011). Energy cost of exergaming: A comparison of the energy cost of 6 forms of exergaming. *Archives of Pediatrics & Adolescent Medicine, 165*(7), 597–602.

Bravata, D. M., Smith-Spangler, C., Sundaram, V., Gienger, A. L., Lin, N., Lewis, R., … & Sirard, J. R. (2007). Using pedometers to increase physical activity and improve health: A systematic review. *JAMA, 298*(19), 2296–2304.

Buchholz, S. W., Wilbur, J., Ingram, D., & Fogg, L. (2013). Physical activity text messaging interventions in adults: A systematic review. *Worldviews on Evidence-Based Nursing, 10*(3), 163–173.

Cadmus-Bertram, L. A., Marcus, B. H., Patterson, R. E., Parker, B. A., & Morey, B. L. (2015). Randomized trial of a Fitbit-based physical activity intervention for women. *American Journal of Preventive Medicine, 49*(3), 414–418.

Cavallo, D. N., Tate, D. F., Ries, A. V., Brown, J. D., DeVellis, R. F., & Ammerman, A. S. (2012). A social media–based physical activity intervention: A randomized controlled trial. *American Journal of Preventive Medicine, 43*(5), 527–532.

Davies, C. A., Spence, J. C., Vandelanotte, C., Caperchione, C. M., & Mummery, W. K. (2012). Meta-analysis of internet-delivered interventions to increase physical activity levels. *International Journal of Behavioral Nutrition and Physical Activity, 9*(1), 52–65.

deJong, A. (2010). Active video gaming: An opportunity to increase energy expenditure throughout aging. *ACSM's Health & Fitness Journal, 14*(6), 44–46.

Duncan, M., Vandelanotte, C., Kolt, G. S., Rosenkranz, R. R., Caperchione, C. M., George, E. S., … & Noakes, M. (2014). Effectiveness of a web-and mobile phone-based intervention to promote physical activity and healthy eating in middle-aged males: Randomized controlled trial of the ManUp study. *Journal of Medical Internet Research, 16*(6), e136.

Freedson, P. S., & Miller, K. (2000). Objective monitoring of physical activity using motion sensors and heart rate. *Research Quarterly for Exercise and Sport, 71*(suppl. 2), 21–29.

Gaggioli, A., Pallavicini, F., Morganti, L., Serino, S., Scaratti, C., Briguglio, M., … Tartarisco, G. (2014). Experiential virtual scenarios with real-time monitoring (interreality) for the management of psychological stress: A block randomized controlled trial. *Journal of Medical Internet Research, 16*(7), e167.

Gao, Z., Hannan P., Xiang, P., Stodden, D. F, & Valdez, V. E (2013). Video game-based exercise, Latino children's physical health, and academic achievement. *American Journal of Preventive Medicine, 44*, 240–246.

Goode, A. D., Reeves, M. M., & Eakin, E. G. (2012). Telephone-delivered interventions for physical activity and dietary behavior change: An updated systematic review. *American Journal of Preventive Medicine, 42*(1), 81–88.

Graham, M., Zook, M., & Boulton, A. (2013). Augmented reality in urban places: Contested content and the duplicity of code. *Transactions of the Institute of British Geographers, 38*(3), 464–479.

Hales, S. B., Davidson, C., & Turner-McGrievy, G. M. (2014). Varying social media post types differentially impacts engagement in a behavioral weight loss intervention. *Translational Behavioral Medicine, 4*(4), 355–362.

Hamel, L. M., Robbins, L. B., & Wilbur, J. (2011). Computer- and web-based interventions to increase preadolescent and adolescent physical activity: A systematic review. *Journal of Advanced Nursing, 67*(2), 251–268.

Hands, B. P., Parker, H., & Larkin, D. (2006). Physical activity measurement methods for young children: A comparative study. *Measurement in Physical Education and Exercise Science, 10*(3), 203–214.

Hasson, R., Haller, J., Pober, D., Staudenmayer, J., & Freedson, P. (2009). Validity of the Omron HJ-112 pedometer during treadmill walking. *Medicine Science in Sports Exercise, 41*(4), 805–809.

Heyward, V. H., & Gibson, A. (2014). *Advanced fitness assessment and exercise prescription* (7th ed.). Champaign, IL: Human Kinetics.

Isaac, J. (2016). Step into a new world – Virtual Reality (VR). Retrieved from www.completegate.com/2016070154/blog/virtual-reality-explained#vrdef.

Jakicic, J. M., Davis, K. K., Rogers, R. J., King, W. C., Marcus, M. D., Helsel, D., … Belle, S. H. (2016). Effect of wearable technology combined with a lifestyle intervention on long-term weight loss: The IDEA randomized clinical trial. *JAMA, 316*(11), 1161–1171.

Kempton, T., Sullivan, C., Bilsborough, J., Cordy, J., & Coutts, A. (2015). Match-to-match variation in physical activity and technical skill measures in professional Australian Football. *Journal of Science and Medicine in Sport, 18*, 109–113.

King, A. C., Glanz, K., & Patrick, K. (2015). Technologies to measure and modify physical activity and eating environments. *American Journal of Preventive Medicine*, *48*(5), 630–638.

Kirwan, M., Duncan, M. J., Vandelanotte, C., & Mummery, W. K. (2012). Using smartphone technology to monitor physical activity in the 10,000 Steps program: A matched case-control trial. *Journal of Medical Internet Research, 14*(2), e55.

Macutkiewicz, D., & Sunderland, C. (2011). The use of GPS to evaluate activity profiles of elite women hockey players during match-play. *Journal of Sports Sciences, 29*(9), 967–973.

Maddison, R., Jiang, Y., Hoorn, S., Exeter, D., Mhurchu, C., & Dorey, E. (2010). Describing patterns of physical activity in adolescents using global positioning systems and accelerometry. *Pediatric Exercise Science, 22*, 392–407.

Man, D. W., Chung, J. C., & Lee, G. Y. (2012). Evaluation of a virtual reality-based memory training programme for Hong Kong Chinese older adults with questionable dementia: A pilot study. *International Journal of Geriatric Psychiatry, 27*(5), 513–520.

McEwen, D., Taillon-Hobson, A., Bilodeau, M., Sveistrup, H., & Finestone, H. (2014). Virtual reality exercise improves mobility after stroke: An inpatient randomized controlled trial. *Stroke*, *45*(6), 1853–1855.

Melton, B. F., Buman, M. P., Vogel, R. L., Harris, B. S., & Bigham, L. E. (2016). Wearable devices to improve physical activity and sleep: A randomized controlled trial of college-aged African American women. *Journal of Black Studies*, published online before print June 8, 2016.

Pasco, D. (2013). The potential of using virtual reality technology in physical activity settings. *Quest, 65*(4), 429–441.

Perrin, A. (2015). Social networking usage: 2005–2015. *Pew Research Center*. Retrieved from www.pewinternet.org/

Rodriguez, D., Brown, A., & Troped, P. (2005). Portable global positioning units to complement accelerometry-based physical activity monitors. *Medicine and Science in Sport and Exercise, 37*(11 (Suppl.)), S572–S581.

Saposnik, G., Cohen, L. G., Mamdani, M., Pooyania, S., Ploughman, M., Cheung, D., … Nilanont, Y. (2016). Efficacy and safety of non-immersive virtual reality exercising in stroke rehabilitation (EVREST): A randomised, multicentre, single-blind, controlled trial. *The Lancet Neurology, 15*(10), 1019–1027.

Sirard, J. R., & Pate, R. R. (2001). Physical activity assessment in children and adolescents. *Sports Medicine, 31*(6), 439–454.

Strekalova, Y. A., & Krieger, J. L. (2015). A picture really is worth a thousand words: Public engagement with the National Cancer Institute on social media. *Journal of Cancer Education*, 1–3.

Sun, H. (2012). Exergaming impact on physical activity and interest in elementary school children. *Research Quarterly for Exercise and Sport, 83*, 212–220.

Sun, H. (2015). Operationalizing physical literacy: The potential of Active Video Games. *Journal of Sport and Health Science, 4*, 145–149.

Thorndike, A. N., Mills, S., Sonnenberg, L., Palakshappa, D., Gao, T., Pau, C. T., & Regan, S. (2014). Activity monitor intervention to promote physical activity of physicians-in-training: Randomized controlled trial. *PloS One, 9*(6), e100251.

Troped, P., Oliveira, M., Matthews, C., Cromley, E., Melly, S., & Craig, B. (2008). Prediction of activity mode with global positioning system and accelerometer data. *Medicine and Science in Sport and Exercise, 40*(5), 972–978.

Tudor-Locke, C., Craig, C., Brown, W., Clemes, S., De Cocker, K., Giles-Corti, B., … Blair, S. (2011). How many steps/day are enough? For adults. *International Journal of Behavioral Nutrition and Physical Activity, 8*(1), 79.

Tudor-Locke, C., Leonardi, C., Johnson, W. D., Katzmarzyk, P. T., & Church, T. S. (2011). Accelerometer steps/day translation of moderate-to-vigorous activity. *Preventive Medicine, 53*(1), 31–33.

Wang, J. B., Cadmus-Bertram, L. A., Natarajan, L., White, M. M., Madanat, H., Nichols, J. F., … & Pierce, J. P. (2015). Wearable sensor/device (Fitbit One) and SMS text-messaging prompts to increase physical activity in overweight and obese adults: A randomized controlled trial. *Telemedicine and e-Health, 21*(10), 782–792.

Wheeler, B., Cooper, A., Page, A., & Jago, R. (2010). Greenspace and children's physical activity: A GPS/GIS analysis of the PEACH project. *Preventative Medicine, 51*, 148–152.

Zhang, J., Brackbill, D., Yang, S., & Centola, D. (2015). Efficacy and causal mechanism of an online social media intervention to increase physical activity: Results of a randomized controlled trial. *Preventive Medicine Reports, 2*, 651–657.

3 Social and behavioral theories in promoting physical activity

Zan Gao and Jung Eun Lee

The health benefits of regular physical activity (PA) participation among various populations has been well documented for several decades. However, the proportions of different age groups meeting the current PA recommendations are relatively low (Blair & Morris, 2009). For example, approximately 21% of adults meet the PA Guidelines of the Centers for Disease Control and Prevention (CDC) of 150 minutes/week moderate-intensity aerobic activity, and less than 30% of high school students have at least 60 minutes of PA every day. Unfortunately, it has been evident that changing individuals' PA behaviors is rather complicated due to the fact that individuals usually encounter considerable barriers and challenges from personal and environmental factors during the behavior change process (Sallis, Cervero, Ascher, Henderson, Kraft, & Kerr, 2006). Oftentimes, however, the barriers and challenges that individuals face when seeking to change PA behavior can be minimized through the application of sound social and behavioral theory (also termed "models").

Notably, early studies intervening to promote PA did not typically embrace social and behavioral theoretical frameworks. Later, as the field developed, it became necessary to employ appropriate theoretical frameworks to better implement effective PA interventions and allow for subsequent intervention replication. As a result of these needs, scholars started to apply social, psychological, behavioral, and even environmental theories to better understand the determinants and correlates of PA behavior (Sutton, 2008). According to King et al. (2015), there are three classifications and seven theories for the types of theories that have been widely applied in the field of PA and health. These classifications are:

1. Personal-level theories: Self-efficacy Theory, Goal Setting Theory, Self-determination Theory, Theory of Planned Behavior, and the Transtheoretical Model.
2. Behavior micro-environmental theories: Social Cognitive Theory.
3. Behavior macro-environmental theories: Social Ecologic Model.

Indeed, over the past 20 years, a burgeoning of theory-based studies in the PA and health promotion field has been observed, with many studies using one or more of the seven theories listed above. Theories and models are important in that: (1) they allow us to better understand and predict individuals' PA behavior; (2) they provide a scientifically validated blueprint from which to formulate effective PA behavioral interventions; and (3) they enable us to organize PA behavior variables in a coherent manner. Simply stated, theories and models can help explain PA behavior, as well as suggest how to develop and implement more effective intervention methodology capable of influencing and changing such behavior to a greater degree. Undoubtedly, the application of the aforementioned theories has tremendously improved our understanding of individuals' PA correlates/determinants that are associated with or impact their PA behavior.

This chapter focuses on behavioral theories for PA promotion—particularly those most pertinent to the integration of emerging technology within PA interventions. First, an overview of widely used behavioral theories for the development, implementation, and evaluation of PA promotion interventions is provided. The following section describes important theories and key concepts/constructs within each theory that are often used to promote PA and health. Immediately following will be a brief summary of the empirical evidence concerning the application of theories in emerging technology-based PA promotion interventions. Finally, a short discussion of the challenges and future directions for the application of theories in technology-based practice and empirical research will be given.

Personal-level theoretical perspectives and PA promotion

Self-efficacy Theory

Self-efficacy Theory originated from the Social Cognitive Theory and includes self-efficacy and outcome expectancy as the two major constructs (Bandura, 1986, 1997). This intrapersonal-level behavioral theory proposes that an individual's behavior can be explained and predicted by the positive relationship between self-efficacy and outcome expectancy. Notably, self-efficacy refers to beliefs about one's capabilities to learn or perform specific behaviors with a certain degree of mastery. Specifically, individuals who feel efficacious are more likely to perform at a higher level, try new behaviors, expend more effort on those behaviors, and persevere longer when they encounter challenges to these behaviors. In PA contexts, evidence has been clear that self-efficacy directly influences or predicts behavior through its effect on goal setting, the capability to persist while facing obstacles, and coping with setbacks and stress.

Outcome expectancy refers to a person's beliefs concerning the likely consequences of a behavior. The importance of an outcome and the degree of its influence may have a great deal of variability among individuals. Thus, it is crucial not to presume that outcomes will always act as incentives for motivated behavior (Rodgers & Brawley, 1991). As a result, Rodgers and Brawley proposed that outcome expectancy is formed by the interaction of two factors: (1) outcome likelihood, which refers to the probability that a certain action will lead to a certain outcome; and (2) outcome values, which refer to the values the individual assigns to the possible outcomes of the behavior. However, relative to self-efficacy, less attention has been paid to outcome expectancy. Of note, in sports and PA contexts, research has shown small or no associations between outcome expectancy and behavior (e.g., Rovniak, Anderson, Winett, & Stephen, 2002).

Research focusing on the ways that self-efficacy and outcome expectancy might operate together to impact individuals' behaviors has produced mixed findings. Bandura (1986, 1997) has proposed that, when one is predicting behaviors in which outcomes are highly contingent on the quality of performance, outcome expectancy does not explain significant variation beyond that explained by self-efficacy. This is evidenced by studies indicating outcome expectancy accounted for little variance in motivational indices or behavior after controlling for self-efficacy (e.g., Gao, Lee, Solmon, & Zhang, 2009; Gao, Lee, Kosma, & Solmon, 2010). Other research work, however, has observed that both self-efficacy and outcome expectancy were independent predictors of behavior in sports and PA (Gao, Xiang, Lee, & Harrison, 2008). Clearly, the predictive attributes of self-efficacy and outcome expectancy require further investigation.

Finally, according to Self-efficacy Theory, an individual's self-efficacy may vary, based upon the dimensions of strength, magnitude, and generality. However, the vast majority of previous studies have only assessed the strength of self-efficacy while neglecting the measurement of magnitude and generality. Additionally, some researchers only measured outcome likelihood for outcome expectancy while omitting the important role that outcome values played. As such, it is possible that the predictive strengths of self-efficacy and outcome expectancy may have been misinterpreted. Consequently, further research is warranted, particularly with regard to the assessment of self-efficacy and outcome expectancy. In sum, research evidence has consistently confirmed self-efficacy to be a reliable and positive predictor of PA behavior. As a result, self-efficacy has been integrated into other social and behavioral theories and models such as the Theory of Planned Behavior and the Transtheoretical Model.

Goal Setting Theory

Over the past few decades, the Goal Setting Theory has been increasingly used as an effective strategy to motivate individuals in many fields, including sports and PA (Locke & Latham, 1990). In particular, goal setting has been proven to be an effective motivational technique for enhancing an individual's productivity and performance (Locke & Latham, 1990). In fact, the Social Cognitive Theory identified goal setting as an important strategy to understand and facilitate behavior change at the intrapersonal level.

According to Locke's mechanistic goal theory, goal setting refers to a process of setting targets as a means of developing and sustaining effort and persistence, mobilizing energy expenditure, developing self-regulation strategies, and directing appropriate attentional focus. Three major aspects of Locke's theory focus on the effects of goal specificity, goal difficulty and goal proximity on performance:

(1) setting specific goals has superior performance effects over setting "do-your-best" goals or no goals; (2) setting difficult but achievable goals has superior performance effects over easy goals; and (3) goals can be set at a distal (long-term) or proximal (short-term) level whereby distal goals make it easy to postpone effort yet proximal goals motivate immediate effort. In addition to the aforementioned goal aspects, namely, goal specificity, goal difficulty, and goal proximity, feedback (i.e., knowledge of personal status concerning one's selected goal) and rewards (i.e., a motivator to continue progress toward a goal) have been added to the Goal Setting Theory to enhance motivation and task performance. These goal aspects and added components (feedback and rewards) are imperative to increase individuals' self-efficacy, motivation, and ultimately PA behavior changes.

Research evidence has strongly supported the effectiveness of these postulations in the industrial and organizational fields. In PA contexts, the majority of research studies have found goal setting to be associated with enhanced performance (Boyce, Wayda, Johnston, & Bunker, 2001; Mooney & Mutrie, 2000). A few studies, however, failed to substantiate the effects of goal specificity, goal difficulty, and goal proximity on performance (Weinberg, Burton, Yukelson, & Weigand, 1993). The inconclusive results have been attributed to several methodological flaws such as failure to control spontaneous goal setting in "do-your-best" (control) groups, failure to make specific goals difficult, and failure to control for social comparisons, which are inherent in sports and PA.

Given these methodological considerations, it is imperative to heed Locke and Latham's suggestions when conducting goal setting research in PA contexts. One possible way to limit spontaneous goal setting is by considering the choice of task relative to the target population completing this task. Specifically, selection of a novel task and/or participants' lack of experience with a task could limit participants' ability to spontaneously set goals (Boyce, 1994). For example, Gao and Podlog (2012) adopted a newly emerged PA, Dance Revolution, and examined the effects of different levels of goal specificity and goal difficulty on Latino children's dance performance and PA levels. They found that easy and difficult goal groups showed significant improvements for dance performance over the "do-your-best" goal group, with the difficult goal group also displaying the highest improvement for PA levels over time. Based upon the findings, Gao and Podlog suggested health professionals should be well versed in appropriate goal setting techniques and implementation in school-based PA interventions—a suggestion which could be applied to other contexts as well. Therefore, it seems vital to incorporate cognitive-behavioral interventions, like goal setting, into a manageable protocol to be implemented by educators and community health professionals, many of whom may not possess (nor require) psychological training.

Self-determination Theory

To promote a continued and physically active lifestyle among individuals who do not meet the current PA recommendations, health professionals must attempt to adopt cognitive theories concerning motivation with the goal of promoting long-term behavior change. Recently, at the intrapersonal level, the application of the Self-determination Theory (Ryan & Deci, 2000) has been fruitful in explaining individuals' situational/proximal motivation for PA and health behaviors.

According to Vallerand (2001), situational motivation refers to the motivation that individuals experience when they are currently engaging in an activity. Situational motivation is comprised of three main types of motivation: (1) intrinsic motivation; (2) extrinsic motivation; and (3) amotivation. Intrinsic motivation refers to an individual's participation in an activity for its own sake (e.g., having fun, feelings of accomplishment), and involves the greatest degree of autonomous self-regulation (Figure 3.1). Extrinsic motivation (i.e., comprised of integrated regulation, identified regulation, introjected regulation, and external regulation) refers to activities that are carried out as a "means to an end" and not for their own sake, and involves less autonomy. With integrated regulation, an individual's behavior has been assimilated into the sense of self by the individual. It represents the highest degree of self-determined regulation within extrinsic motivation. As for identified regulation, behaviors occur when individuals accept certain activities as important to their personal goals and values (e.g., an individual sees exercise as necessary to reach their weight loss goal). Finally, in introjected regulation, an individual's participation in a behavior

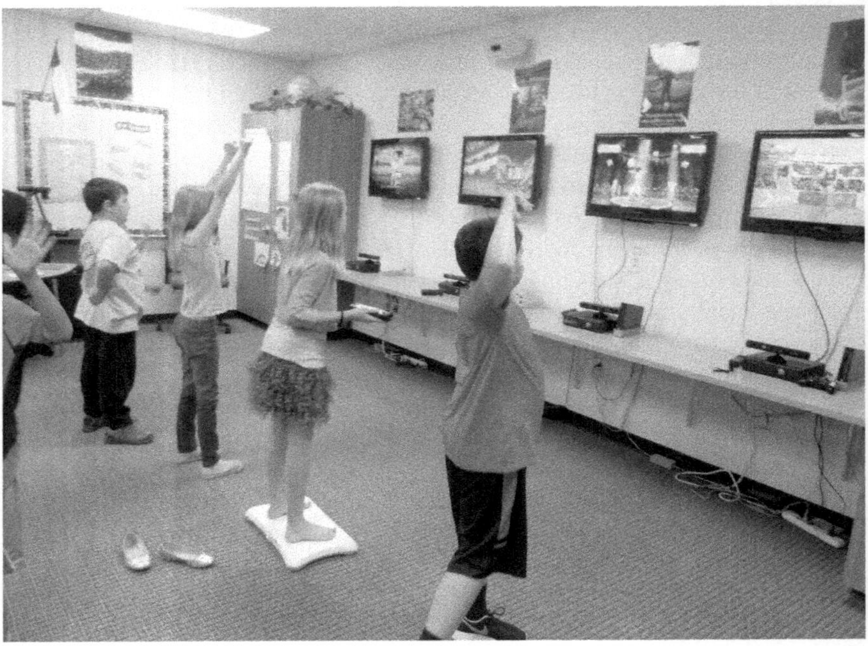

Figure 3.1 Kids playing active video games.

Source: Photo by Zan Gao.

occurs primarily out of a sense of compulsion and duress/guilt, among other external factors, while individuals in external regulation carry out behaviors in order to gain an external reward or avoid punishment. Notably, amotivation refers to a lack of intention and a relative absence of motivation (Ryan & Deci, 2000). These motivation types lie on a self-determination continuum with individuals becoming increasingly self-determined as one moves from amotivation to intrinsic motivation. Along the continuum, intrinsic motivation, integrated regulation, and identified regulation represent higher levels of self-determined motivation and lead to more positive behavioral consequences (Gao, 2012a; Gao, Podlog, & Harrison, 2012).

Indeed, the Self-determination Theory proposes that an individual's behavioral regulation of an activity varies to the extent to which the behavior is self-determined or controlling. Generally, individuals with higher intrinsic motivation, integrated regulation, and identified regulation demonstrate better effort and engagement in PA contexts. Introjected regulation, external regulation, and amotivation represent lower levels of self-determined motivation and lead, most often, to negative consequences. For example, individuals with dominant amotivation display boredom and more readily opted out of PA (Gao, 2012a; Gao, Hannon, Newton, & Huang, 2011). Further, the Self-determination Theory posits that an individual has three basic psychological needs: (1) autonomy (i.e., beliefs about one's choice regarding his or her own behavior); (2) competence (i.e., beliefs about one's capabilities to learn a task or perform a behavior); and (3) relatedness (i.e., feeling connected to others, an organization, or a community). These psychological needs are deemed to be essential to an individual, as an individual may be increasingly intrinsically motivated to perform a behavior if he or she perceives the behavior as important to satisfy one or more of these needs. Hence, if these needs are satisfied, an individual will demonstrate optimal motivation, producing positive behavioral outcomes; and vice versa (Ryan & Deci, 2000).

In the field of PA and health, researchers are seeking to understand the mechanism that supports need satisfaction and the subsequent optimal motivation using the Self-determination Theory as a framework, and are increasingly applying this theoretical framework in guiding PA interventions (Gao, 2012a; Gao, Hannon, Newton, & Huang, 2011; Gao, Podlog, & Harrison, 2012). Yet, further studies are warranted in applying this theory to guide PA behavior change as, due to its comprehensive nature, the Self-determination Theory has the potential to facilitate further understanding of behavioral mechanisms; thus aiding in the design of effective and appropriate interventions targeting PA promotion.

Theory of Planned Behavior

To increase individuals' PA levels, identifying factors that influence the decision-making process is critical. A model that has been used to understand this process is the Theory of Planned Behavior (Ajzen, 1991) (Figure 3.2). The Theory of Planned Behavior was developed on the basis of an earlier work, the

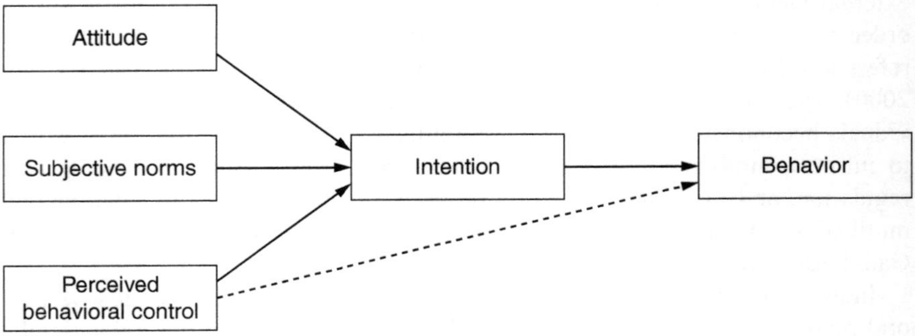

Figure 3.2 Theory of Planned Behaviour.
Source: Photo by Zan Gao.

Theory of Reasoned Action (Ajzen & Fishbein, 1980). The Theory of Reasoned Action emphasized intention as the most immediate or proximal factor of the desired behavior change—a factor influenced by two constructs: attitudes and subjective norms. However, the theory was later expanded to include the construct of perceived behavioral control, in what we now know as the Theory of Planned Behavior. Specifically, the Theory of Planned Behavior (Ajzen, 1991) postulates that attitudes, subjective norms, and perceived behavioral control jointly influence intention which still serves as the most proximal determinant of behavior. Notably, perceived behavioral control is also hypothesized to directly affect behavior.

According to the Theory of Planned Behavior, PA intention is defined as an individual's desire and motivation to be active. Attitude refers to the perceived consequences (positive or negative) of PA participation—representing a function of behavioral beliefs (i.e., perceived advantages and disadvantages of PA participation and evaluation of behavioral outcomes). Subjective norms reflect the perceived social pressure from significant others to engage in an active lifestyle and functions on the basis of normative beliefs (i.e., perceptions about whether certain individuals encourage or discourage PA participation). Lastly, perceived behavioral control reflects both self-efficacy (i.e., situational self-confidence for initiating and maintaining physically active behavior) and controllability of the behavior (i.e., perceived ability to overcome PA barriers). As a result of the aforementioned considerations, a basic hypothesis can be postulated for the Theory of Planned Behavior. Namely, an individual's intention to perform a behavior increases if they possess favorable attitudes and subjective norms, with concurrently strong perceived behavioral control.

Overall, the predictive strength of Theory of Planned Behavior for PA has been supported. Specifically, in two meta-analyses regarding the use of the Theory of Planned Behavior (Hagger, Chatzisarantis, & Biddle, 2002; Symons Downs & Hausenblas, 2005), the most important predictor of PA was observed to be intention, while the most significant predictors of intention were attitude and perceived behavioral control; generally, subjective norms demonstrated small or no significant effects on PA intention. Empirical studies indicate that the Theory of Planned Behavior is useful in explaining behavioral intentions in various populations (Chatzisarantis, Frederick, Biddle, Hagger, & Smith, 2007). However, there may be some limitations for the Theory of Planned Behavior with regard to explaining PA behaviors.

Most notably, results regarding the effect of the time interval between increased intention and subsequent behavior change is inconclusive. According to one previous meta-analysis (Hausenblas, Carron, & Mack, 1997), the strength of the intention–behavior relationship did not weaken over time, which contradicts the findings of other literature (Chatzisarantis, Hagger, Biddle, & Smith, 2005). However, Downs and Hausenblas (2005), when examining the predictive utility of intention on behavior change, suggested that to improve the predictive utility of intention on subsequent behavior change, it is necessary to assess intention as close as possible to the initiation of required behavior. The preceding temporal consideration needs to be considered by health professionals desiring to implement the Theory of Planned Behavior within PA and health promotion interventions. Furthermore, the large amount of unexplained variance between intention and behavior still remains problematic and raises questions regarding whether researchers should solely rely on this theory for future interventions. In summary, although the application of the Theory of Planned Behavior has strong support for understanding PA behavior, the implementation of the theory in future interventions warrants caution—particularly with respect to the temporal assessment of its construct.

Transtheoretical Model

In addition to a number of social cognitive behavioral theories, stage-based behavioral models have also been considered when wishing to understand the adoption of health behaviors. The most popular stage-based approach applied in PA contexts is the Transtheoretical Model (Prochaska & DiClemente, 1982). Within the Transtheoretical Model, individuals are posited to progress through a series of stages, with each stage consisting of different behavioral and psychological patterns regarding the adoption of a health behavior. Specifically, individuals are classified into one of the following six stages as assessed by their readiness to engage in behavior change: (1) precontemplation; (2) contemplation; (3) preparation; (4) action; (5) maintenance; and (6) termination (Prochaska & DiClemente, 1982).

In the precontemplation stage, a person does not intend to make any behavioral change. This reluctance to make a behavior change may be due to lack of information and/or motivation. Regarding the second stage, contemplation, we see an individual beginning to think about changing their behavior within the next six months—often weighing the pros and cons of changing the behavior. Of note, individuals in the contemplation stage are not yet ready to take action to change the behavior. An individual is ready to take action to change a behavior within the next month after progression to the preparation stage, and typically have a plan for how they intend to change the behavior. Action represents the fourth stage of behavior change and refers to an individual using their previously developed behavior change plan to begin actively changing a behavior. Notably, the action stage is the most variable, with individuals at greatest risk of regressing to an early stage. If an individual does not regress to an earlier stage when in the action stage and successfully adheres to their behavior change plan for six months or longer, these individuals will then be classified as being in the maintenance stage. The major focus of the maintenance stage is relapse prevention. Only when and if relapse is successfully prevented and the individual states they have no desire to go back to their old behavior and are comfortable engaging in their new behavior, is the individual said to be in the termination stage. However, most individuals who have changed their behavior stay somewhere in the maintenance stage (Edberg, 2007).

According to Transtheoretical Model, as individuals progress through each stage, it is important to tailor intervention strategies to address the different psychological and cognitive needs characterized by each stage. Notably, however, the model is not linear, meaning individuals do not progress systematically from one stage to the next. Rather, individuals may enter at any stage but relapse to an earlier stage, beginning the process again. Thus, designing stage-tailored interventions which meet the stage-specific needs of individuals will not only increase intervention adherence, but will also alleviate reluctance to initiate participation in the desired behavior(s) (Prochaska & Marcus, 1994).

Literature regarding the effectiveness of interventions using the Transtheoretical Model have demonstrated mixed findings. In a systematic review by van Sluijs and colleagues (2006), the authors did not find any favorable effects of Trantheoretical Model-based interventions on PA compared to other alternative theories or models. Additionally, Adams and White (2003) found that despite more than two-thirds of short-term (<6 months) studies indicating positive effects of Transtheoretical Model-based interventions compared to control, the number of long-term studies reporting the positive effect of the Transtheoretical Model-based interventions was small.

There may be two main reasons why Transtheoretical Model-based interventions demonstrated a lack in effectiveness over time in previous literature. First, the criteria used for assessing the methodological quality of empirical studies seems to vary from study to study. Indeed, while some empirical studies utilized a randomized controlled trial design, others lacked a control group (e.g., cross-sectional design) (West, 2005). Consequently, deciding upon the inclusion and exclusion criteria in reviews could have significantly impacted the analysis and subsequent conclusions regarding the effectiveness of the Transtheoretical Model. Second, the lack of strong evidence may be due to the fact that some health behaviors are simply more conducive to Transtheoretical Model-based interventions (Bridle et al., 2005). Undoubtedly, fundamental differences exist between some health behaviors, such as PA, and the addictive behavior upon which the theory was originally developed (i.e., smoking; Prochaska & DiClemente, 1982). Indeed, PA is a multifaceted and complex behavior, with health professionals who favor the model possibly focusing too much on the individual while underestimating the multiple external factors affecting individuals' PA behavior.

Behavior micro-environment theoretical perspectives and PA promotion

Social Cognitive Theory

At the behavior micro-environment level, it is assumed that an individual's beliefs, thoughts, social support, and the external environment influence his or her behavior, with reciprocal effects observed between these factors. The Social Cognitive Theory (Bandura, 1986, 1997) is one of the most frequently used theoretical frameworks used at this level of PA and health promotion to explain individuals' PA correlates and behaviors. This theory proposes that the behavior, the individual's environment, and the individual continuously change and simultaneously influence each other in a relationship termed reciprocal determination (Figure 3.3). Specifically, reciprocal determinism means that an individual can be both an agent for change and also a responder to change. Therefore, three factors (personal factors, environmental factors, and behavior) must be considered when trying to understand individuals' PA behaviors (Gao, 2012b).

According to the Social Cognitive Theory (Bandura, 1986), self-efficacy, goals, outcome expectancy, socioeconomic status, age, and gender, represent

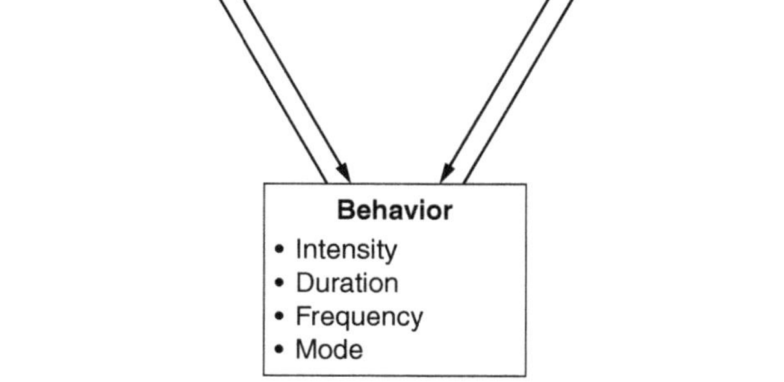

Figure 3.3 Social Cognitive Theory.

Source: Photo by Zan Gao.

major constructs of personal factors, among others. For example, in PA contexts, high self-efficacy positively relates to the adoption of and adherence to PA behavior among a wide range of populations (Gao, 2012b; Gao, Lee, & Harrison, 2008; Gao, Xiang, Lee, & Harrison, 2008). As self-efficacy, goals, and outcome expectancy were described in great detail in the previous sections (Gao, 2012b; Gao, Huang, Liu, & Xiong, 2012; Gao, Lochbaum, & Podlog, 2011), this terminology and their relationships with PA behavior are not reiterated here.

Environmental factors include, but are not limited to, social support and physical/social environmental factors. Social support refers to the physical and emotional comfort given by family, friends, co-workers and others. A number of studies have documented that social support, especially support from family and peers, plays an important role in promoting adolescents' PA levels (Davison, 2004; Hohepa, Scragg, Schofield, Kolt, & Schaaf, 2007). Particularly, parents have been observed to influence adolescents' PA participation by providing transportation and encouragement, as well as participating in PA with their children (Dowda, Dishman, Pfeiffer, & Pate, 2007). In terms of peer support, it has been evident that the frequency of individuals' participation in PA with friends, especially in shared PA, has a positive association with their overall frequency of PA (Beets, Pitetti, & Forlaw, 2007; Voorhees et al., 2005). Moreover, other research has also indicated that social support, coupled with self-efficacy, had a significant association with students' moderate and vigorous PA (Gao et al., 2012; Martin & McCaughtry, 2008a). Physical and social environmental factors, on the other hand, include physical opportunities for PA, access to safe PA environments, and social restrictions. Substantial evidence supports that physical and social environmental factors seems to hold great promise for understanding PA behavior (Sallis, Prochaska, & Taylor, 2000). However, more research is needed.

In conclusion, the Social Cognitive Theory describes factors that may influence behavior while also identifying the reciprocal mechanisms regarding how these factors interactively affect one another to lead to behavior change. Within this theory, the intrapersonal, interpersonal, sociocultural, and environmental factors function interactively to facilitate or inhibit an individual's PA behavior. As a result, this theory has emerged as one of the most popular theoretical frameworks used in the field of PA and health.

Behavior macro-environment theoretical perspectives and PA promotion

Social Ecologic Model

To better understand PA behavior change, researchers have also incorporated the influence of an individual's environment at all levels of society in the analysis and promotion of behavior change—thus adopting the Social Ecological Model in the study of PA behaviors (Addy et al., 2004). The Social Ecological Model is a multilevel theoretical approach that introduces social-environmental factors such as social support from friends, and physical environmental factors such as convenient access to PA facilities (Zhang, Solmon, Gao & Kosma, 2012) while also emphasizing the influence of organizations, the community, and public policy as important vehicles in the shaping of behavior.

The basic assumption of the Social Ecological Model is that individuals' behaviors are the results of interactions among individual, interpersonal, organizational, societal, and community-level factors occurring within a specific behavioral setting (Stokols, 2000). Guided by the Social Ecological Model, researchers have systematically investigated the individual, social, and physical environmental correlates of PA in a variety of populations (Addy et al., 2004; Sallis et al., 2008). Notably, using the social ecological perspective in this manner to promote PA can provide useful insights concerning effective interventions to increase PA participation at the population-level.

The use of this ecological approach has been widely accepted as a method to guide interventions tackling public health concerns in the United States (U.S. Department of Health and Human Services, 2010). However, there are some challenges for researchers relying on this ecological approach to inform interventions within the domain of PA behavior. Specifically, while ecological models may have great strength in providing overarching frameworks to guide interventions, these models are sometimes inadequate at discerning specific mechanisms by which one level influences or interacts with other factors at different levels to explain individual behavior. Thus, it is understandable why researchers within the PA domain are still in favor of the previously reviewed cognitive-based theories. Indeed, these cognitive-based theories satisfy the researchers' traditional desire to infer causality when solving problems at the individual level. That said, PA is a complex behavior. Due to the preceding fact, researchers are becoming aware that this behavior cannot be explained as a linear process happening exclusively at the individual level. As such, the ecological approaches are becoming more widely accepted and integrated, in order to better understand how complex interactions between multiple levels of influence may impact PA determinants and the mediating role of these determinants (Bronfenbrenner, 2005; McLaren & Hawe, 2005). Another important aspect to acknowledge is that the influence of determinants may not be the same over time and that the determinants may also have direct influence on behavior (Plsek & Wilson, 2001). The traditional research approach proposes that the measurement of social cognitive factors such as attitudes, efficacy, and beliefs will determine the effectiveness of interventions in improving participation in a specific behavior. This approach may be flawed, however, as it fails to appreciate the complexities involved in human behavior (Resnicow & Page, 2008)—yet another potential advantage of incorporating the Social Ecological Model.

In conclusion, the Social Ecological Model recently has been accepted in PA settings due to the appreciation of the multilevel factors that may directly or indirectly impact complex PA behavior. However, despite its success in incorporating various determinants into the explanation of PA behaviors, lack of information regarding specific mechanisms for the relationship between factors at different levels of this model may be noted as a limitation. Future endeavors to integrate some of the cognitive theories with this ecological model may be necessary to overcome this shortcoming.

Application of behavior theories using emerging technologies

Knowing the various influences of interventions on individuals' PA correlates and determinants is an important first step in designing intervention programs to promote PA participation and health. Throughout the chapter, we have reviewed the details of seven theoretical frameworks that have been widely employed in the field of PA and health: (1) Self-efficacy Theory; (2) Goal Setting Theory; (3) Self-determination Theory; (4) Theory of Planned Behavior; (5) Transtheoretical Model; (6) Social Cognitive Theory; and (7) the Social Ecological Model. Studies to date using emerging technologies have typically addressed the feasibility or efficacy of such technologies, or have simply used these technologies as motivational tools or incentives for PA behavior change. However, researchers have applied some of the preceding social and behavioral theories in many projects integrating emerging technologies, such as computers and the Internet, online social media, active video games, and mobile device apps. Some exceptions are studies using newly-available emerging technologies such as health wearable devices, GPS/GIS, and virtual reality.

The aforementioned social and behavioral theories have been extensively used as the theoretical frameworks for numerous observational and experimental studies involving phone-based, computer-based, and Internet-based PA interventions a decade ago (Lewis et al., 2008; Lewis, Marcus, Pate, & Dunn, 2002). For example, Lewis et al. (2008) investigated differences in use patterns and perceived website usefulness between stage-tailored Internet and standard Internet groups using the Transtheoretical Model and Social Cognitive Theory as theoretical frameworks, finding that the stage-tailored Internet group logged onto their website significantly more than the standard Internet group. They also indicated goal setting and self-monitoring to be most useful for PA behavior change (Lewis et al., 2008). In another example, Papandonatos and colleagues (2012) adopted the Transtheoretical Model in a 12-month randomized controlled trial using both print-based and phone-based Transtheoretical Model intervention strategies, and found statistically significant changes in the self-efficacy, decisional balance, and cognitive and behavior processes of change at the 6-month post-intervention assessment. These authors also suggested that the magnitude of these changes increased during the 6–12-month intervention follow-up in the group receiving print materials. Among children, Pope et al. (2016) investigated the effects of an active video game program on children's Transtheoretical Model-based PA determinants and PA levels. At pre-test and post-test, elementary children were administered measures regarding stages of change for PA behavior, decisional balance for PA behaviors, PA self-efficacy, and self-reported PA levels. Following the pretest, a weekly 30-minute, 18-week Dance Revolution intervention was implemented. Children were classified into three groups: progressive children (i.e., progressed to a higher stages of change); stable children (i.e., remained at the same stages of change); and regressive children (i.e., regressed to a lower stages of change). The researchers found that progressive children had more improvements in self-efficacy, decisional balance, and PA levels than regressive children over time.

Generally speaking, Social Cognitive Theory has been widely applied in studies using emerging technology such as active video games and online social media. For example, in a longitudinal intervention study with active video games, Gao and associates indicated that an active video game intervention had a positive impact on children's self-efficacy and social support but not outcome expectancy over the course of one year (Gao, Huang, Liu, & Xiong, 2012). Pope and Gao (2017) also used this theory as a guide to examine the effectiveness of a smartphone exercise app (i.e., MapMyFitness) on college students' sedentary behavior and PA, as well as social cognitive beliefs and identified differences on some social cognitive outcomes.

As one major component of this theory, social support has also been studied in numerous projects—particularly those interventions using online social media and games. Verheijden et al. (2005), for instance, investigated the role of social support in lifestyle-focused weight management interventions using online social media. Social support among children and teachers (Fogel et al., 2010) and between player and peers (Paw et al., 2008) have also been investigated. The findings of these studies unanimously support the use of social support in the regulation of individuals' PA behavior when integrating emerging technology.

Other theories, such as the Self-determination Theory and the Theory of Planned Behavior, are also used in this area of inquiry. To examine the extent to which children's self-determined motivation predicted children's moderate-to-vigorous PA when playing active video games, Gao and his research team conducted a number of observational studies (Gao et al., 2011; Gao, 2012b; Gao, Podlog, & Huang, 2013). They found that children's intrinsic motivation positively predicted children's moderate-to-vigorous PA while amotivation was a negative predictor; thus recommending professionals offer such games in an interesting and enjoyable way to foster children's intrinsic motivation. Further, in a study by Maddison et al. (2007), the Theory of Planned Behavior was utilized as the theoretical framework with researchers reporting active video game play significantly affected children's PA attitudes, subjective norms, intention, and strenuous exercise behavior.

Finally, the Goal Setting Theory has been used as either a stand-alone theory or as a major component incorporated into other theories like the Social Cognitive Theory. Recently, Gao and Podlog (2012) used the Goal Setting Theory in their active video game study. In particular, they instructed children to set different goals—specific goals (difficult goal, easy goal) and a "do-your-best" goal in the intervention—finding children who set specific goals had better outcomes than those who set vague and the "do-your-best goal," hence recommending specific goals be set to improve children's sustained PA behavior. Notably, the Social Ecological Model has rarely been used in the previously mentioned experimental or observational studies. Yet, with the prevalence of GPS/GIS use in people's daily life, the application of the Social Ecological Model in PA behavior changes interventions shows promise.

Opportunities and challenges moving forward

In this chapter, seven social and behavioral theories have been elaborated upon while numerous other theories (e.g., achievement goal theory, motivation protection theory, etc.) were neglected. However, the selection of the theories included in this chapter is based upon the popularity and application of these theories in the field of PA and health. Furthermore, it should be reiterated that the aforementioned theories also demonstrate the complex interplay of behavioral determinants of PA behavior at different levels. For example, PA behavior is influenced by a number of personal factors including self-efficacy, motivation, goal setting, intention and behavioral stages at the intrapersonal (individual) level, social support from family and friends at the interpersonal level, and environment, policy, as well as perceptions of crime and safety at the community/regional level.

Traditionally, intervention strategies to change PA behaviors have focused on intrapersonal factors such as beliefs, cognition, knowledge, and movement skills. In doing so, researchers and health professionals usually select from intrapersonal-level theories such as the Self-efficacy Theory, the Goal Setting Theory, the Self-determination Theory, the Theory of Planned Behavior, and the Transtheoretical Model. Indeed, these theories correctly target behavior change at the intrapersonal level by manipulating constructs such as: self-efficacy, goal setting, stages of change, attitudes, outcome expectancy, and intrinsic motivation. For example, enhancing an individual's self-efficacy has been proposed by many theories to promote PA behavior. That is, health professionals may make deliberate efforts to enhance individuals' self-efficacy using such effective strategies such as: (1) helping individuals successfully complete the task to foster a sense of accomplishment; (2) providing timely and accurate feedback on a task; (3) setting small, incremental, and achievable goals; (4) using good role models for behavioral change; and (5) monitoring and reinforcing behavior by keeping records.

Commonly used cost-effective strategies at the interpersonal level include establishing social support programs and building accommodating social environments—strategies accomplished more easily using online social media and online communities for active video games and apps. These behavior change strategies utilize the Social Cognitive Theory which explains human behavior through a three-way, dynamic, reciprocal model in which personal factors, environmental factors, and behavior continually interact with one another (Figure 3.4). From a behavior micro-environment theoretical perspective, key constructs of this theory that are relevant to behavior change interventions include not only intrapersonal factors (e.g., self-efficacy, self-regulation), but also social environmental factors (e.g., social support, social environment, and social networks).

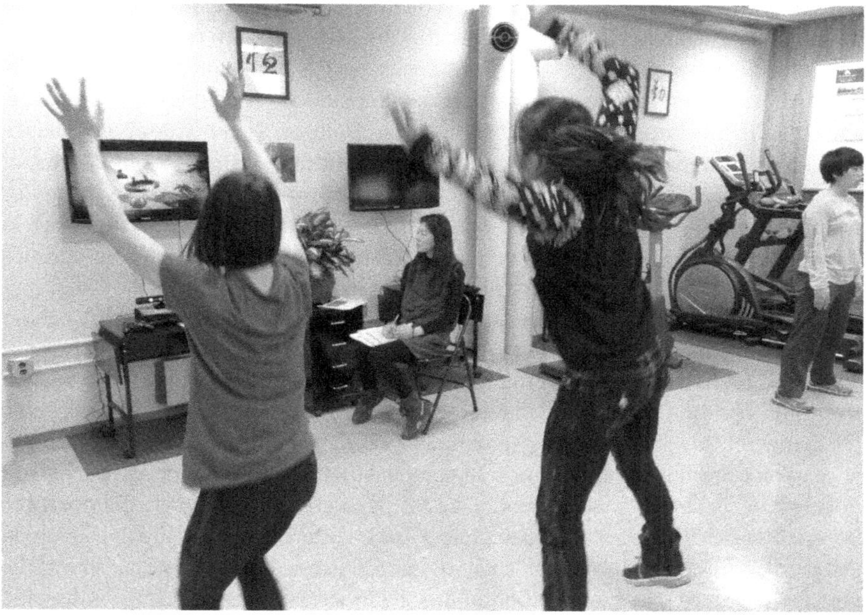

Figure 3.4 Elite athletes playing active video games.
Source: Photo by Zan Gao.

Aside from the above approaches to PA behavioral change, it has been shown that approximately 50% of individuals who initiate a PA program drop out within the first six months, and without successful intervention at multiple levels of the environment impacting behavioral change, the retention rate drops dramatically post-intervention (Dishman & Buckworth, 1996). Thus, ecological models have gained credibility over the past decade as there is now consensus that PA behavior change is a complicated and multifaceted phenomenon with multiple levels of factors affecting intervention outcomes. In response, the Social Ecological Model, a behavior macro-environment theory, has been increasingly used to explain the impact of individuals, social environments, physical environments, and policies on individuals' PA behavior change. To achieve enduring changes as a result of PA behavior change interventions from a multilevel perspective, researchers should continue to embrace the use of this theory to inform behavioral interventions (Humpel, Owen, & Leslie, 2002; Stokols, 2000). Notably, however, this shift to the examination of a complex range of factors which shape PA behaviors might make the selection of behavioral change intervention strategies daunting.

With the preceding point in mind, the fact remains that the choice of effective behavioral intervention strategies depends upon the selection of which theory is most appropriate under specific circumstances in a target population. Despite the great potential that the Social Ecological Model may hold to change complex behaviors (such as PA) through multilevel interventions, certain issues exist regarding the extent to which particular factors from various levels interact and influence PA behavior in a given context. This calls for more research to investigate the factors that exert the most influence on PA behavior under certain circumstances before an agreed consensus is reached. Meanwhile, researchers should still rely heavily upon other theories, such as Social Cognitive Theory and Transtheoretical Model, to make up for the limitations present in the Social Ecological Model and best assess factors related to individuals' PA behavior change. Simply stated, different theories are best suited to different problems at various levels of intervention, such as individuals, groups, and/or communities — a fact that health professionals should keep in mind.

Theory, research, and practice are part of a continuum to understand PA behavior correlates and determinants, to test the effectiveness of behavior change strategies, and to disseminate cost-effective and efficacious interventions. What is clear from this review is that PA behavior change is a complicated and multifaceted phenomenon that is affected by numerous factors at multiple levels. Simple reliance upon certain intrapersonal or interpersonal theories does not necessarily result in effective behavior change among target populations. Moreover, although the Social Ecological Model includes factors from different environmental levels in the prediction and influence of an individual's PA behavior, caution should be noted with regard to the application of this theory at the individual level in specific situations. Meanwhile, emerging technologies, such as online social media, active video games and health wearable devices, have expanded the range of theory-based strategies available for effective PA behavior change over the past decade. That said, more research is needed to develop and test theories (and the integration of multiple theories) to create evidence-based, theory-backed PA intervention guidelines using emerging technologies.

References

Adams, J. & White, M. (2003). Are activity promotion interventions based on the transtheoretical model effective? A critical review. *British Journal of Sports Medicine, 37*(2), 106–114.

Addy, C., Wilson, D., Kirtland, K., Ainsworth, B., Sharpe, P., & Kimsey, D. (2004). Association of perceived social and physical environmental supports with physical activity and walking behavior. *American Journal of Public Health, 94*, 440–443.

Ajzen, I. (1991). The theory of planned behavior. *Organizational Behavior and Human Decision Processes, 50*(2), 179–211.

Ajzen, I., & Fishbein, M. (1980). *Understanding attitudes and predicting social behavior*. Englewood Cliffs, NJ: Prentice-Hall.

Bandura, A. (1986). *Social foundations of thought and action: A social cognitive theory*. Englewood Cliffs, NJ: Prentice Hall.

Bandura, A. (1997). *Self-efficacy: The exercise of control.* New York: Freeman.

Beets, M. W., Pitetti, K. H., & Forlaw, L. (2007). The role of self-efficacy and referent specific social support in promoting rural adolescent girls' physical activity. *American Journal of Health Behavior, 31*(3), 227–237.

Blair, S. N., & Morris, J. N. (2009). Healthy hearts—and the universal benefits of being physically active: Physical activity and health. *Annals of Epidemiology, 19*(4), 253–256.

Boyce, B. A. (1994). Effects of goal setting on performance and spontaneous goal setting behavior of experienced pistol shooters. *Sport Psychologist, 8*, 87–93.

Boyce, B. A., Wayda, V. K., Johnston, T., & Bunker, L. K. (2001). The effects of three types of goal setting conditions on tennis performance: A field-based study. *Journal of Teaching Physical Education, 20*, 188–200.

Bridle, C., Riemsma, R. P., Pattenden, J., Sowden, A. J., Mather, L., Watt, I. S., & Walker, A. (2005). Systematic review of the effectiveness of health behavior interventions based on the transtheoretical model. *Psychology and Health, 20*(3), 283–301.

Bronfenbrenner, U. (2005). *Making human beings human: Bioecological perspectives on human development.* Thousand Oaks, CA: Sage.

Chatzisarantis, N. L., Frederick, C., Biddle, S. J., Hagger, M. S., & Smith, B. (2007). Influences of volitional and forced intentions on physical activity and effort within the theory of planned behaviour. *Journal of Sports Sciences, 25*(6), 699–709.

Chatzisarantis, N. L. D., Hagger, M. S., Biddle, S. J. H., & Smith, B. (2005). The stability of the attitude–intention relationship in the context of physical activity. *Journal of Sports Sciences, 23*, 49–61.

Davison, K. K. (2004). Activity-related support from parents, peers and siblings and adolescents' physical activity: Are there gender differences? *Journal of Physical Activity and Health, 1*(4), 263–276.

Dishman, R. K., & Buckworth, J. (1996). Increasing physical activity: A quantitative synthesis. *Medicine and Science in Sports and Exercise, 28*(6), 706–719.

Dishman, R. K., Motl, R. W., Saunders R., Felton, G., Ward, D. S., Dowda, M., & Pate, R. R. (2004). Self-efficacy partially mediates the effect of a school-based physical-activity intervention among adolescent girls. *Preventive Medicine, 38*, 628–636.

Dowda, M., Dishman, R. K., Pfeiffer K. A., & Pate, R. R. (2007). Family support for physical activity in girls from 8th to 12th grade in South Carolina. *Preventive Medicine, 44*(2), 153–159.

Dowda, M., Pfeiffer, K., Brown, W., Mitchell, J., Byun, W., & Pate, R. (2011). Parental and environmental correlates of physical activity of children attending preschool. *Archives of Pediatrics and Adolescent Medicine, 165*(10), 939–944.

Downs, D. S., & Hausenblas, H. A. (2005). The theories of reasoned action and planned behavior applied to exercise: A meta-analytic update. *Journal of Physical Activity and Health, 2*, 76–80.

Edberg, M. (2007). *Essentials of health behavior: Social and behavioral theory in public health.* Sudbury, MA: Jones & Bartlett Learning, LLC.

Fogel, V. A., Miltenberger, R. G., Graves, R., & Koehler, S. (2010). The effects of exergaming on physical activity among inactive children in a physical education classroom. *Journal of Applied Behavior Analysis, 43*(4), 591–600. http://doi.org/10.1901/jaba.2010.43-591.

Gao, Z. (2012a). Motivated but not active: The dilemmas of incorporating interactive dance into gym class. *Journal of Physical Activity and Health, 9*, 794–800.

Gao, Z. (2012b). Urban Latino school children's physical activity correlates and daily physical activity participation: A social cognitive perspective. *Psychology, Health and Medicine, 17*(5), 542–550.

Gao, Z., Hannon, J. C., Newton, M., & Huang, C. (2011). Effects of curricular activity on students' situational motivation and physical activity levels. *Research Quarterly for Exercise and Sport, 82*(3), 536–544.

Gao, Z., Huang, C., Liu, T., & Xiong, W. (2012). Impact of interactive dance games on urban children's physical activity correlates and behavior. *Journal of Exercise Science and Fitness, 10*, 107–112.
Gao, Z., & Kosma, M. (2008). Intention as a mediator of weight training behavior among college students: An integrative framework. *Journal of Applied Sport Psychology, 20*, 1–12.
Gao, Z., Lee, A. M., & Harrison, L. Jr. (2008). Understanding students' motivation in sport and physical education: From the expectancy-value model and self-efficacy theory perspectives. *Quest, 60*, 236–254.
Gao, Z., Lee, A. M., Kosma, M., & Solmon, M. A. (2010). Understanding students' motivation in middle school physical education: Examining the mediating role of self-efficacy on physical activity. *International Journal of Sport Psychology, 41*, 199–215.
Gao, Z., Lee, A. M., Solmon, M. A., & Zhang, T. (2009). Changes of middle school students' motivation toward physical education over one school year. *Journal of Teaching in Physical Education, 28*, 378–399.
Gao, Z., Lochbaum, M., & Podlog, L. (2011). Self-efficacy as a mediator of children's achievement motivation and in-class physical activity. *Perceptual and Motor Skills, 113*(3), 969–981.
Gao, Z., Lodewyk, K., & Zhang, T. (2009). The role of ability beliefs and incentives in middle school students' intentions, cardiovascular fitness, and effort. *Journal of Teaching in Physical Education, 28*, 3–20.
Gao, Z., & Podlog, L. (2012). Urban Latino children's physical activity levels and performance in interactive video dance games: Effects of goal difficulty and goal specificity. *Archives of Pediatrics and Adolescent Medicine, 166*(10), 933–937.
Gao, Z., Podlog, L., & Harrison, L. (2012). College students' goal orientations, situational motivation and effort/persistence in physical activity. *Journal of Teaching in Physical Education, 31*, 246–260.
Gao, Z., Podlog, L., & Huang, C. (2013). Associations among children's situational motivation, physical activity participation, and enjoyment in an active dance video game. *Journal of Sport and Health Science, 2*(2), 122–128.
Gao, Z., Xiang, P., Lee, A. M., & Harrison, L. Jr. (2008). Self-efficacy and outcome expectancy in beginning weight training class: Their relations to behavioral intentions and actual behavior. *Research Quarterly for Exercise and Sport, 79*, 92–100.
Gao, Z., Zhang, T., & Stodden, D. (2013). Children's physical activity levels and psychological correlates in interactive dance versus aerobic dance. *Journal of Sport and Health Science, 2*(3), 146–151.
Hagger, M. S., Chatzisarantis, N. L. D., & Biddle, S. J. H. (2002). A meta-analytic review of the theories of reasoned action and planned behavior in physical activity: Predictive validity and the contribution of additional variables. *Journal of Sport & Exercise Psychology, 24*, 3–32.
Hausenblas, H. A., Carron, A. V., & Mack, D. E. (1997). Application of the theories of reasoned action and planned behavior to exercise behavior: A meta-analysis. *Journal of Sport and Exercise Psychology, 19*, 36–51.
Hohepa, M., Scragg, R., Schofield, G., Kolt, G. S., & Schaaf, D. (2007). Social support for youth physical activity: Importance of siblings, parents, friends and school support across a segmented school day. *International Journal of Behavioral Nutrition and Physical Education, 4*, 54–59.
Humpel, N., Owen, N., & Leslie, E. (2002). Environmental factors associated with adults'

participation in physical activity. A review. *American Journal of Preventive Medicine, 22*, 188–199.

King, A., Stokols, D., Talen, E., & Brassington, G. S. (2002). Theoretical approaches to the promotion of physical activity: Forging a transdisciplinary paragidgm. *American Journal of Preventive Medicine, 23*(2S), 15–25.

Lewis, B. A., Marcus, B. H., Pate, R. R., & Dunn, A. L. (2002). Psychosocial mediators of physical activity behavior among adults and children. *American Journal of Preventive Medicine, 23*, 26–35.

Lewis, B. A., Williams, D., Dunsiger, S., Sciamanna, C., Whiteley, J., Napolitano, M., … Marcus, B. (2008). User attitudes towards physical activity websites in a randomized controlled trial. *Preventive Medicine, 47*, 508–513.

Locke, E. A., & Latham, G. P. (1900). *A theory of goal setting and task performance.* Englewood Cliffs, NJ: Prentice Hall.

Maddison, R., Mhurchu, C. N., Jull, A., Prapavessis, H., & Rodgers, A. (2007). Energy expended playing video console games: An opportunity to increase children's physical activity? *Pediatric Exercise Science, 19*, 334–343.

Martin, J. J., & McCaughtry, N. (2008). Predicting physical activity in inner-city Hispanic American children. *Hispanic Health Care International, 6*(3), 150–158.

McLaren, L., & Hawe, P. (2005). Ecological perspectives in health research. *Journal of Epidemiology and Community Health, 59*, 6–14.

Mooney, R. P., & Mutrie, N. (2000). The effects of goal specificity and goal difficulty on the performance of badminton skills in children. *Pediatric Exercise Science, 12*, 270–283.

Papandonatos, G., George, D., Williams, D., Jennings, E., Napolitano, M., Bock, B., … Maucus, B. (2012). Mediators of physical activity behavior change: Findings from a 12-month randomized controlled trial. *Health Psychology, 31*(4), 512–520.

Paw, M. C. A., Jacobs, W., Vaessen, E., Titze, S., & van Mechelen, W. (2008). The motivation of children to play an active video game. *Journal of Science and Medicine in Sport, 11*, 163–166.

Plsek, P. E., & Wilson, T. (2001). Complexity science: Complexity, leadership, and management in healthcare organizations. *British Medical Journal, 323*, 746–749.

Pope, Z., Lewis, B., & Gao, Z. (2016). Using the Transtheoretical Model to examine the effects of exergaming on physical activity among children. *Journal of Physical Activity and Health, 12*, 1205–1212.

Pope, Z., & Gao, Z., (2017). *Effectiveness of smartphone-based physical activity intervention on college student health: Randomized-controlled trial.* Presented at Society for Health and Physical Educators annual meeting in Boston, MA, March 2017.

Prochaska, J. O. & DiClemente, C. C. (1982). Transtheoretical therapy: Toward a more integrative model of change. *Psychotherapy: Theory, Research and Practice, 19*(3), 276–288.

Prochaska, J. O. & DiClemente, C. C. (1984). *The transtheoretical approach: Crossing traditional boundaries of therapy.* Homewood, IL: Dow Jones-Irwin.

Prochaska, J. O., & Marcus, B. (1994). The transtheoretical model: Application to exercise. In R. K. Dishman (ed.), *Advances in exercise adherence* (pp. 161–180). Champaign, IL: Human Kinetics.

Resnicow, K., & Page, S. E. (2008). Embracing chaos and complexity: A quantum change for public health. *American Journal of Public Health, 98*, 1382–1389.

Rodgers, W. M., Wilson, P. M., Hall, C. R., Fraser, S. N., & Murray, T. C. (2008). Evidence for a multidimensional self-efficacy for exercise scale. *Research Quarterly for Exercise and Sport, 79*, 222–234.

Rodgers, W. M., & Brawley, L. R. (1991). The role of outcome expectations in participation motivation. *Journal of Sport and Exercise Psychology, 13*, 411–427.
Rovniak, L. S., Anderson, E. S., Winett, R. A., & Stephens, R. S. (2002). Social cognitive determinants of physical activity in young adults: A prospective structural equation analysis. *Annals of Behavioral Medicine*, *24*(2), 149–156
Ryan, R. M., & Deci, E. L. (2000). Self-determination theory and the facilitation of intrinsic motivation, social development, and well-being. *American. Psychology, 55*, 68–78.
Sallis, J. F., Cervero, R. B., Ascher, W., Henderson, K. A., Kraft, M. K., & Kerr, J. (2006). An ecological approach to creating active living communities. *Annual Review of Public Health, 27*, 297–322.
Sallis, J. F., Owen, N., & Fisher, E. B. (2008). Ecological models of health behavior (4th ed.). In K. Glanz, B. K. Rimer, & K. Viswanath (Eds.), *Health behavior and health education: Theory, research and practice* (pp. 465–485). San Francisco: Jossey-Bass.
Sallis, J. F., Prochaska, J. J., & Taylor, W. C. (2000). A review of correlates of physical activity of children and adolescents. *Medicine and Science in Sport and Exercise, 32*(5), 963–975.
Stokols, D. (2000). Social ecology and behavioral medicine: Implications for training, practice, and policy. *Behavioral Medicine, 26*(3), 129–138.
Sutton, S. (2008). How does the Health Action Process Approach (HAPA) bridge the intention-behavior gap? An examination of the model's causal structure. *Applied Psychology, 57*, 66–74.
Symons Downs, D., & Hausenblas, H. A. (2005). The theories of reasoned action and planned behavior applied to exercise: A meta-analytic update. *Journal of Physical Activity and Health, 2*, 76–97.
U.S. Department of Health and Human Services. (2010). Healthy People 2020. Retrieved from www.healthypeople.gov/2020/.
Vallerand, R. J. (2001). A hierarchical model of intrinsic and extrinsic motivation in sport and exercise. In G. C. Roberts (Ed.), *Advances in motivation in sport and exercise* (pp. 263–320). Champaign, IL: Human Kinetics.
van Sluijs, E. M. F., van Poppel, M. N. M., Twisk, J. W. R., & van Mechelen, W. (2006). Physical activity measurements affected participants' behavior in a randomized controlled trial. *Journal of Clinical Epidemiology, 59*(4), 404–411.
Verheijden, M. W., Bakx, J. C., van Weel, C., Koelen, M. A., & van Staveren, W. A. (2005). Role of social support in lifestyle-focused weight management interventions. *European Journal of Clinical Nutrition, Supplement 1*, S179–S186.
Voorhees, C. C., Murray, D., Welk, G., Birnbaum, A., Ribisl, K. M., Johnson, C. C., … Jobe, J. B. (2005). The role of peer social network factors and physical activity in adolescent girls. *American Journal of Health Behavior, 29*(2), 183–190.
Voorhees, C., & Young, D. (2003). Personal, social and physical environmental correlates of physical activity levels in young, urban Latinas. *American Journal of Preventive Medicine, 25*, 61–67.
Weinberg, R. S., Burton, D., Yukelson, D., & Weigand, D. (1993). Goal setting in competitive sport: An exploratory investigation of practices in collegiate athletes. *Sport Psychologist, 7*, 275–289.
West, R. (2005). Time for a change: Putting the transtheoretical (Stages of Change) model to rest, *Addiction, 100*, 1036–1039.
Zhang, T., Solmon, M. A., Gao, Z., & Kosma, M. (2012). Promoting school students' physical activity: A social ecological perspective. *Journal of Applied Sport Psychology, 24*, 92–105. doi: 10.1080/10413200.2011.627083.

Part II

Emerging technologies in physical activity and health

4 Computer and Internet use in enhancing physical activity

Jung Eun Lee and Zan Gao

Despite national physical activity (PA) recommendations of at least 150 minutes per week of moderate-to-vigorous PA (MVPA), less than one-third of American adults (21%) meet this recommendation (Centers for Disease Control and Prevention, 2014). As a result, innovative and effective approaches to promote PA and health have been investigated. As of January of 2014, 87% of the U.S. adults (231 million) use the Internet (Perrin & Duggan, 2015), with Internet users similar across age, gender, and ethnicity (Perrin & Duggan, 2015). For example, it has been reported that Internet use is most popular among individuals aged between 18 and 64 years—demonstrating the Internet's ability to aid a wide range of individuals in accessing information (Carr et al., 2013). Due to the aforementioned wide-ranging use of the Internet, Internet-based PA interventions are among the most promising channels of health promotion in the present day.

Increasing the attractiveness of Internet-based PA interventions is the ability to use this mode of intervention delivery to reduce some of the barriers that traditional face-to-face intervention delivery poses to participants (e.g., transportation, increased time requirements, etc.; Napolitano et al., 200 3). Indeed, Internet-based PA interventions can deliver individually tailored PA and health-related messages, enhancing access to expert feedback regarding numerous PA modalities. Individually tailored interventions are appealing, given the fact that tailored messages are easier to read/remember and are more relevant and effective in promoting health behavior changes than non-tailored interventions (Hamel, Robbins, & Wilbur, 2010). Finally, Internet-based PA interventions offer researchers and health professionals the ability to implement interventions any time/any place and often at a lower cost (Joseph, Durant, Benitez, & Pekmezi, 2014). Throughout the remainder of this chapter, the reader will be treated to a review of the extant literature regarding Internet-based PA interventions, with the greatest attention given to the health benefits arising from these interventions. Following this discussion, the limitations of Internet-based PA interventions will be reviewed, after which, directions for future research and the proper application of Internet-based interventions will be presented.

Components of Internet-based PA interventions

Delivery methods for Internet-based PA interventions vary from study to study. Most frequently, Internet-based PA interventions have been delivered by email-only or website portal-only or via a combined approach (Figure 4.1). Further, some Internet-based PA studies have also included non-Internet components, including face-to-face and/or telephone-based counseling, as well as concurrently using mobile device applications in the tracking and uploading of PA statistics (Joseph et al., 2013).

Internet-based PA interventions using website portals to engage participants and deliver intervention content have used message boards/chat rooms. For example, in a study by Carr et al. (2013), participants were asked to post any health-related questions to the researchers on a message board placed on a study-related website. The message board's main purpose was to encourage participant's PA participation. Message boards/chat rooms have also been used to promote social support among study participants. Specifically, in some studies, message boards/chat rooms allowed participants to interact with one another—exchanging ideas, sharing information, and receiving support for PA participation (Grim, Hortz, & Petosa, 2011; Morgan et al., 2011; Reid et al., 2012; Wadsworth & Hallam, 2010). Another prominent strategy employed via website-based interventions has been the use of educational modules (Bennett, Broome, Schwab-Pilley, & Gilmore, 2011; Glasgow et al., 2010; Lachausse, 2012;

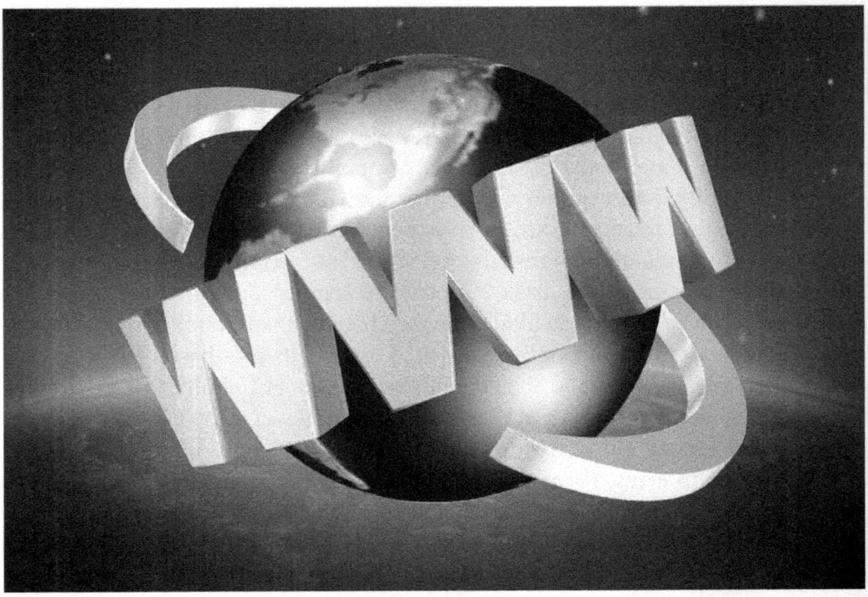

Figure 4.1 World Wide Web.

Source: pixabay.com.

Magoc, Tomaka, & Bridges-Arzaga, 2011; Motl, Dlugonski, Wójcicki , McAuley, & Mohr, 2011). For example, Magoc and colleagues (2011) used Internet-based educational modules to deliver structured, theory-based health information to promote PA. Over the course of the intervention, these modules asked participants to complete tasks regarding various PA-related topics such as self-monitoring, goal setting, and barriers. Other studies (e.g., Marcus et al., 2007; Slootmaker, Chinapaw, Schuit, Seidell, & Van Mechelen, 2009; Wanner et al., 2009; Watson, Bickmore, Cange, Kulshreshtha, & Kvedar, 2012) used computer-generated, individually tailored feedback to further increase the effectiveness of Internet-based PA interventions. In the Step into Motion trial (Marcus et al., 2007), participants completed monthly online questionnaires throughout the intervention that provided individually tailored feedback to participants regarding increasing their PA participation using computer algorithms.

Finally, some Internet-based PA interventions have also incorporated the concurrent use of mobile device applications for goal-setting and self-monitoring purposes (e.g., Bennett et al., 2011; Booth, Nowson, & Matters, 2008; Carr et al., 2013; Glasgow et al., 2010; Magoc et al., 2011; Morgan et al., 2011; Pellegrini et al., 2012; Wadsworth & Hallam, 2010; Watson et al., 2012). For example, participants have been asked to record their daily PA or step counts and upload these results to an online system which provides timely feedback in relation to the number of steps taken (Booth et al., 2008).

Effectiveness of Internet-based PA interventions

According to a meta-analysis regarding the effectiveness of Internet-based PA interventions, a small yet significant short-term effect is present when this intervention modality is implemented (Davies, Spence, Vandelanotte, Caperchione, & Mummery, 2012). Notably, this effect was stronger when structured educational PA information was provided to participants (Davies et al., 2012). However, researchers indicated a need for future studies to explore the long-term effect of this type of intervention. Another review also discussed factors which might influence the effectiveness of Internet-based PA interventions (Vandelanotte et al., 2007). Among the most notable factors that could influence the effectiveness of such an intervention, the frequency of contact that participants had over the Internet via emails, education modules, chat rooms, or online coach had the highest association with positive outcomes. Indeed, Internet-based PA interventions with five or more routes of communication between study participants and/or researchers demonstrated more favorable PA behavior changes than those with five or less (Vandelanotte et al., 2007). Vandelanotte and colleagues also found the use of theory during Internet-based PA interventions to influence study outcomes. In a study by Carr et al. (2013), several components of an Internet-based PA intervention were employed using the Social Cognitive Theory as a theoretical framework. Participants in the intervention group were included in a researcher-developed "Step into Motion" PA website, while control participants used publicly available PA websites. Findings indicated the intervention group using the researcher-developed, "Step into Motion" website, which was backed by theory, had significantly greater increased PA levels at three months compared to the control group—demonstrating that Internet-based PA interventions that are backed by theory may be more effective than those devoid of theory.

According to Joseph et al. (2013), studies comparing the delivery of PA interventions via Internet-based platforms as compared to in-person (Pellegrini et al., 2012; Touger-Decker, Denmark, Bruno, O'Sullivan-Maillet, & Lasser, 2010) or print-based platforms (Cook, Billings, Hersch, Back, & Hendrickson, 2007; Marcus et al., 2007) observed that these delivery methods yielded approximately identical results. These findings indicate that Internet-based PA interventions may be equally effective in promoting PA behavior change compared to more traditional PA intervention delivery methods (i.e., in-person or print-based delivery). However, it is noteworthy that Internet-based PA interventions are capable of achieving these results in a more cost-effective and accessible manner among a wider range of populations—making Internet-based PA interventions a promising method of intervention delivery (Joseph et al., 2013). Further, pairing Internet-based PA interventions with other emerging technologies being used more frequently to promote health (e.g., mobile device apps, health wearables) may further enhance the effectiveness of Internet-based PA interventions. More research is needed to investigate these statements.

Behaviors targeted and theories used

Internet-based PA interventions have sought to target a number of specific health outcomes. In a review by Joseph and colleagues (2013) regarding Internet-based PA interventions, it was found that while PA was often the primary outcome of the interventions, many studies incorporated other health-related outcomes affected by or related to PA such as weight loss and healthy eating indices in addition to risk factors for cardiovascular disease, diabetes, arthritis, or depression. Notably, approximately 70% of the Internet-based PA interventions included in the preceding review used an established theoretical framework. Theories are useful while planning, implementing, and evaluating interventions (Glanz, Rimer, & Viswanath, 2008). Indeed, interventionists can use theories to target specific health behavior determinants (e.g., self-efficacy) and develop intervention strategies to improve these determinants. As different theories are best suited to different health behavior determinants, choice of a suitable theory usually begins with identifying the problem, goal, and unit of study (e.g., individual, group, and organization level). For example, when researchers attempt to develop smoking cessation interventions at the individual level, the Transtheorectical Model may be useful (Glanz et al., 2008). While select studies may choose to develop and implement interventions using more than one health behavior theory (see Chapter 3), most interventions employ a single theory for this purpose.

Assessment of PA in Internet-based interventions

Various measures have been used to assess PA during Internet-based PA interventions. Given the fact that the majority of Internet-based PA interventions do not have a vast number of face-to-face interaction, most studies have used self-reported PA measures to assess this health behavior (Joseph et al., 2013). The three most frequently used subjective measures have been the International PA Questionnaire (Craig et al., 2003), the Godin Leisure Time Exercise Questionnaire (Godin & Shephard, 1985), and the Seven-Day PA Recall (Sallis et al., 1993). That said, a few studies used either objective measures such as pedometers or accelerometers, or both subjective and objective measures (Joseph et al., 2013).

Internet-based PA interventions in the healthcare field

An increased proportion of the population is now using the Internet to acquire health information. Resulting from increased use of the Internet to acquire health information, greater-diversity has been seen in the populations seeking this information. The healthcare field is mirroring these trends, with Internet-based PA interventions implemented among patients with: cardiovascular disease, type 2 diabetes, and other clinical diagnoses such as arthritis/rheumatism, angina, cancer, chronic obstructive pulmonary disease, and depressive symptoms. In this section of the chapter, a brief review of the effectiveness of Internet-based PA interventions for these populations will be provided.

Patients with cardiovascular disease

A systematic review examining the effect of Internet-based PA interventions in patients with diagnosed cardiovascular disease highlighted five well-designed randomized controlled trials (Pietrzak et al., 2014). The settings for these interventions varied from an interactive health management program (Southard, Southard, & Nuckolls, 2003) to cardiac rehabilitation programs (Devi, Powell, & Singh, 2014; Zutz, Ignaszewski, Bates, & Lear, 2007) or self-management programs (Blasco et al., 2012; Vernooij et al., 2012). Most often, these Internet-based PA interventions asked participants to self-monitor their disease symptoms and risk factors, engage in online communication with nurses or health experts, set treatment goals, and participate in online educational sessions (Figure 4.2).

The findings from these studies were promising. Southard et al. (2003) observed body mass index in the intervention group to decrease compared to a control group, but no differences were seen between groups on PA, blood pressure, lipid levels, and dietary habits. During two self-management programs, heart attack risk was lower in the intervention group compared to the controls, with individual risk factors favoring the intervention group patients as well (Blasco et al., 2012; Vernooij et al., 2012). Finally, two studies demonstrated

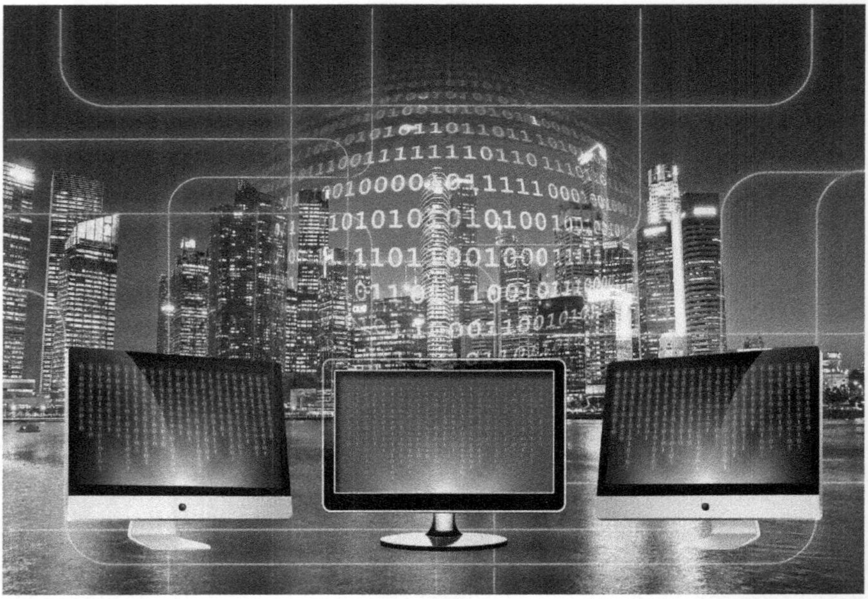

Figure 4.2 Internet use in physical activity promotion.
Source: pixabay.com.

that a higher proportion of patients enrolled in an Internet-based PA intervention met treatment goals for blood pressure compared to standard care control groups (Blasco et al., 2012, Goessens et al., 2008). A major limitation of these studies, however, was that only one study (Zutz et al., 2007) included PA as the primary outcome. Given the paucity of literature regarding the effectiveness of Internet-based PA interventions in patients with cardiovascular disease, more studies in this line of inquiry are warranted.

Populations with diagnosed diabetes

Internet-based PA interventions have also been used among patients with diabetes, with mostly positive results. Specifically, among diabetes patients, most Internet-based PA interventions were found to improve blood pressure and lipid profiles, with weight loss frequently observed as well. Notably, all studies implemented some type of interactive self-management program with study staff to aid in improving blood pressure, blood glucose, PA participation, weight loss, and medication adherence.

In a study by Bond et al. (2007), nurse provided feedback was provided to diabetic patients via instant messaging emails, with online educational discussion sessions also held—each with the objective to aid diabetic patients' management of their disease. In two studies by Glasgow et al. (2010, 2012), participants were asked to upload their health goals for medication adherence and exercise/food choices to the program websites after which they received feedback on whether they met their goals. Participants also had access to blood test results and educational modules. Findings from both studies indicated improvements in healthy eating and PA at four months, with the intervention group's improvements being maintained at 12 months—a finding not seen in the control group. Van der Weegen et al. (2015) also observed greater PA post-intervention and at a 3-month follow-up in the group receiving the Internet-based PA intervention compared to the partial intervention or usual care groups. Finally, Pietrzak et al. (2014) indicated a majority of studies using Internet-based PA interventions among patients with type 2 diabetes observed decreased blood pressure and improved glycosylated hemoglobin levels.

Other clinical populations

Internet-based PA interventions have been used in numerous other clinical populations in the healthcare field. In a study by Bosak, Yates, and Pozehl (2010), the feasibility of delivering an Internet-based PA intervention was examined in adults with metabolic syndrome. They found that the website was accessed a total of two hours over six weeks—greater than the time spent delivering usual care—with participants' evaluations of the intervention being positive. A similar feasibility trial found Internet-based PA interventions more favorable among young adult cancer survivors comparted to Internet-based interventions exclusively reviewing cancer-related topics (Rabin et al., 2012).

Effectiveness research has also been completed on populations with clinically physical and psychological diagnoses. For example, one study randomly assigned patients with rheumatoid arthritis to an Internet-based PA intervention providing individualized feedback and group contacts or a comparison group receiving an Internet-based PA intervention providing general PA information only (van den Berg et al., 2006). At the 6- and 9-month assessments, a greater proportion of intervention participants engaged in requisite amounts of moderate- and vigorous-intensity PA compared to comparison participants, with significantly higher vigorous-intensity PA seen in the intervention group at 12 months as well. However, no group differences were observed for objectively measured PA levels, self-reported quality of life, or disease progression. Regarding psychological diagnoses, Strom et al. (2013) found an Internet-based PA intervention to significantly reduce the presence of depressive symptoms among the intervention group as compared to a waitlist control. Unfortunately, no group differences were seen with regard to PA. As mental illnesses affect millions of people daily, more research into the use of Internet-based PA interventions to improve PA and depression symptoms is required.

Internet-based PA interventions among various populations

Children and adolescents

Not surprisingly, adolescents spend a great deal of time engaging in computer-based activities (Hamel, Robbins, & Wilbur, 2010). Recent reports state that children aged between 8 and 18 years spend approximately an hour a day, on average, engaged in non-work-related computer activity (Rideout, Roberts, & Foehr, 2005). That said, data also shows that adolescents prefer obtaining health information online when compared to printed materials or other traditional modalities (e.g., face-to-face interventions) (Hamel et al., 2010). As such, researchers have begun to implement Internet-based PA interventions among youth populations, with the aim of promoting PA and other proper health habits—potentially mitigating poor health outcomes in adolescence and adulthood.

Three studies were among the earliest randomized controlled trials completed on the use of Internet-based PA interventions among youth (Jago et al., 2006; Marks et al., 2006; Williamson et al., 2006). Jago et al. (2006) implemented an Internet-based PA intervention in 473 10- to 14-year-old Boy Scouts in Texas, which used role-modeling, goal setting, and problem-solving to improve children's accelerometer-determined PA levels. Compared to a control group receiving a nutritional intervention, significantly greater increased light PA was observed among the intervention children. Conversely, Marks et al. (2006) found increased PA only among adolescents within a control group receiving a print-based PA intervention compared to an intervention group receiving Internet-based interactive games, quizzes, and charts developed with the purpose of improving adolescent PA levels—perhaps due to the short duration of the intervention. Finally, Williamson et al. (2006) compared an Internet-based PA intervention to an Internet-based health education intervention in African American female adolescents. After the first six months, girls in the intervention group lost more mean body fat (1.12%) compared to the control group. However, over the next 18 months, both groups regained all weight lost, with no difference between group at this time point. Unfortunately, no PA data was provided. Other interventions have incorporated parental feedback and have been implemented in school-based settings.

Haerens and colleagues (2007a, 2007b) implemented an 8-month randomized controlled trial among adolescents, wherein the adolescents were placed within an intervention or control group receiving identical Internet-based PA interventions. However, only the intervention group received parental feedback. Researchers observed that the intervention adolescents increased moderate-to-vigorous PA by 4 minutes/day while the control group's moderate-to-vigorous PA decreased 7 minutes/day indicating parental feedback/support may still be needed among younger populations, likely due to the fact PA and eating-related behaviors are not solely at the discretion of youth populations—influenced heavily by their parents. The same researchers also compared a shorter school-based 3-month individually tailored Internet-based PA intervention to a non-individually tailored, paper-based PA intervention (Haerens et al., 2009), with findings indicating no significant differences between groups. The preceding findings are in contrast to the findings of Bourdeaudhuij et al. (2010). These researchers conducted a school-based randomized-controlled trial in a group of 12–17-year-olds from six European countries investigating the short-term (1 month) and mid-term (3 months) effectiveness of an individually tailored Internet-based PA intervention compared to a non-individually tailored Internet-based PA intervention. As a result of targeting adolescents' determinants of PA (e.g., self-efficacy, social support), it was observed that the intervention group more frequently cycled for transportation, walked more in leisure time, and participated in greater durations of total moderate-to-vigorous PA at three months in comparison to controls. Potential moderators and limitations of the studies reviewed must be kept in mind, however.

Investigations into the moderators which influence the effectiveness of Internet-based PA interventions in youth indicate Internet-based PA interventions might be more effective in youth when the participant is male, is older, has higher baseline intentions to increase PA, and possesses higher perceived social support for or modeling of PA by siblings. Regarding the limitations of the literature to date on the use of Internet-based PA interventions, it is clear that the majority of the studies regarding the effectiveness of Internet-based PA interventions were designed exclusively for or had a majority sample of girls. According to recent data, as of 2011, only 38.3% of males in grades 9–12 met the national 60 minutes per day recommendation for moderate-to-vigorous PA (Healthy People 2020, 2016). Furthermore, according to Ogden et al. (2014), prevalence of overweight or obese boys aged between 12 years and 19 years are higher (35.1%) than for girls (33.8%). Thus, developing appropriate PA interventions for boys is imperative. Internet-based PA interventions targeting youth were also found to be most effective when taking a multi-factorial approach—incorporating parent/sibling support and modeling and the use of a theoretical framework to guide the development, implementation, and analysis of the intervention (Cook et al., 2014). However, only a small proportion of the literature reviewed individually tailored the Internet-based PA intervention to the youth. As we know, individually tailored interventions are more productive than non-individually tailored interventions (see Lewis et al., 2006), more Internet-based PA interventions need to strive to individually tailor content and feedback to each participant. Finally, the setting in which the Internet-based PA intervention is implemented is important (Hamel et al., 2010). Indeed, according to Hamel and colleagues (2010), school-based interventions may be more effective than home-based interventions, with school-based interventions often demonstrating greater increases in PA and reductions in weight loss than home-based interventions—perhaps due to the integration of these interventions into the school curriculum and with teacher/peer support. Given the paucity of literature that have implemented Internet-based PA interventions in the school setting, a concerted effort is needed to integrate this type of PA intervention in this setting.

Young adults

Most studies of Internet-based PA interventions among young adults reported positive results (Joseph et al., 2014; Mailey et al., 2010; Okazaki et al,. 2014; Sriramatr et al., 2014) except for one (Franco et al., 2008). In an earlier study by Mailey et al. (2010), researchers examined the effects of an Internet-based PA intervention on self-efficacy, depression, anxiety, and objectively measured PA in college students receiving mental health counseling. At the conclusion of the 10-week intervention, the intervention group showed increased PA, self-efficacy, and improvements in depression and anxiety—suggesting Internet-based PA interventions are an efficacious supplement to face-to-face psychological counseling. Specific populations of young adults have also been examined.

Joseph et al. (2014) examined the feasibility of a culturally relevant Internet-based PA intervention predicated upon the Social Cognitive Theory in the promotion of PA among overweight/obese African American female college students, observing initially increased PA at the 3-month assessment, but decreased PA back to baseline levels at the 6-month assessment. In a study among female college students in Thailand, Sriramatr et al. (2014) also used the Social Cognitive Theory to guide the implementation of an Internet-based PA intervention. Resulting from tracking PA and setting PA-related self-efficacy and outcome expectancy goals, findings indicated that the Internet-based PA program was effective at promoting and allowing for the maintenance of increased PA at 3- and 6-month assessments when comparing the intervention group to the control group. Finally, Okazaki et al. (2014) investigated the effectiveness of an Internet-based PA intervention in the promotion of increased PA and energy expenditure among college students. Participants used the online website portal to set weekly PA goals and were asked to send a weekly email to the researchers reviewing their progress toward achievement of these goals in addition to providing a statement of new goals for the coming week. Individually tailored feedback was given regarding their goal achievement. Findings revealed the intervention group to engage in significantly higher PA levels when compared to the control group—highlighting once more the importance of individually tailoring Internet-based PA interventions to participants.

However, not all Internet-based PA interventions in young adults have been successful. In 2008, Franco and colleagues conducted a study investigating the effects of an Internet-based PA intervention on college students' PA and nutrition-related behaviors. Participants were randomly assigned to either two different Internet-based intervention groups or an attention placebo control group. While both intervention groups significantly increased fruit and vegetable intake compared to the control group, no increase in PA levels were seen among intervention groups. Researchers commented that the results seen were likely a result of the fact the emphasis on PA was not as high as it could have been and that the baseline PA among the student participants was already high—suggesting again that attention needs to be paid to how to best target certain health behaviors regardless of the population of interest.

Much like studies of Internet-based PA interventions among youth, a major limitation of literature concerning this PA intervention delivery method among young adults was the fact the samples were largely comprised of women. Further, some interventions were offered as part of a college course—perhaps biasing the results in a favorable manner. Finally, conflicting findings were seen regarding whether or not greater baseline PA influences intervention effectiveness (Joseph et al., 2014; Okazaki et al., 2014). Thus, future studies need to design Internet-based PA interventions that appeal to both genders, are not part of a college course, and are individually tailored to ensure a participant's baseline PA levels do not bias the results.

Adults and older adults

Studies on Internet-based PA interventions among adults and older adults have revealed mixed findings (Broekhuizen et al., 2016; Hargreaves, Mutrie, & Fleming, 2016; Marsaux et al., 2015; Zacharia et al., 2013). Specifically, Broekhuizen et al. (2016) tested the effectiveness of an Internet-based PA intervention in inactive older adults (60–70 years) with the aim of improving participants' PA levels and quality of life. Participants were placed in an intervention or control group. The intervention group was given DirectLife (Philips, Consumer Lifestyle, Amsterdam, the Netherlands) which consisted of an accelerometer-based activity monitor, a personal website, and a personal e-coach. Participants wore the activity monitor with data uploaded to an online database. Notably, individually tailored goals were set by the DirectLife program based on participants' baseline assessment while uploaded data from the activity monitor was used for the provision of regular feedback on their progress toward goals. Findings indicated that 42% of the intervention group participants reached their PA goals in addition to significantly improving their quality of life compared to the control group. Similarly, positive findings were seen in the StepWise study by Hargreaves et al. (2016), with intervention participants tracking and receiving positive and supportive feedback regarding their walking activity, increasing and maintaining their daily step count at 11,000 steps higher than seen at baseline, with concomitant improvements observed for blood pressure, resting heart rate, and motivation to be physically active. Finally, some systematic reviews have suggested Internet-based PA interventions to be effective when implemented among adults in the workplace (Zacharia et al., 2013). Nonetheless, the literature regarding the use of Internet-based PA interventions among older adults is sparse—likely because the current generation of older adults is not as technologically adept as the current youth generation. That said, concerted efforts must be made to increase the ease of use of Internet-based PA interventions among this population as preliminary findings look promising.

Opportunities and challenges

Many PA interventions incorporated theoretical models into their interventions. However, it is hard to conclude whether the interventions which incorporated theories were more effective in promotion of PA (van den Berg, Schoones, Vliet Vlieland, 2007). One of the biggest future challenges, therefore, will be to conduct larger, high-quality randomized controlled trials to discern the increased effects of theory-based Internet-based PA interventions above and beyond that of non-theory-based interventions. Other challenges for future Internet-based PA interventions are related to the limitations seen most frequently in the literature. To begin with, few Internet-based PA interventions included objective PA measurements. To generate strong conclusions, it is important to determine PA in relation to PA levels assessed via objective measures (e.g., accelerometers and pedometers). Second, there needs to be uniformity in measuring PA outcomes. In particular, empirical studies most often measured PA in time, energy expenditure, and/or proportions of people meeting PA recommendations. Other studies used indirect measures such as weight loss, heart rate, or stages of motivational readiness to measure PA instead of directly measuring changes in PA levels. Consensus measurement protocol will be paramount to the future of this field.

Practical implications

To enhance the effectiveness of Internet-based PA intervention, it is crucial to engage participants by introducing them to intervention materials and increasing their Internet use. It may be possible that participants who are motivated to change their behavior are more likely to use the Internet more than those who lack motivation. However, empirical data indicates that participants who logged on more often had greater exposure to intervention material and demonstrated more positive outcomes. One way to increase the interactivity may be through the use of computer algorithms to provide participants with immediate and tailored feedback about their PA behavior. Providing participants with adapted tips and suggestions may increase their engagement and retention in the program. Researchers have also suggested interventions that stimulate active participant interaction and use behavioral modification techniques might be helpful in eliciting more participant engagement and retention.

Future research regarding the use of Internet-based PA interventions should also make the following considerations before implementation. When working with children, Internet-based PA interventions should be implemented in the school setting, given the fact the large majority of children can be reached in this context. Second, using established theory as an intervention framework is also vital in the development and planning of effective programs, given the fact that theory allows researchers to more effectively implement methodology capable of targeting certain health behaviors in addition to allowing for better interpretation of the findings (Brug, Oenema, & Ferreira, 2005).

References

Ajzen, I. (1991). The theory of planned behavior. *Organizational Behavior and Human Decision Processes, 50*(2), 179–211.

Bennett, J. B., Broome, K. M., Schwab-Pilley, A., & Gilmore, P. (2011). A web-based approach to address cardiovascular risks in managers: Results of a randomized trial. *Journal of Occupational and Environmental Medicine, 53*, 911–918.

Bensley, R. J., Brusk, J. J., & Rivas, J. (2010). Key principles in internet-based weight management systems. *American Journal of Health Behaviors, 34*(2), 206–214.

Blasco, A., Carmona, M., & Fernandez-Lozano, I. (2012). Evaluation of a telemedicine service for the secondary prevention of coronary artery disease. *Journal of Cardiopulmonary Rehabilitation and Prevention, 32*, 25–31.

Bond, G. E., Burr, R., Wolf, F. M., Price, M., McCurry, S. M. ... Teri, L. (2007). The effects of a Web-based intervention on the physical outcomes associated with diabetes among adults age 60 and older: A randomized trial. *Diabetes Technology Therapy, 9*, 52–55.

Booth, A. O., Nowson, C. A., & Matters, H. (2008). Evaluation of an interactive, internet-based weight loss program: A pilot study. *Health Education Research, 23*, 371–381.

Bosak, K. A., Yates, B., & Pozehl, B. (2010). Effects of an internet physical activity intervention in adults with metabolic syndrome. *Western Journal of Nursing Research, 32*(1), 5–22. http://doi.org/10.1177/0193945909333889.

Bourdeaudhuij, I. de, Maes, L., Henauw, S. de, Vriendt, T. De, Moreno, L. A., Kersting, M., et al.(2010). Evaluation of a computer-tailhored physical activity intervention in adolescents in six European countries: The Activ-O-Meter in the HELENA intervention study. *Journal of Adolescent Health, 46*, 458–466. http://doi.org/10.1016/j.jadohealth.2009.10.006.

Broekhuizen, K., Gelder, J. De, Wijsman, C. A., Wijsman, L. W., Westendorp, R., Verhagen, E., et al.(2016). An internet-based physical activity intervention to improve quality of life of inactive older adults: A randomized controlled trial. *Journal of Medical Internet Research, 18*, 1–11. http://doi.org/10.2196/jmir.4335.

Bronfenbrenner, U. (1979). *The ecology of human development*. Cambridge, MA: Harvard University Press.

Brouwer, W., Oenema, A., Raat, H., Crutzen, R., Nooijer, J. De, Vries, N. K. De, & Brug, J. (2010). Characteristics of visitors and revisitors to an Internet-delivered computer-tailored lifestyle intervention implemented for use by the general public. *Health Education Research, 25*(4), 585–595. http://doi.org/10.1093/her/cyp063.

Brug, J., Oenema, A., & Ferreira, I. (2005). Theory, evidence, and intervention mapping to improve behavior, nutrition, and physical activity interventions. *International Journal of Behavioral Nutrition and Physical Activity, 2*(2), 1–14.

Carlson, J. A., Sallis, J. F., Ramirez, E. R., Patrick, K., & Norman, G. J. (2012). Physical activity and dietary behavior change in Internet-based weight loss interventions: Comparing two multiple-behavior change indices. *Preventive Medicine, 54*(1), 50–54. http://doi.org/10.1016/j.ypmed.2011.10.018.

Carr, L. J., Lewis, B., Ciccolo, J. T., Hartman, S., Bock, B., Dominick, G., & Marcus, B. H. (2013). Randomized controlled trial testing an internet physical activity intervention for sedentary adults. *Health Psychology, 32*(3), 328–336. http://doi.org/10.1037/a0028962.

Centers for Disease Control and Prevention. (2014). Facts about physical activity. Retrieved from www.cdc.gov/physicalactivity/data/facts.htm.

Ciccolo, J. T., Lewis, B., & Marcus, B. (2008). Internet-based physical activity interventions. *Current Cardiovascular Risk Reports, 2*, 299–304.

Cook, R. F., Billings, D. W., Hersch, R. K., Back, A. S., & Hendrickson, A. (2007). A field test of a web-based workplace health promotion program to improve dietary practices, reduce stress, and increase physical activity: Randomized controlled trial. *Journal of Medicine and Internet Research, 9*(2), e17.

Cook, T., Bourdeaudhukj, I., Maes, L., Haerens, L., Grammatikaki, E., Widhalm, K., … Manios, Y. (2014). Moderators of the effectiveness of a web-based tailored intervention promoting physical activity in adolescents: The HELENA Active-O-Meter. *Journal of School Health, 84*(4), 256–266.

Craig, C. L., Marshall, A. L., Sjostrom, M., Bauman, A., Booth, M. L., Ainsworth, B. E., … Oja, P. (2003). International Physical Activity Questionnaire: 12-country reliability and validity. *Medicine and Science in Sports and Exercise, 35*, 1381–1395.

Davies, C. A., Spence, J. C., Vandelanotte, C., Caperchione, C. M., & Mummery, W. K. (2012). Meta-analysis of internet-delivered interventions to increase physical activity levels. *International Journal of Behavioral Nutrition and Physical Activity, 9*, 52–65.

Devi, R., Powell, J., & Singh, S. (2014). A web-based program improves physical activity outcomes in a primary care angina population: Randomized controlled trial. *Journal of Medical Internet Research, 16*(9), e186. http://doi.org/10.2196/jmir.3340.

Franco, D. L., Cousineau, T. M., Trant, M., Craig, T., Rancourt, D., Thompson, D., … Ciccazzo, M. (2008). Motivation, self-efficacy, physical activity and nutrition in college students: Randomized controlled trial of an internet-based education program. *Preventive Medicine, 47*, 369–377. http://doi.org/10.1016/j.ypmed.2008.06.013.

Glanz, K., Rimer, B. K., Viswanath, K. (2008). Theory, research, and practice in health behavior and health education. In K. Glanz, B. K. Rimer & K. Viswanath (Eds.), *Health behavior and health education* (pp. 24–43). San Francisco, CA: John Wiley & Sons, Inc.

Glasgow, R. E., Kurz, D., King, D. K., Dickman, J. M., Faber, A. J., & Halterman, E. (2010). Outcomes of a minimal versus moderate support versions of an internet-based diabetes self-management support program. *Journal of General Internal Medicine, 25*, 1315–1322.

Glasgow, R. E., Kurz, D., King, D., Dickman, J. M., Faber, A. J., Halterman, E., … Ritzwoller, D. (2012). Twelve-month outcomes of an Internet-based diabetes self-management support program. *Patient Education and Counseling, 87*, 81–92. http://doi.org/10.1016/j.pec.2011.07.024.

Godin, G., & Shephard, R. J. (1985). A simple method to assess exercise behavior in the community. *Canadian Journal of Applied Sport Science, 10*, 141–146.

Goessens, B. M., Visseren, F. L., & de Nooijer, J. (2008). A pilot-study to identify the feasibility of an Internet-based coaching program for changing the vascular risk profile of high-risk patients. *Patient Education Counseling, 73*, 67–72.

Grim, M., Hortz, B., & Petosa, R. (2011). Impact evaluation of a pilot web-based intervention to increase physical activity. *American Journal of Health Promotion, 25*, 227–230.

Haerens, L., Bourdeaudhuij, I. De, Maes, L., Cardon, G., & Deforche, B. (2007a). School-based randomized controlled trial of a physical activity intervention among adolescents. *Journal of Adolescent Health, 40*, 258–265. http://doi.org/10.1016/j.jadohealth.2006.09.028.

Haerens, L., Deforche, B., Vandelanotte, C., Maes, L., & Bourdeaudhuij, I. De. (2007b). Acceptability, feasibility and effectiveness of a computer-tailored physical activity intervention in adolescents. *Patient Education and Counseling, 66*, 303–310. http://doi.org/10.1016/j.pec.2007.01.003.

Haerens, L., Maes, L., Vereecken, C., Henauw, S. De, Moreno, L., & Bourdeaudhuij, I. De. (2009). Effectiveness of a computer tailored physical activity intervention in adolescents compared to a generic advice. *Patient Education and Counseling, 77*, 38–41. http://doi.org/10.1016/j.pec.2009.03.020.

Hamel, L. M., Robbins, L. B., & Wilbur, J. (2010). Computer- and web-based interventions to increase preadolescent and adolescent physical activity: A systematic review. *Journal of Advanced Nursing, 67*(2), 251–268. http://doi.org/10.1111/ j.1365-2648.2010.05493.x.

Hargreaves, E. A., Mutrie, N., & Fleming, J. D. (2016). A web-based intervention to encourage walking (StepWise): Pilot randomized controlled trial. *JMIR Research Protocols, 5*(1), 1–17. http://doi.org/10.2196/resprot.4288.

Hartman, S. J., Marinac, C. R., Marcus, B. H., Rosen, R. K., & Gans, K. M. (2015). Internet-based physical activity intervention for women with a family history of breast cancer. *Health Psychology, 34*, 1296–1304.

Harvey-Berino, J., West, D., Krukowski, R., Prewitt, E., Vanbiervliet, A., Ashikaga, T., & Skelly, J. (2010). Internet delivered behavioral obesity treatment. *Preventive Medicine, 51*(2), 123–128. http://doi.org/10.1016/j.ypmed.2010.04.018.

Healthy People 2020 (2016). *Physical Activity*. Office of Disease Prevention and Health Promotion. Retrieved from www.healthypeople.gov/2020/topics-objectives/topic/physical-activity/national-snapshot.

Hill, C., Ã, C. A., & Wright, D. B. (2007). Can theory-based messages in combination with cognitive prompts promote exercise in classroom settings ? *Social Science & Medicine, 65*, 1049–1058. http://doi.org/10.1016/j.socscimed.2007.04.024.

Huberty, J., Dinkel, D., Beets, M., & Coleman, J. (2013). Describing the use of the internet for health, physical activity, and nutrition information in pregnant women. *Maternal and Child Health Journal, 17*, 1363–1372. http://doi.org/10.1007/s10995-012-1160-2.

Hurkmans, E. J., Berg, M. H. Van Den, Ronday, K. H., Peeters, A. J., Cessie, S., & Vlieland, T. P. M. V. (2010). Maintenance of physical activity after Internet-based physical activity interventions in patients with rheumatoid arthritis. *Rheumatology, 49*, 167–172. http://doi.org/10.1093/rheumatology/kep285.

Jago, R., Baranowski, T., Baranowski, J. C., Thompson, D., Cullen, K. W., Watson, K., & Liu, Y. (2006). Fit for Life Boy Scout badge: Outcome evaluation of a troop and Internet intervention. *Preventive Medicine, 42*, 181–187. http://doi.org/10.1016/j.ypmed.2005.12.010.

Joseph, R. P., Durant, N. H., Benitez, T. J., & Pekmezi, D. W. (201 4). Internet-based physical activity interventions. *American Journal of Lifestyle Medicine, 8*(1), 42–67. http://doi.org/10.1177/1559827613498059.

Joseph, R. P., Dutton, G. R., Cherrington, A., Fontaine, K., Baskin, M., Casazza, K., … Durant, N. H. (2015). Feasibility, acceptability, and characteristics associated with adherence and completion of a culturally relevant internet-enhanced physical activity pilot intervention for overweight and obese young adult African American women enrolled in college. *BMC Research Notes*, 1–10. http://doi.org/10.1186/s13104-015-1159-z.

Joseph, R. P., Pekmezi, D., Dutton, G. R., Cherrington, A. L., Kim, Y., Allison, J. J., & Durant, N. H. (2016). Results of a culturally adapted Internet-enhanced physical activity pilot intervention for overweight and obese young adult African American women. *Journal of Transcultural Nursing, 27*(2), 136–146. http://doi.org/10.1177/1043659614539176.

Lachausse, R. G. (2012). My student body: Effects of an internet-based prevention program to decrease obesity among college students. *Journal of American College Health, 60*, 324–330.

Lewis, B., Forsyth, L., Pinto, B., Bock, B., Roberts, M., & Marcus B. (2006). Psychosocial mediators to physical activity in a randomized controlled intervention trial. *Journal of Sport Exercise Psychology, 28,* 193–204.

Lustria, M. L. A., Cortese, J., Noar, S. M., & Glueckauf, R. L. (2009). Computer-tailored health interventions delivered over the web: Review and analysis of key components. *Patient Education and Counseling, 74*, 156–173. http://doi.org/10.1016/j.pec.2008.08.023.

Magoc, D., Tomaka, J., & Bridges-Arzaga, A. (2011). Using the web to increase physical activity in college students. *American Journal of Health Behavior, 35*, 142–154.

Mailey, E. L., Wójcicki, T. R., Motl, R. W., Hu, L., Strauser, D. R., Collins, K. D., & McAuley, E. (2010). Internet-delivered physical activity intervention for college students with mental health disorders: A randomized pilot trial. *Psychology, Health & Medicine, 15*(6), 646–659.

Marcus, B. H., Lewis, B. A., Williams, D. M., Dunsiger, S., Jakicic, J. M., Whiteley, J. A., Albrecht, A. E., Napolitano, A. A., Bock, D. E. & Tate, D. F. (2007). A comparison of Internet and print-based physical activity interventions. *Archives of Internal Medicine, 167*(9), 944–949.

Marcus, B. H., Nigg, C. R., Riebe, D., & Forsyth, L. H. (2000). Implications for population-based physical-activity promotion. *American Journal of Preventive Medicine, 19*(2), 121–126.

Marks, J. T., Campbell, M. K., Ward, D. S., Ribisl, K. M., Wildemuth, B. M., Symons, M. J., & Carolina, N. (2006). A comparison of web and print media for physical activity promotion among adolescent girls. *Journal of Adolescent Health, 39*, 96–104. http://doi.org/10.1016/j.jadohealth.2005.11.002.

Marsaux, C. F. M., Celis-morales, C., Fallaize, R., Macready, A. L., Manios, Y., Traczyk, I., … Saris, W. H. M. (2015). Effects of a web-based personalized intervention on physical activity in European adults: A randomized controlled trial. *Journal of Medical Internet Research, 17*(10), 1–17. http://doi.org/10.2196/jmir.4660.

Mehta, P., & Sharma, M. (2011). Internet and cell phone-based physical activity interventions in adults. *Archives of Exercise in Health and Disease, 2*(2), 108–113. http://doi.org/10.5628/aehd.v2i2.49.

Morgan, J. P., Collins, C. E., Plotnikoff, R. C., Cook, A. T., Berthon, B., Mitchell, S., & Casllister, R. (2011). Efficacy of a workplace-based weight loss program for overweight male shift workers: The Workplace POWER (Preventing Obesity Without Eating like a Rabbit) randomized controlled trial. *Preventive Medicine, 52,* 317–325.

Motl, R. W., Dlugonski, D., Wo, T. R., Mcauley, E., & Mohr, D. C. (2011). Internet intervention for increasing physical activity in persons with multiple sclerosis. *Multiple Sclerosis Journal, 17*(1), 116–128. http://doi.org/10.1177/1352458510383148.

Motl, R. W., Hu, L., Mailey, E. L., Wo, T. R., Strauser, D. R., Collins, K. D., & Mcauley, E. (2010). Internet-delivered physical activity intervention for college students with mental health disorders: A randomized pilot trial. *Psychology, Health & Medicine, 15*(6), 646–659. http://doi.org/10.1080/13548506.2010.498894.

Napolitano, M. A., Fotheringham, M., Tate, D., Sciamanna, C., Leslie, E., Owen, N., … Marcus, B. (2003). Evaluation of an internet-based physical activity intervention: A preliminary investigation. *Annual Behavioral Medicine, 25*(2), 92–99.

Norman, G. J., Zabinski, M. F., Adams, M. A., Rosenberg, D. E., Yaroch, A. L., & Atienza, A. A. (2007). A review of eHealth interventions for physical activity and dietary behavior change. *American Journal of Preventive Medicine, 33*(4), 336–345. http://doi.org/10.1016/j.amepre.2007.05.007.

Ogden, C., Carroll, M., Kit, B., & Flegal, K. (2014). Prevalence of childhood and adult obesity in the United States, 2011–2012. *Journal of the American Medical Association, 311*(8), 806–814.

Okazaki, K., Okano, S., Haga, S., & Seki, A. (2014). One-year outcome of an interactive internet-based physical activity intervention among university students. *International Journal of Medical Informatics, 83*(5), 354–360. http://doi.org/10.1016/j.ijmedinf.2014.01.012.

Perrin, A., & Duggan, M. (2015). *Americans' internet access, 2000–2015*. Pew Research Center. Retrieved from www.pewinternet.org/2015/06/26/Americans-internet-access-2000-2015/.

Pellegrini, C. A., Verba, S. D., Otto, A. D., Helsel, D. L., Davis, K. K., & Jakicic, J. M. (2012). The comparison of a technology-based system and an in-person behavioral weight loss intervention. *Obesity (Silver Spring), 20*, 356–363.

Pew Internet (2013). *Majority of adults look online for health information*. Pew Research Center. Retrieved from www.pewresearch.org/daily-number/majority-of-adults-look-online-for-health-information/.

Pekmezi, D. W., Williams, D. M., Jennings, E. G., Lewis, B. A., Jakicic, J. M., & Marcus, B. H. (2010). Feasibility of using computer-tailored and internet-based interventions to promote physical activity in underserved populations. *Telemedicine and E-Health, 16*(4), 498–504.

Pietrzak, E., Cotea, C., & Pullman, S. (2014). Primary and secondary prevention of cardiovascular disease. *Journal of Cardiopulmonary Rehabilitation and Prevention, 34*, 303–317. http://doi.org/10.1097/HCR.0000000000000063.

Poirier, J., Bennett, W., Jerome, G., Shah, N., Lazo, M., Yeh, H., ... Cobb, N. (2016). Effectiveness of an activity tracker and internet-aased Adaptive walking program for adults: A randomized controlled trial. *Journal of Medical Internet Research, 18*(2), 1–13. http://doi.org/10.2196/jmir.5295.

Portnoy, D. B., Scott-sheldon, L. A. J., Johnson, B. T., & Carey, M. P. (2008). Computer-delivered interventions for health promotion and behavioral risk reduction: A meta-analysis of 75 randomized controlled trials, 1988–2007. *Preventive Medicine, 47*, 3–16. http://doi.org/10.1016/j.ypmed.2008.02.014.

Rabin, C., Dunsiger, S., Ness, K. K., & Marcus, B. H. (2012). Internet-based physical activity intervention targeting young adult cancer survivors. *Journal of Adolescent and Young Adult Oncology, 1*(4), 188–194. http://doi.org/10.1089/jayao.2011.0040.

Reid, R. D., Morrin, L. I., Beaton, L. J., Papadakis, S., Kocourek, J., McDonnell, L., ... Pipe, A. L. (2012). Randomized trial of an internet-based computer-tailored expert system for physical activity in patients with heart disease. *European Journal of Preventive Cardiology, 19*, 1357–1364.

Rideout, V., Roberts, D. F. & Foehr, U. G. (2005) *Generation M: Media in the lives of 8–18 year-olds. A Kaiser Family foundation study*. Menlo Park, CA: The Henry J. Kaiser Family Foundation.

Sallis, J. F., Buono, M. J., Roby, J. J., Micale, F. G., & Nelson, J. A. (1993). Seven-day recall and other physical activity self-reports in children and adolescents. *Medicine and Science in Sports and Exercise; 25*, 99–108.

Slootmaker, S. M., Chinapaw, M. J., Schuit, A. J., Seidell, J. C., & Van Mechelen, W. (2009). Feasibility and effectiveness of online physical activity advice based on a personal activity monitor: Randomized controlled trial. *Journal of Medicine and Internet Research, 11*(3), e27.

Soetens, K. C. M., Vandelanotte, C., Vries, H. De, & Mummery, K. W. (2014). Using online computer tailoring to promote physical activity: A randomized trial of text,

video, and combined intervention delivery modes. *Journal of Health Communication, 19*(12), 1377–1392. http://doi.org/10.1080/10810730.2014.894597.
Southard, B. H., Southard, D. R., & Nuckolls, J. (2003). Clinical trial of an internet-based case management system for secondary prevention of heart disease. *Journal of Cardiopulmonary Rehabilitation, 23*, 341–348.
Sriramatr, S., Berry, T. R., & Spence, J. C. (2014). An internet-based intervention for promoting and maintaining physical activity: A randomized controlled trial. *American Journal of Health Behaviors, 38*(3), 430–439.
Strom, M., Uckelstam, C., Andersson, G., Hassm, P., Umefjord, G., & Carlbring, P. (2013). Internet-delivered therapist-guided physical activity for mild to moderate depression: A randomized controlled trial. *PeerJ, 1*, 1–17. http://doi.org/10.7717/peerj.178.
Touger-Decker, R., Denmark, R., Bruno, M., O'Sullivan-Maillet, J., & Lasser, N. (2010). Workplace weight loss program: Comparing live and internet methods. *Journal of Occupational and Environmental Medicine, 52*, 1112–1118.
Vandelanotte, C., Spathonis, K. M., Eakin, E. G., & Owen, N. (2007). Website-delivered physical activity interventions: A review of the literature. *American Journal of Preventive Medicine, 33*(1), 54–64. http://doi.org/10.1016/j.amepre.2007.02.041.
Van den Berg, M., Ronday, H. K., Peeters, A., Cessie, S., van der Giesen, F. J., Breedveld, F. C., & Vlieland, T. P. M. V. (2006). Using internet technology to deliver a home-based physical activity intervention for patients with rheumatoid arthritis: A randomized controlled trial. *Arthritis & Rheumatism, 55*(6), 935–945. http://doi.org/10.1002/art.22339.
Van den Berg, M. H., Schoones, J. W., & Vlieland, T. P. V. (2007). Internet-based physical activity interventions: A systematic review of the literature. *Journal of Medical Internet Research, 9*(3), e26.
van der Weegen, S., Verwey, R., Spreeuwenberg, M., Tange, H., van der Weijden, T., & de Witte, L. (2015). It's LiFe! Mobile and web-based monitoring and feedback tool embedded in primary care increases physical activity: A cluster randomized controlled trial. *Journal of Medical Internet Research, 17*(7), 1–14. http://doi.org/10.2196/jmir.4579.
Vernooij, J. W., Kaasjager, H. A., & van der Graaf, Y. (2012). Internet based vascular risk factor management for patients with clinically manifest vascular disease: Randomized controlled trial. *British Medical Journal, 344*, e3750.
Wadsworth, D. D., & Hallam, J. S. (2010). Effect of a website intervention on physical activity of college females. *American Journal of Health Behavior, 34*, 60–69.
Wanner, M., Martin-Diener, E., Braun-Fahrlander, C., Bauer, G., & Martin, B. W. (2009). Effectiveness of active-online, an individually tailored physical activity intervention, in a real-life setting: Randomized controlled trial. *Journal of Medicine and Internet Research, 11*(3), e23.
Wantland, D. J., Portillo, C. J., Holzemer, W. L., Slaughter, R., & McGhee, E. (2004). The effectiveness of web-based vs. non-web-based interventions: A meta-analysis of behavioral change outcomes. *Journal of Medical Internet Research, 6*(4), 1–20. http://doi.org/10.2196/jmir.6.4.e40.
Watson, A., Bickmore, T., Cange, A., Kulshreshtha, A., & Kvedar, J. (2012). An internet-based virtual coach to promote physical activity adherence in overweight adults: Randomized controlled trial. *Journal of Medicine and Internet Research, 14*(1), e1.
Weinstein, P. K. (2006). A review of weight loss programs delivered via the internet. *Journal of Cardiovascular Nursing, 21*(4), 251–258.

Whittemore, R., Chao, A., Jang, M., Jeon, S., Liptak, T., Popick, R., & Grey, M. (2016). Implementation of a school-based internet obesity prevention program for adolescents. *Journal of Nutrition Education and Behavior, 45*(6), 586–594. http://doi.org/10.1016/j.jneb.2013.03.012.

Williamson, D. A., Walden, H. M., White, M. A., York-crowe, E., Newton, R. L., Alfonso, A., … Parkes, D. R. (2006). Two-year internet-based randomized controlled trial for weight loss in African-American girls. *Obesity, 14*(7), 1231–1243.

Yoo, H. J., Park, M., & Kim, T. N. (2009). A ubiquitous chronic disease care system using cellular phones and the internet. *Diabetic Medicine, 26*, 628–635.

Zacharia, S., Funk, M., Gwin, S., Taylor, E. L., & Branscum, P. (2013). Internet-based physical activity interventions at the worksite: A systematic review. *American Journal of Health Studies, 28*(3), 114–126.

Zutz, A., Ignaszewski, A., Bates, J., & Lear, S. A. (2007). Utilization of the internet to deliver cardiac rehabilitation at a distance: A pilot study. *Telemedicine Journal and E-Health, 13*, 323–330.

5 Online social media and physical activity promotion

Jung Eun Lee and Zan Gao

The turn of the century ushered in a new age of Internet connectivity with the advent of social media sites such as MySpace in 2003. Today social media sites abound, with sites such as Wechat, Facebook, Twitter, Snapchat and Instagram among the most popular. Recent data (Perrin & Duggan, 2015) indicated that 78% of adults access the Internet and, of this proportion of adults accessing the Internet, 65% use online social media like Facebook and Twitter. Facebook, for example, is the world's largest and most frequently used social media site, with 1.32 billion users as of June 2014 (Maher et al., 2014). Moreover, a recent poll revealed 50% of the Facebook users visit the website everyday (Statistics Brain, 2013). Indeed, Internet users are spending one-quarter of all time spent on online using social media (Maher et al., 2014). Social media sites are popular as they allow users to create an online profile to connect with friends/family, opine on current events, and access/view information presented in various media formats (i.e., text-, video-, or audio-based content) within their network (Greene, Sacks, Piniewski, Kil, & Hahn, 2013). Recently, social media sites have become an avenue through which researchers/health professionals are promoting physical activity (PA) and health.

Social media is being targeted as a PA intervention delivery approach due to these sites' ability to do the following: (1) reach large and diverse populations; (2) present health messages using video and auditory-based formats of media as opposed to only traditional text-based media formats; and (3) maintain high levels of user engagement and retention (Maher et al., 2015). Indeed, in the past decade, individuals have been seeking easily accessible, low-cost, online technologies to address their health needs (Fallows, 2005). Notably, social media sites have been shown to be an important component in altering social norms related to certain health outcomes such as obesity—potentially increasing individuals' awareness of the need to be physically active and, therefore, promoting weight loss (Leahey, Gokee LaRose, Fava, & Wing, 2011). For example, placing intervention participants in a private group on a social media site such as Facebook allows researchers/health professionals to deliver empirically valid health information to these individuals in a cost-effective manner. Delivering health information via groups created on social media sites also allows for interventionists and participants to interact with one another—changing PA-related attitudes and social norms and increasing the likelihood of engaging in PA participation by as much as 45% (Nakhasi, Shen, Passarella, Appel, & Anderson, 2014). Finally, social media-based PA interventions also reduce the participant burden associated with traditional face-to-face wellness counseling (e.g., transportation, missed time at work, etc.).

Throughout this chapter, we will review the current status of social media-based PA interventions, critique the effects of this intervention modality on various health outcomes and discuss the negative issues related to social media, as well as the practical implications and directions for future studies.

Implementation of social media-based interventions on behavior change

According to a review by Maher et al. (2014), social media-based interventions demonstrate small to moderate effects in promoting health behavior (e.g., PA, healthy eating) and related outcomes (e.g., weight loss, more favorable body composition). The demonstrated effectiveness of social media-based interventions is likely due to social media's ability to address the research-related issues of reach (the extent to which the population of interest is exposed to the content), engagement (the degree to which participants get involved and participate in the interventions), and retention (how many people are retained at the end of intervention).

Despite its capability of reaching large and diverse populations, social media-based health interventions do not always achieve high levels of engagement—limiting the effectiveness of the intervention due to the small level of participation by participants following intervention protocols. Aside from one social media-based health intervention which achieved a decent rate of engagement (see Foster, Linehan, Kirman, Lawson, & James, 2010), most studies have reported engagement levels between 5% and 15% (Maher et al., 2014). The aforementioned engagement rates were in spite of researchers' attempts to continuously interact with participants, provide prompts, and send reminder emails regarding the research's protocols. Differences between studies with regard to participant recruitment might also explain some differences in engagement. For example, in the above study reporting higher participant engagement, Foster et al. (2010) recruited participants who already knew each other and created a friendly, competitive environment with an online ranking board of each participant's step counts—contrasting with other studies which achieved low engagement while striving to use Facebook and Twitter to promote PA social support among individuals with no previous relationship (Napolitano Hayes, Bennett, Ives, & Foster, 2013; Valle, Tate, Mayer, Allicock, & Cai, 2013). Indeed, it might be argued that the higher engagement rates seen by Foster and colleagues (2010) were attributable to the fact that the researchers' approach was better aligned with how people use social media (Figure 5.1). Specifically, individuals more commonly use sites like Facebook to interact with people with whom they share an offline connection as well, rather than using Facebook to interact with new people (Ellison, Steinfield, & Lampe, 2007).

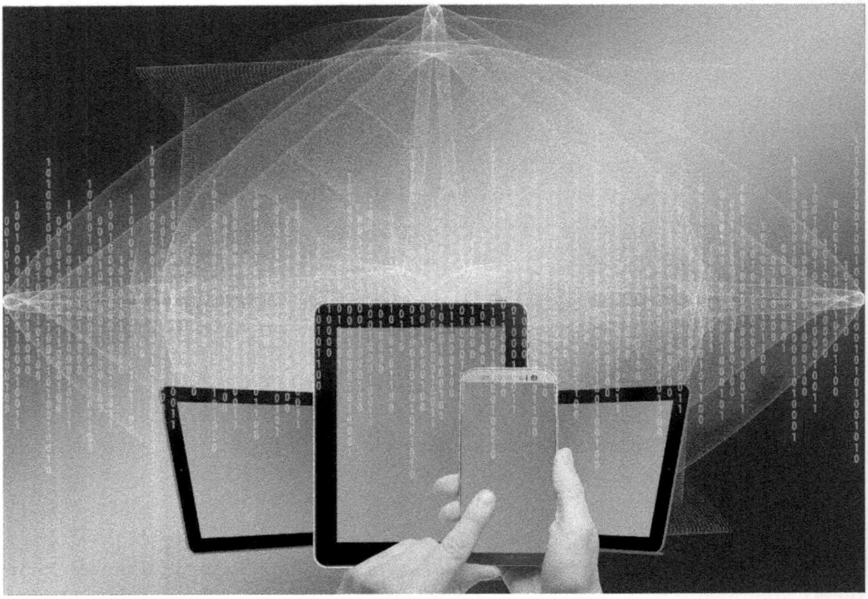

Figure 5.1 Social network on mobile devices.

Source: pixabay.com.

Finally, with regard to retention, social media-based health studies have most frequently used Facebook, as this social media site reports 61% of regular users access the site daily (Kaushal, 2013). Researchers using Facebook to implement health interventions frequently managed to retain a high proportion of participants across the study period (77–96% of users) (Cavallo et al., 2012; Foster et al., 2010; Napolitano et al., 2013; Valle et al., 2013). High retention is important, given the fact that health behavior interventions with higher retention rates are vital to the overall effectiveness of the intervention (Thomas, Nelson, & Silverman, 2011). Stated simply, if individuals cannot stick with an intervention, health behavior change is not able to take place.

Social media-based PA interventions in the healthcare field

Social media-based PA interventions have also been implemented in the healthcare field. This intervention delivery modality is desirable in the healthcare field as it reduces participant burden—an important fact as many patients may have diseases or treatment limitations that make tasks such as transporting themselves to and from a clinic difficult. Below, major studies in the healthcare field which have used social media-based PA interventions will be introduced, with their findings highlighted.

Individuals with mental disorder

Mental disorders have an influence on a person's thoughts, mood, and feelings. As a result, these conditions can have a major impact on an individual's quality of life as they affect relationships and the functions of everyday life. Approximately 46% of the U.S. population has a diagnosed mental disorder, with anxiety disorders being the most common (Kessler et al., 2005). Social media-based PA interventions have been implemented in patients with mental disorders. For example, Aschbrenner Naslund, Shevenell, Mueser, & Bartels (2015) investigated the feasibility of a weight loss program with peer support mobile technology and social media interaction for obese individuals with mental illnesses. The 24-week intervention consisted of: (1) once-weekly 90-minute weight management group sessions taught by two lifestyle coaches and supported by a wellness peer; (2) twice-weekly optional 1-hour group exercise sessions led by a certified fitness trainer; and (3) continuous mHealth technology and social media interaction to increase motivation, facilitate self-monitoring of diet/PA behavior, and promote peer support outside of treatment sessions. While attendance at the weekly sessions was low (56%), findings indicated that 45% of participants had lost weight at the 6-month follow-up, with the same percentage of individuals demonstrating improved fitness. Notably, participants suggested future interventions should include more active learning, a simplified dietary component, more in-depth technology training, and greater attention to mental health. As this study represents the one of few exemplar investigations into the delivery of a social media-based PA intervention among individuals with mental disorders, researchers should build upon the suggestions made by the participants.

Cancer survivors

Social media-based PA interventions have also been used among young adult cancer survivors. In a 12-week feasibility study, Valle et al. (2013) implemented an intervention called FITNET via Facebook with 86 young adult cancer survivors, aimed at increasing moderate-to-vigorous-intensity PA (Figure 5.2). Participants in the FITNET intervention group received PA-related Facebook messages and tips and tracked and recorded pedometer steps on the site, after which personalized feedback was provided. Additionally, researchers facilitated social support via Facebook by posting discussion questions, PA-related videos/articles, and prompts related to the tracking of PA and progress toward personal goals. The FITNET intervention group was compared with a self-help comparison (SC) group having all of the preceding intervention components delivered via Facebook but no access to the goal setting and feedback tools. Findings revealed both groups to have increased self-reported weekly minutes of MVPA over the course of the 12-week intervention, with no significant difference between groups. However, increases in light PA were greater in the FITNET group relative to the SC group. Researchers speculated the lack of an intervention effect on MVPA relative to the SC group might have been due to: (1) insufficient power to detect a significant difference as a result of a small sample size and large

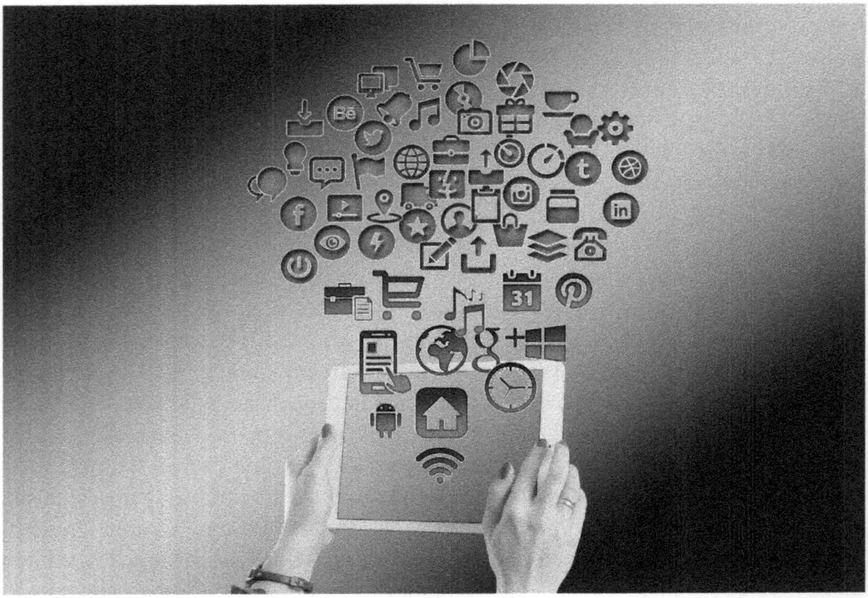

Figure 5.2 Online social media on a mobile device.
Source: pixabay.com.

within-group variance; and (2) the simultaneous targeting of multiple psychosocial constructs precluded researchers from determining the extent to which specific strategies within the program accounted for group changes in PA. Again, as this study represents one of few exemplar studies using a social media-based PA intervention among cancer survivors, future studies should improve upon the methodology.

Effectiveness of social media-based PA interventions

Studies exploring the feasibility/effectiveness of social media-based PA interventions have also been completed among healthy, but inactive populations. Of these studies, a majority recruited adults, with a paucity of research targeting adolescents. In this section, these studies and their noteworthy findings, strengths, and limitations will be highlighted. Implications for future research and practice will also be discussed.

Adolescents

Few studies have addressed the effectiveness of social media-based PA interventions in adolescents. Ruotsalainen and colleagues (2015) evaluated the effects of a 12-week, Facebook-delivered intervention on PA and body mass index in overweight/obese Finnish 13–16-year-olds. Participants were randomly assigned to one of three groups: (1) lifestyle and self-monitoring intervention group: received Facebook-delivered lifestyle counselling and PA self-monitoring tools; (2) lifestyle-only group: received the same Facebook-delivered lifestyle counselling but no PA self-monitoring tools; and (3) control group: received post-intervention feedback on their PA. Findings revealed no significant differences between the two intervention groups or control group over time for PA levels or body mass index. Notably, however, the lifestyle and self-monitoring group demonstrated lower sedentary time on weekdays at post-intervention compared to the control group, with no significant within-group changes seen in any study group. That said, focus group research among adolescent females found PA intervention components to be most appealing to adolescents when emphasizing sport, exercise, and fitness, in addition to providing opportunities for socialization with friends and self-improvement strategies, with Facebook representing the most widely desired social media site for this type of intervention. Conversely, cartoon imagery, humor, a school-based intervention, and a protocol which only gave advice on increasing walking behaviors were undesirable features of social media-based PA interventions (van Kessel, Kavanagh, & Maher 2016). Researchers should take note of features desired most by adolescents to increase the effectiveness of their social media-based PA interventions as this intervention modality holds great promise among this technologically advanced generation.

Young adults

Delivering a social media-based PA intervention in college students has high potential effectiveness beacause of two factors. First, this population demonstrates a high usage rate of social media sites. Second, college students are at great risk of overweight and obesity, given the fact that many college students are making PA and nutritional choices autonomously for the first time. Indeed, high rates of physical inactivity and obesity have been seen among this demographic (Desai, Miller, Staples, & Bravender, 2008; Nelson, Gortmaker, Subramanian, Cheung, & Wechsler, 2007; Sira & Pawlak, 2010). Therefore, college students are another population in which such interventions have been implemented—often with more frequency than other populations.

Merchant et al. (2014) conducted a randomized controlled trial to examine the effectiveness of a social media-based PA intervention in the promotion of weight loss among overweight/obese college students. Participants used their personal accounts to access a health page moderated by a health coach. Researchers concluded that Facebook can be used to remotely deliver health content within a PA intervention to promote weight loss with the help of a health coach who can iteratively tailor content and interact with participants. Notably, however, engagement with the study's Facebook page was highly variable and declined over time—an area of concern for future studies. An earlier study by

Napolitano et al. (2013) also targeted college students with a social media-based intervention, using different combinations of Facebook and/or text messaging to implement the intervention. At 8 weeks, the Facebook plus text messaging group had significantly greater weight loss than the Facebook-only group and waitlist controls—with a large majority of the participants finding the intervention content helpful and stating they would recommend the intervention to others. Given the results of both of the studies reviewed, it is clear that innovative social media-based PA and weight loss interventions can be effectively implemented via platforms such as Facebook given social media's integration into college students' lives.

Adults

Social media-based PA intervention studies conducted on adults have explored features of social media that might have the most influence on intervention effectiveness. For example, social media sites can function as support groups, educational modules, and/or a space to keep track of PA records—all of which could lead to changes in PA behaviors. Thus, findings and strengths of the studies that examined these features will be discussed in the following subsections.

Information vs. support

Brindal et al. (2012) compared the effectiveness of a 12-week social media-based PA intervention to promote weight loss. Eligible individuals were randomly allocated to one of three groups—each with an associated social media site: (1) an information-based group; (2) a supportive group; or (3) an individualized-supportive group. Both of the latter two supportive social media sites included weight tracking and meal planning tools, in addition to allowing participants to interact and support one another. However, the individualized-supportive site also included a meal planner which offered individually tailored dietary recommendations using an algorithm based on a user's preferences for certain foods. Findings demonstrated higher retention for the supportive groups compared to the information-based group at 12 week, but no differences in weight loss between the intervention groups and control group.

Peer encouragement and pedometer use

Maher and colleagues (2015) conducted a study using the Facebook app "Active Team" to implement a social media-based PA intervention. Participants were provided a pedometer and encouraged to achieve the recommended 10,000 steps per day (see Tudor-Locke et al., 2011) using the social media-based Active Team to form groups of between three and eight existing Facebook friends. The Active Team intervention included a calendar to log daily step counts; a dashboard showing step-logging progress, awards, and gifts; a team tally board to allow users to monitor their own and their teammates' progress; a team message board for team members to communicate with one another; daily tips for increasing PA; gamification features, such as awards for individual and team step-logging and step-count achievements; and the ability to send virtual gifts to teammates. At the 8-week follow-up, the Active Team intervention participants had significantly increased overall PA time by 135 minutes relative to the control group. The main component of the increased PA time was walking time. Researchers concluded that a social media-based PA intervention with concurrent pedometer use can produce sizable short-term PA increases.

Promotional messages vs. peer support

A number of features of social media lend themselves well to the enhancement of social support and provision of empirically-based information. To investigate which features of social media demonstrate the greatest ability to increase PA, Zhang and colleagues (2015) conducted a study to compare the ability of health promotion messages or the creation of peer networks to increase PA in 217 graduate students. A 13-week social media-based PA program was implemented, with participants randomized to two social media-based groups (i.e., a peer support-oriented group or health message-oriented group) or a control group. Findings indicated participants in the peer support group reported exercising moderately for an additional 1.6 days each week compared to baseline measurements—an increase significantly greater than seen in the control group. Researchers concluded that even social support from anonymous individuals was more successful than health messages for improving PA. Explicitly, this study used real-time signals about peers' exercise behaviors (i.e., number of PA classes within which a peer is enrolled) as the main form of social support/influence. Zhang and colleagues stated the strength of the effect peer support had on PA in the current study is striking, given the conservative aspect of the peer network.

Education-only vs. self-monitoring on Facebook

In contrast to the other studies of social media-based PA interventions in adults reviewed previously, results in favor of social media-based interventions were not found by Cavello and colleagues (2012). Specifically, these researchers randomized female college students into two groups: (1) Facebook intervention group: placed on a Facebook page for social support and given access to a PA-related website; and (2) control group: only received access to the aforementioned PA-related website. Findings indicated that while intervention participants experienced increased social support and PA over time, no differences in these outcomes were seen between groups over time. Researchers concluded that a social media-based PA intervention may not have any greater effects on social support or PA when compared to traditional Internet-based approaches to PA promotion (Figure 5.3).

Figure 5.3 Online social media on a computer.
Source: pixabay.com.

Podcast vs. mobile communication

Turner-McGrievy and Tate (2011) examined whether a combination of podcasts, mobile support communication and diet monitoring can promote weight loss. In this 6-month, minimal-contact intervention, overweight (n=96) adults were randomly assigned to a podcast and mobile group or podcast-only group. The podcast and mobile group was provided podcast which reviewed nutrition and PA information while also using a PA/diet monitoring mobile app to track the health behaviors and communicate with study researchers and participants via the social media site, Twitter. Only podcasts were provided to the podcast-only group participants. Findings indicated weight loss and days per week participants engaged in diet monitoring did not differ significantly at 6 months between groups. However, participants in the podcast and mobile group were 3.5 times more likely than participants in the podcast-only group to use an app to monitor dietary intake, with the number of podcasts participants reported downloading over the 6-month period significantly moderately correlated with weight loss in both groups. Finally, significant differences were reported for sources of social support, with the podcast group participants relying more on friends, and the podcast and mobile group participants relying to a greater degree on online resources, however, the PA measured by energy expenditure was not significantly different between groups. Noteworthy is the fact that the numerous components common to face-to-face interventions that the researchers tried adding to this study (i.e., self-monitoring, group support, and contact with study counselors) were seldom used by participants and may have detracted from what was already a successful podcast intervention. Moreover, the components may have detracted from the podcast and mobile group participants seeking social support from friends and family—support which is imperative for behavior change.

Offline social support

While social media-based PA interventions have often attempted to encourage use of this platform to facilitate online social support for PA, few attempts have been made using these sites to facilitate offline social support for PA in the real world. Indeed, for participants with little offline social support, modest online increases in social media-based support social support may not be sufficient to increase PA.

To address this issue regarding offline social support for PA, Schneider and colleagues (2015) used the free, commercially available "Meetup," an online social media site used commonly to schedule community event locations and times, to examine if creating walking groups for dog owners on the site might facilitate increased offline social support for PA and PA participation. Participants from two cities enrolled in the 6-month study. Findings revealed no differences for PA between the Meetup intervention group and the control condition wherein participants only received emails with content regarding increasing PA. Further, while participants in the Meetup condition reported an increase in the perceived positive outcomes of dog walking compared to the control group, social support, sense of community, and dog walking barriers did not change appreciably over time or in comparison to the control group. More research is needed to discern how to promote offline social support via social media-based PA interventions.

Negative aspects of online social media

While social media does offer numerous benefits in its ability to reach large and diverse segments of population and deliver content in multiple media formats (e.g., video, audio, and text-based formats), there are negative aspects of social media worth noting that might influence social media-based PA interventions. While the list below is not exhaustive, the list does discuss the negative aspects most pertinent to social media-based intervention delivery.

Social overload

Social media users are asked to respond to increasing numbers of messages and social relationships when using social media sites. Consequently, some users may feel that too much social support is required for them to engage with other online friends—which results in driving these individuals away from using the said social media site. This situation has been termed "social overload," and is influenced by the extent of usage, number of online friends, subjective social norms, and type of relationships (being online-only friends vs. being online and offline friends). An individual experiencing social overload often reports exhaustion and low user satisfaction which then increases the intentions of users to reduce or stop social media use (Bouc, 2013). Therefore, the challenge for researchers/health professionals is how to engage individuals in social media-based PA interventions without contributing to social overload and driving these individuals away from social media and, more specifically, the online intervention.

Online bullying and trolling

Through social media, individuals sometimes feel they have the power to post offensive remarks, pictures, or video clips that could potentially cause a great amount of emotional pain for another individual. Online bullying, (i.e., cyber-bullying) occurs relatively often, with 39% of social media users admitting to being cyber-bullied (Turkle, 2011). Currently, there are few limitations regarding the content individuals can post online. As such, researchers/health professionals need to be sure to promote a positive and supportive social media-based intervention environment which does not condone offensive or judgmental remarks. If a participant is posting disparaging content which is diminishing the morale/confidence of other participants, the ill-mannered participant should be dropped from the program.

The action of actually bullying someone online and continuing to engage in these actions is referred to as trolling. Trolling can take many different forms, including, but not limited to: persistent name-calling, regularly playing online pranks on volatile individuals, and continually posting controversial comments with the intention of causing anger and arguments. As trolling has become commonplace online, it is important for researchers/health professionals to find ways in which they can protect their participants' identity. On a site like Facebook, an intervention group can be implemented using a "Secret Group." These Secret Groups are invitation-only and cannot be searched by anyone on Facebook. This ensures that no one looking to troll can access the group and disrupt the positive, socially supportive environment that researchers are striving to create in order to promote PA and health.

Internet addiction

Social networking can also have an impact on individual's loneliness. Social-networking sites like Facebook and MySpace may provide people with a false sense of connection that ultimately increases the sense of loneliness in people who feel alone (Cornblatt, 2009). It is also possible that social networking can foster feelings of sensitivity to disconnection, which also leads to loneliness. Online social networking plays a positive role in subjective well-being when the networking is used to facilitate physical interactions, but networking activities that do not facilitate face-to-face interactions tend to diminish trust, which ultimately results in negative subjective well-being. As such, it is important for researchers/health professionals to find ways to create social media-based PA interventions that do not promote these type of negative psychological effects, but to possibly design interventions which facilitate online and offline connections.

Privacy issues

Sharing of personal identifying information and the control of information posted on social media sites—even after this type of information has been deleted—have raised privacy concerns among social media site users as this information has in some cases been illegally given to third parties for their use. A good example was when the controversial social media site "Quechup" gathered users' social media account information for use in a spamming operation (Barnes, 2006). Further, in spring 2015, a news radio piece entitled "Weighing Privacy Vs. Rewards of Letting Insurers Track Your Fitness" introduced how life insurance companies are now offering lower insurance premiums to people who are willing to report their activity tracker data to the company (Farr, 2015). This may sound like a good deal, but this could be an example of a privacy trade-off between confidentiality and improved personal finances. Finally, another example was observed in the fall of 2015 when Facebook used their newsfeed to do a study on how different types of posts could impact mood without informing its members. This experiment by Facebook may not have caused any harm to its members, but people were furious when they discovered that they had been experimented on without being informed. Thus, the fact that social media sites can use personal data in this manner raises red flags.

With regard to scientific research and medical treatments desiring to use social media-based intervention methods, privacy concerns among intervention participants are somewhat mitigated by the fact that information gathering and data collection procedures are heavily scrutinized by institutional or Medical Review Boards. Specifically, these committees ensure that participants are adequately and fully informed of study procedures and that each participant knows they have a right to discontinue participation for any reason at any time. That said, enrolling participants in a social media-based intervention presents unique challenges to review boards as social media sites contain a large amount of personal information about participants. Notably, while the information on social media sites is considered public, it is not yet known whether republishing this information in a research paper is considered an invasion of privacy (Lowry, Cao, & Everard, 2011).

Practical implications

Currently available empirical studies have shown that social media-based PA interventions can be useful in promoting health in various populations. Indeed, such interventions have the following benefits with regard to implementation: (1) researchers/health professionals can tailor information to individual or groups of participants; (2) social media sites offer intervention participants a source of social support which can act as a motivation to continue engaging in PA and other health behaviors; and (3) social media sites allow for improved reach, engagement, and retention of participants.

To more effectively capitalize on the aforementioned advantages of social media-based PA interventions, the use of theory in interventions is paramount if researchers/health professionals wish to develop and implement interventions which are capable of targeting specific health behaviors (e.g., PA) with a high degree of effectiveness. Little use of behavioral theory was seen among the social media-based PA interventions. Theories, such as the Social Cognitive Theory and the Transtheoretical Model, are behavioral theories which can be used to tailor interventions to participants. These theories have been used with success in many PA interventions and should be considered for social media-based PA interventions as well—particularly as research shows tailored interventions to be more effective than non-tailored interventions in the promotion of weight loss, healthy eating, and PA (Khaylis, Yiaslas, Bergstrom, & Gore-Felton, 2010). Moreover, as social support is often a component in PA interventions, research should also consider grouping individuals in social media-based PA intervention groups with individuals whom they already know. Greater effectiveness of social media-based PA interventions has been demonstrated when participants were grouped with individuals whom they already knew. Finally, researchers need to be vigilant about keeping users engaged, as user engagement can slip during social media-based PA interventions. Oftentimes "gamification" (i.e., the act of offering small rewards for meeting intervention goals) of interventions works best to increase user engagement in online forms of intervention delivery (Jepson, Harris, Platt, & Tannahill, 2010).

A final area of concern when implementing social media-based PA intervention lies in the need for researchers and health professionals to keep in mind how they might need to orient social media-based PA interventions toward specific populations. For example, walking may be the preferred exercise type among cancer survivors (Jones & Courneya, 2002; Karvinen et al., 2006; Vallance, Courneya, Jones, & Reiman, 2006; Valle et al., 2013). Indeed, Valle et al. (2013) reported that cancer survivors managed to increase only their walking time but not any other PA of higher intensity. When implementing weight loss programs among overweight or obese populations, it has also been found that social support might be the most important component (Verheijden, Bakx, van Weel, Koelen, & van Staveren, 2005). Finally, while little research has been conducted on the use of social media-based PA interventions among adolescents, researchers and health professionals need to be aware that overweight/obese adolescents may have significantly more negative views of PA than their normal weight counterparts (Deforche, de Bourdeaudhuij, & Tanghe, 2006). Additionally, as a result of their poorer health, overweight or obese adolescents may have a unique barrier to PA participation (e.g., reduced motor skill) which need to be kept in mind (Kantomaa, Stamatakis, & Kankaanpaetal, 2013; Zabinski, Saelens, Stein, Hayden-Wade, & Wilfley, 2003). Therefore, it is important to encourage these populations to first reduce their daily sedentary behaviors after which small, incremental changes can be made to facilitate more PA (Ruotsalainen et al., 2015).

Directions for future studies

Although the majority of studies report the positive effects of social media-based PA interventions to improve health, some limitations of the current literature should be noted. First, given the high number of quasi-experimental and non-experimental study designs used in the literature, the lack of a control group in these studies prevents researchers from discerning causal (e.g., direct) effects of such interventions on health outcomes. Furthermore, given the fact that social media represent a new field of inquiry with regard to PA intervention, the majority of studies had small sample sizes, resulting in an inability to detect differences between groups due to low study power. Additionally, some studies did not use objective PA measures, limiting the validity of PA outcomes (Valle et al., 2013).

According to Maher et al. (2014), social networking-based health interventions may be effective in changing behavior. However, this field of research is still in its infancy and it is unclear whether social networking-based interventions are equally useful for all health behaviors or whether they may be more effective for some more than others. Given that many of the health benefits of health behavior are achieved over a long-term period, further research is needed to examine whether the short-term behavior change achieved can be sustained over a longer period. More studies are also needed to determine whether sustained interaction with the user interface is required to sustain behavior change or whether behavior change may persist after interaction with intervention materials ceases (Maher et al., 2014). Additionally, existing online social networks such as Facebook and Twitter appear to offer promise for sustained engagement, however, whether retention and engagement with specific aspects of these platforms would match the intervention engagement or retention is unclear. Thus, innovative approaches reflecting the way people use online social networks (with existing friends and for entertainment) are warranted.

Finally, future work is also needed to determine how to maintain behavior change in the longer term, how to reach at-need populations, and how to disseminate such interventions on a mass scale. For logistical reasons, researchers used self-reported measures of PA which are typically considered to be susceptible to social desirability bias (Motl, McAuley, & DiStefano, 2005). Interestingly, Crutzen and Goritz (2011) recently examined this issue in over 5000 participants, and found social desirability bias was, in fact, unrelated to web-based self-reported PA, suggesting that web-based self-reports of PA are more trustworthy and useful. An advantage of self-reported PA, as opposed to objectively measured PA, is the considerably lower participant assessment burden, which arguably enhances the study's ecological validity (Maher et al., 2015).

References

Aschbrenner, K. A., Naslund, J. A., Shevenell, M., Mueser, K., & Bartels, S. (2015). Feasibility of behavioral weight loss treatment enhanced with peer support and mobile health technology for individuals with serious mental illness. *Psychiatric Quarterly, 87,* 401.

Barnes, S. B. (2006). A privacy paradox: Social networking in the United States. Retrieved from http://firstmonday.org/ojs/index.php/fm/article/viewArticle/1394/1312.

Bouc, A. (2013, September 28). NSA collecting social media information from citizens. *Liberty Voice*. Retrieved from http://guardianlv.com/2013/09/nsa-collecting-social-media-information-from-citizens/.

Brindal, E., Freyne, J., Saunders, I., Berkovsky, S., Smith, G., & Noakes, M. (2012). Features predicting weight loss in overweight or obese participants in a web-based intervention: Randomized trial. *Journal of Medical Internet Research, 14*(6), e173–e189.

Cavallo, D. N., Tate, D. F., Ries, A. V, Brown, J. D., Devellis, R. F., & Ammerman, A. S. (2012). A social media-based physical activity intervention: A randomized controlled trial. *American Journal of Preventive Medicine, 43*(5), 527–532.

Centola, D. (2013). Social media and the science of health behavior. *Circulation, 127*(21), 2135–2144.

Cialdini, R. B. (2007). Descriptive social norms as underappreciated sources of social control. *Psychometrika, 72*(2), 263–268.

Cornblatt, J. (2009, August 21). Lonely planet: Isolation increases in US. *Newsweek.* Retrieved from www.newsweek.com/lonely-planet-isolation-increases-us-78647.

Crutzen R. & Göritz, A. S. (2011). Does social desirability compromise self-reports of physical activity in Web-based research? *International Journal of Behavioral Nutrition and Physical Activity, 8*(31), 1–15.

Deforche, B. I., De Bourdeaudhuij, I. M., & Tanghe, A. P. (2006). Attitude toward physical activity in normal-weight, overweight and obese adolescents. *Journal of Adolescent Health, 38*(5), 560–565.

Desai, M., Miller, W., Staples, B., & Bravender, T. (2008). Risk factors associated with overweight and obesity in college students. *Journal of American College Health, 57*(1), 109–114.

Ellison, N. B., Steinfield, C., & Lampe, C. (2007). The benefits of Facebook "friends": Social capital and college students' use of online social network sites. *Journal of Computer-Mediated Communication, 12*(4), 1143–1168.

Fallows, D. (2005). How women and men use the Internet, In *Pew Internet & American Life Project*. Retrieved from www.pewinternet.org/pdfs/PIP_Women_ and_Men_ online.pdf.

Farr, C. (2015, April 9) Weighing privacy vs. rewards of letting insurers track your fitness. *NPR.* Retrieved from www.npr.org/sections/alltechconsidered/2015/04/09/398416513/weighing-privacy-vs-rewards-of-letting-insurers-track-your-fitness.

Foster, D., Linehan, C., Kirman, B., Lawson, S., & James, G. (2010). *Motivating physical activity at work: Using persuasive social media for competitive step counting*. Paper presented at 14th International Academic MindTrek Conference: Envisioning Future Media Environments (pp. 111–116).

Fox, J. (2014). Why the online trolls troll. *Psychology Today*. Retrieved from www.psychologytoday.com/blog/better-living-technology/201408/why-the-online-trolls-troll.

Greene, J., Sacks, R., Piniewski, B., Kil, D., & Hahn, J. S. (2013). The impact of an online social network with wireless monitoring devices on physical activity and weight loss. *Journal of Primary Care & Community Health*, *4*(3), 189–194.

Jepson, R. G., Harris, F. M., Platt, S., & Tannahill, C. (2010). The effectiveness of interventions to change six health behaviors: A review of reviews. *BMC Public Health, 10*(1), 538–544.

Jones, L. W. & Courneya, K. S. (2002). Exercise counseling and programming preferences of cancer survivors. *Cancer Practice, 10*, 208–15.

Kantomaa, M. T. Stamatakis, E. & Kankaanpaetal, A. (2013). Physical activity and obesity mediate the association between childhood motor function and adolescents' academic achievement, *Proceedings of the National Academy of Sciences of the United States of America, 110*(5), 1917–1922.

Karvinen, K. H., Courneya, K. S., & Campbell, K. L. (2006). Exercise preferences of endometrial cancer survivors: A population-based study. *Cancer Nursing, 29*, 259–265.

Kaushal, N. (2013) Facebook to roll-out countrywise metrics of monthly active users & daily active users! In *PageTraffic Buzz*. Retrieved from www.pagetrafficbuzz.com/facebook-rollout-country-wise-metrics-monthly-active-users-daily-active-users/17486.

Kessler, R. C., Berglund, P., Demler, O., Jin, R., Merikangas, K. R. & Walters, E. E. (2005). Lifetime prevalence and age-of-onset distributions of DSM-IV disorders in the national comorbidity survey replication. *Archives of General Psychiatry, 62*(6), 593–602.

Khaylis, A., Yiaslas, T., Bergstrom, J., & Gore-Felton, C. (2010). A review of efficacious technology-based weight-loss interventions: Five key components. *Telemedicine Journal and e-Health, 16*(9), 931–938.

Kumanyika, S. K., Wadden, T. A., Shults, J., Fassbender, J. E., Brown, S. D., & Bowman, M. A. (2009). Trial of family and friend support for weight loss in African American adults. *Archives of Internet Medicine, 169*(19), 1795–1804.

Leahey, T. M., Gokee LaRose, J., Fava, J. L., & Wing, R. R. (2011). Social influences are associated with BMI and weight loss intentions in young adults. *Obesity (Silver Spring), 19*, 1157–1162.

Lefebvre, R. C., & Bornkessel, A. S. (2013). Digital social networks and health. *Circulation, 127*(17), 1829–1836.

Lowry, B., Cao, J., & Everard, A. (2011). Privacy concerns versus desire for interpersonal awareness in driving the use of self-disclosure technologies: The case of instant messaging in two cultures. *Journal of Management Information Systems. 27*(4): 163–200.

Maher, C. A., Ferguson, M., Vandelanotte, C., Plotnikoff, R., Bourdeaudhuij, I. De, Thomas, S., … Olds, T. (2015). A web-based, social networking physical activity intervention for insufficiently active adults delivered via Facebook app: Randomized controlled trial. *Journal of Medical Internet Research, 17*(7), e174. http://doi.org/10.2196/jmir.4086.

Maher, C. A., Lewis, L. K., Ferrar, K., Marshall, S., Bourdeaudhuij, I. De, & Vandelanotte, C. (2014). Are health behavior change interventions that use online social networks effective? A systematic review. *Journal of Medical Internet Research, 16*(2), 1–13.

Merchant, G., Weibel, N., Patrick, K., Fowler, J. H., Norman, G. J., Gupta, A., … Merchant, G. (2014). Click "Like" to change your behavior: A mixed methods study of college students' exposure to and engagement with Facebook content designed for weight loss. *Journal of Medical Internet Research, 16*(6), e158.

Middelweerd, A., Laan, D. M. Van Der Stralen, M. M. Van, Mollee, J. S., Stuij, M., Velde, S. J., & Brug, J. (2015). What features do Dutch university students prefer in a smartphone application for promotion of physical activity? A qualitative approach. *International Journal of Behavioral Nutrition and Physical Activity, 12*(31), 1–11.

Motl, R. W., McAuley, E., & DiStefano, C. (2005). Is social desirability associated with self-reported physical activity? *Preventive Medicine, 40*(6), 735–739.

Nakhasi, A., Shen, A. X., Passarella, R. J., Appel, L. J., & Anderson, C. (2014). Online social networks that connect users to physical activity partners: A review and descriptive analysis. *Journal of Medical Internet Research, 16*(6), e153–e167. http://doi.org/10.2196/jmir.2674.

Napolitano, M. A., Hayes, S., Bennett, G. G., Ives, A. K., & Foster, G. D. (2013). Using Facebook and text messaging to deliver a weight loss program to college students. *Obesity, 21*(1), 25–31.

Nelson, T., Gortmaker, S., Subramanian, S., Cheung, L., & Wechsler, H. (2007). Disparities in overweight and obesity among U.S. college students. *American Journal of Health Behavior, 31*(4), 363–373.

Perrin, A., & Duggan, M. (2015). *American's internet access: 2000–2015*. Pew Research Center. Retrieved from www.pewinternet.org/2015/06/26/Americans-internet-access-2000-2015/.

Ruotsalainen, H., Kyngäs, H., Tammelin, T., Heikkinen, H., & Kääriäinen, M. (2015). Effectiveness of Facebook-delivered lifestyle counselling and physical activity self-monitoring on physical activity and body mass index in overweight and obese adolescents: A randomized controlled trial. *Nursing Research and Practice, 2015*, 159205. http://doi.org/10.1155/2015/159205.

Schneider, K. L., Murphy, D., Ferrara, C., Oleski, J., Panza, E., Savage, C., … Lemon, S. C. (2015). An online social network to increase walking in dog owners: A randomized trial. *Medicine and Science in Sports and Exercise, 27*, 631–639.

Sira, N., & Pawlak, R (2010). Prevalence of overweight and obesity, and dieting attitudes among Caucasian and African American college students in Eastern North Carolina: A cross-sectional survey. *Nutrition Research and Practice,4*(1), 36–42.

Statistic Brain. (2013). *Facebook Statistics*. Retrieved from www.statisticbrain.com/facebook-statistics/.

Thomas, J. R., Nelson, J. K., & Silverman, S. J. (2011). *Research methods in physical activity* (pp. 307–327). Champaign, IL: Human Kinetics.

Tudor-Locke, C., Craig, C. L., Aoyagi, Y., Bell, R. C., Croteau, K. A., De Bourdeaudhuij, I., … Blair, S. (2011). How many steps/day are enough? For older adults and special populations. *International Journal of Behavioral Nutrition and Physical Activity, 8*(80), 1–19.

Turkle, S. (2011). *Alone together: Why we expect more from technology and less from each other*. New York: Basic Books.

Turner-McGrievy, G., & Tate, D. (2011). Tweets, apps, and pods: Results of the 6-month mobile Pounds Off Digitally (Mobile POD) Randomized weight-loss intervention among adults. *Journal of Medical Internet Research, 13*(4), e120.

Vallance J. K. H., Courneya, K. S., Jones, L. W., & Reiman, T. (2006). Exercise preferences among a population-based sample of Non-Hodgkin's lymphoma survivors. *European Journal of Cancer Care, 15*, 34–43.

Valle, C. G., Tate, D. F., Mayer, D. K., Allicock, M., & Cai, J. (2013). A randomized trial of a Facebook-based physical activity intervention for young adult cancer survivors. *Journal of Cancer Survivors, 7*, 355–368.

Van Kessel, G., Kavanagh, M., & Maher, C. (2016). A qualitative study to examine feasibility and design of an online social networking intervention to increase physical activity in teenage girls. *PloS One, 11*(3), e0150817.

Verheijden, M. W., Bakx, J. C., van Weel, C., Koelen, M. A., & van Staveren, W. A. (2005). Role of social support in lifestyle-focused weight management interventions. *European Journal of Clinical Nutrition, Supplement 1*, S179-S186.

Zabinski, M. F. Saelens, B. E. Stein, R. I. Hayden-Wade, H. A., & Wilfley, D. E. (2003). Overweight children's barriers to and support for physical activity. *Obesity Research, 11*(2), 238–246.

Zhang, J., Brackbill, D., Yang, S., & Centola, D. (2015). Efficacy and causal mechanism of an online social media intervention to increase physical activity: Results of a randomized controlled trial. *Preventive Medicine Reports, 2*(2015), 651–657.

6 Mobile device apps in enhancing physical activity

Zachary Pope and Zan Gao

It is a beautiful sunny day—not one you intend to waste. You call your friends and ask them what they are up to—inquiring if they would like to go catch some Pokémon using the Pokémon Go application (a.k.a., app). Armed with nothing more than your smartphones, you and your friends spend the next several hours traversing around town to local landmarks which also serve as Pokéstops—hotspots where Pokémon are most likely to be located in the augmented reality world created by the Pokémon Go app. Not only do you and your friends enjoy an active day together catching Pokémon, you also manage to make friends with other fellow Pokémon players also playing the game. Notably, mobile device apps like Pokémon Go, which augment the real world in a virtual reality game-based manner, are starting to become available to the consumer. The objective of these games is to get individuals outside and moving, with the intended outcome being long-term health.

Indeed, with the advent of the iPhone 3 and the iPad, along with other subsequent smart mobile devices, computer software programmers have developed thousands of apps for use by individuals to monitor their physical activity (PA), fitness, health and wellness over the past several years. These apps include both simple (e.g., providing information on steps and estimated distance) and complex programs (e.g., providing information on vital signs and physiological indices such as heart rate and energy expenditure). To describe the ever-growing field of health-oriented apps, these mobile device health apps have been termed "mHealth apps."

Nowadays it is uncommon to meet an individual who does not possess a mobile device. The most recent Pew Research Center report indicated an astounding 64% of Americans now own a smartphone, with 88–97% of respondents using their smartphone for texting, email, voice/video calls, and internet access (Pew Research Group, 2015). As a result of their deep integration into our lives, smartphones have revolutionized nearly every aspect of our daily lives over the past decade. From education and business to social life and health, the impact of the smartphone can be felt (Sarwar & Soomro, 2013). Yet, smartphones are not the only mobile devices transforming our everyday lives. The rise in popularity of the smartphone has given rise to the tablet market as well. Tablets are typically larger and offer more computing power than smartphones—

computing power sometimes equivalent to that of smaller laptop computers—making these devices ideal for those who desire/need more computing capabilities than a smartphone provides, but who also prefer lightweight portability.

Furthering the impact of smartphones and tablets are these devices' ability to provide users access to millions of downloadable apps. In 2015, the number of apps available on Google Play (for Android-based phones/tablets) and the Apple App Store (for iOS-based phones/tablets) totaled 1.6 and 1.5 million, respectively (Statista, 2016). Of these apps, 165,000 were considered mHealth applications—a term used to describe health apps which, through mobile phones, personal digital assistants (PDAs), patient monitoring devices, and other wireless device platforms (e.g., tablets) aid in medical and public health practices (Intercontinental Marketing Services Institute of Health Informatics, 2015). Presently, the Intercontinental Marketing Services Institute of Health Informatics (2015) indicates 59,400 (36%) of the available "Wellness Management" mHealth apps are geared toward "fitness," with 28,050 (17%) and 19,800 (12%) mHealth apps created for "lifestyle and stress" and "diet and nutrition" purposes, respectfully. These apps are timely, given the fact that the most recent estimates state the prevalence of obesity among individuals 20 years or older in the United States to be approximately 35%, with the combined prevalence of overweight and obesity among American adults at a staggering 67% (Ogden, Carroll, Kit, & Flegal, 2014). As overweight/obesity and physical inactivity contribute to a higher likelihood of chronic diseases (Field et al., 2001), mHealth apps are poised to play a major role in the primary prevention of these conditions via PA promotion.

Given the large amount of available mHealth apps currently on the market, many of which were developed to help consumers improve or maintain their health and wellness, knowledge of these apps' use in the promotion of PA is vital to help ameliorate and possibly reverse the overweight and obesity trends seen in the United States and around the globe—potentially mitigating the poorer health outcomes resulting from overweight/obesity (Reilly & Kelly, 2011). As such, this chapter will provide readers with an overview of the use of mHealth apps for PA promotion in various populations after which the use of mHealth apps in different contexts and for Big Data analysis will be reviewed (Figure 6.1). The chapter will conclude by discussing the development and implementation of effective mHealth PA interventions and the practical implications the use of mHealth apps have for PA promotion and, more generally, health promotion. Given smartphones' higher frequency among the mHealth literature to date, the chapter's emphasis will lean more towards a discussion of smartphone apps in the promotion of PA and health. However, where high-quality research regarding the promotion of PA is available using other mobile devices (e.g., tablet-based apps), this research will be reviewed as well.

mHealth apps and health promotion in various populations

While the widespread presence of smartphones and tablets has been mentioned as contributing to these devices' ability to impact our daily lives, the fact these

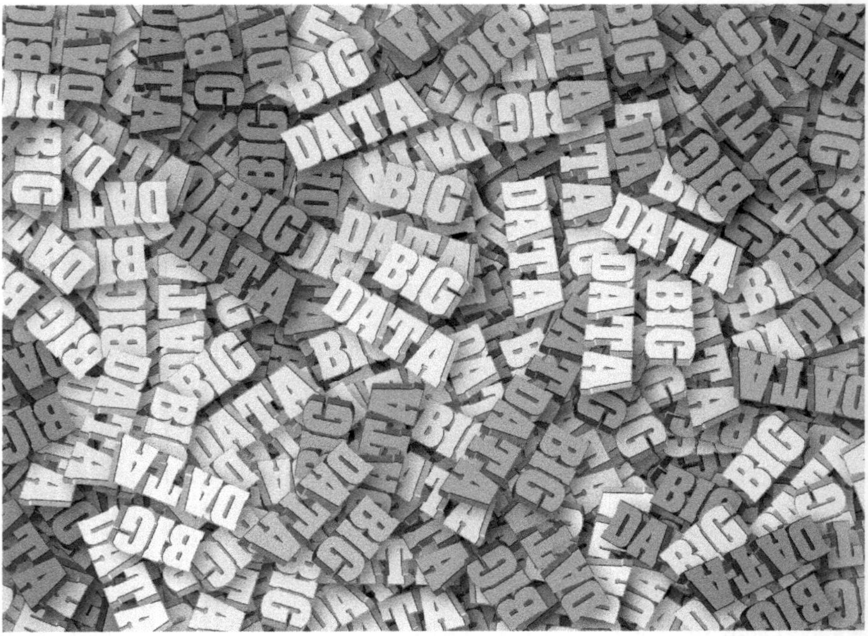

Figure 6.1 Big Data in GPS and GIS.
Source: pixabay.com.

devices and their apps are easy to use further contributes to these devices' popularity. Within the mHealth literature, the ease with which the apps on these devices can be used has made mHealth interventions for improving PA participation and related behaviors possible among many different populations. Not only have mHealth interventions been implemented among individuals of varying age, these interventions have been used among individuals of different race/ethnicity, socioeconomic status, and disease states (e.g., healthy, non-clinical populations versus clinical populations). In what follows, the reader will be treated to a review of these mHealth interventions by age group with differences in race/ethnicity, socioeconomic status, and disease states highlighted throughout. Notably, two types of mHealth apps exist: (1) mHealth apps designed by researchers specifically for research projects and not for consumer download; and (2) commercially designed mHealth apps designed for consumer download which may or may not have had researcher input in the development of said app. When necessary, differences in the literature between the two preceding app types will be made.

Youth (2–19 years old)

PA among U.S. youth is poor, with only 42% of children and 8% of adolescents (Troiano et al., 2008) meeting the PA guidelines of 60 minutes of moderate-to-vigorous PA per day (U.S. Department of Health and Human Services, 2008). As the current generation of youth have grown up with ever-expanding technological power, this generation is very interested in technology and a prime target for mHealth interventions.

Despite this generation's great interest in technology, mHealth studies of youth younger than 19 years of age are scarce in the literature and have typically been conducted among adolescents. Toscos, Faber, Connelly, & Upoma (2008) were among the first to investigate the use of app-based PA promotion among adolescents—in this case, teenage girls—finding that over the course of a brief 2-week trial, all participants increased their step counts while also decreasing perceived PA barriers—with social support provided via the app found to be most important. Notably, more recent, methodologically rigorous studies have been conducted.

In a recent 8-week randomized controlled trial by Direito, Jiang, Whittaker, & Maddison (2015), the effects of two commercially available apps ("Zombies, Run! 5K Training" and the "Get Running-Coach to 5K" apps) on European adolescents' cardiorespiratory fitness were evaluated, with findings indicating that, compared to the control group, the mile times of adolescents randomized into either of the app-based interventions were approximately 25–30 seconds faster at posttest, but that no significant differences between the app-based groups and control were seen for the secondary psychosocial outcomes or objectively determined PA—likely due to the study's lack of a theoretical framework (Brug, Oenema, & Ferreira, 2005). Fortunately, a pair of randomized controlled trials among underserved adolescent boys of low socioeconomic status (Lubans, Smith, Skinner, & Morgan, 2014; Smith et al., 2014) was more effective in implementing theory as part of a mHealth app-based PA intervention. Utilizing the Self-Determination Theory and Social Cognitive Theory, the app-based Active Teen Leaders Avoiding Screen-time (ATLAS) intervention observed significantly reduced screen-time and sugar-sweetened beverage consumption and significantly improved muscular fitness and resistance training abilities among intervention boys compared to controls. Notably, while improvements in PA and BMI favored boys in the intervention group, no significant intervention effects were seen for either variable—a finding attributed to poor accelerometry compliance by the boys and the use of BMI for body composition (Smith et al., 2014). Nonetheless, the findings of this trial highlight not only the potential efficaciousness of an app-based PA intervention among underserved adolescents of low socioeconomic status, but also the importance of theory in developing an effective intervention.

As seen, of the scant high-quality literature available regarding the use of apps in PA promotion among youth, results are mixed regarding the effectiveness of mHealth interventions. Reasons for these mixed findings might be attributable, in part, to: (1) the lack of a guiding theoretical framework within some of the literature; and (2) the moderate intervention compliance among the adolescents in the studies. That said, given the high rates of obesity seen among youth globally, mHealth interventions need to use a theoretical framework to guide the development of multi-component studies, which use several methods to intervene to promote PA and health (e.g., parent involvement, teacher reinforcement, etc.). Finally, these future studies need to ensure that intervention fidelity procedures are in place to ensure youths' compliance with data collection protocols.

Young adults and adults (20–39 years old)

Contrary to youth aged 2–19 years, numerous literature is present regarding the integration of mHealth apps among young adults and adults (aged 20–39 years) to promote PA. The greater amount of literature is likely attributable to the fact that this age range represents a period during which individuals are most likely to possess a mobile device of their own—dissimilar to youth who may or may not possess a mobile device like a smartphone. Given the fact many individuals 20–39 years old are mobile device owners and well aware of the benefits of PA, this cohort might represent one of the most receptive populations for mHealth interventions.

Early investigations into the use of mHealth apps in individuals aged 20–39 years focused on participants' ability to integrate apps into their daily routine to monitor health behaviors, with findings indicating smartphone apps to be easier for participants to use for behavior tracking than alternatives such as web applications (Gasser et al., 2006). Tsai et al. (2007) also conducted a preliminary trial among overweight or obese adults which allowed participants to monitor exercise and caloric balance in real time using a smartphone app, observing good compliance with the app and changes in PA and eating behavior as a result of app use. However, studies on mHealth interventions for the self-regulation of health behavior prior to 2010 were exploratory in nature—investigating mHealth app intervention feasibility (i.e., whether or not these apps would work in the "real world"), but providing little data on the effectiveness of mHealth apps for PA and health promotion. Subsequent mHealth studies among young adults and adults have investigated the effectiveness of mHealth app intervention and participants' ability to self-regulate PA and associated behaviors given the importance of self-regulation in behavior change (Bandura, 1991).

One of the first mHealth app effectiveness trials among the age group was conducted by Mattila, Lappalainen, Parkka, Salminen, and Korhonen (2010) using a researcher-developed smartphone app, The Wellness Diary, in which 27 overweight or obese male and females tracked their weight and related behaviors (e.g. steps, food intake). Findings indicated a strong correlation between diary use and weight loss over the course of the course of the 12-week study. Several studies suggested mHealth app interventions resulted in significantly higher light PA and more steps (Hebden, Cook, van der Ploeg, & Allman-Farinelli, 2012; Hebden et al., 2014; Kirwan, Duncan, Vandelanotte, & Mummery, 2012).

Finally, other researchers have also evaluated whether social support might also facilitate health behavior change. During a 6-week randomized controlled trial, Harries, Eslambolchilar, Stride, Rettie, and Walton (2013) found step counts among the individual app and social feedback app conditions to be 59% and 69% higher, respectively, than controls, with this research highlighting the potential effect that integrating social feedback into mHealth app interventions may have on desired outcomes.

As reviewed, numerous research has been completed among young adults and adults given this cohort's high likelihood of mobile device ownership (Pew Research Center, 2015). Nevertheless, most research among this age group has been conducted among healthy, but overweight or obese individuals in order to begin to reverse and/or prevent the disease and disability overweight and obesity can lead to in middle age and older adulthood (An & Shi, 2015).

Middle-aged adults (40–65 years old)

Middle-aged adults represent one of the most important populations of interest for the implementation of effective mHealth app interventions. Field et al. (2001) state that the risk of developing chronic diseases increases substantially among this population with increased overweight and obesity. Given that fact, calls have been made for innovative and multi-factorial interventions to attenuate and perhaps reverse the overweight/obesity epidemic and reduce long-term health consequences associated with the epidemic (Wyatt, Winters, & Dubbert, 2006). Therefore, many innovative and multi-factorial interventions in middle-aged adults have concentrated on reversing the trends of high physical inactivity in this cohort (Hallal et al., 2012). mHealth interventions have been one such approach, with mHealth app interventions proven to be versatile (e.g., capable of being employed in numerous contexts) and efficacious in middle-aged adults for PA promotion.

Early studies examined the effectiveness of mobile device apps in the self-regulation and promotion of PA in healthy, but sedentary, minority populations within the workplace. In a mHealth study of minority healthy, but sedentary, middle-aged women, Fukuoka, Vittinghoff, Jong, and Haskell (2010) observed a significant increase of approximately 800 steps per day in the sample—suggesting, again, mHealth apps' effectiveness across diverse populations. Additionally, as most middle-aged adults have steady careers, Carter, Burley, Nykjaer, and Cade (2013) implemented an mHealth app intervention, My Meal Mate, in the workplace to promote PA and weight loss, finding significantly higher intervention adherence and weight loss among the app-based group compare to groups using a website or paper diary—attributable to the ability to track PA-related energy expenditure with the app. Yet, this represents one of the few mHealth studies done within the workplace—indicating the need for more investigation of mHealth in promoting middle-aged adults' PA and health.

Clinical populations are also of concern among this age cohort. In a study of 12 type 2 diabetes patients, the effectiveness of a smartphone app over a 6-month period in the self-regulation of blood glucose, PA, and nutrition habits was examined (Arsand, Tatara, Ostengen, & Hartvigsen, 2010). After 6 months, researchers observed a mean decrease in blood glucose levels of 2 mg/dL and an increase in steps per day, with 58% of the participants also increasing their fruit and vegetable consumption. Other early studies among diabetic middle-aged patients have found similarly positive results for improvement of BMI, total cholesterol, steps per day, diastolic blood pressure, and weight loss (Stuckey et al., 2011; Thomas & Wing, 2013). Primary care patients have also been of interest to researchers implementing mHealth app interventions. Findings from mHealth app studies in primary care indicated significantly improved daily step counts among patients with acute psychiatric conditions (Glynn et al., 2014) and significant improvements in daily PA and quality of life in patients with type 2 diabetes and/or cardio-obstructive pulmonary disease (Verwey et al., 2014).

Clearly, mHealth interventions have been put forward as an innovative solution to help this cohort become more aware of, and positively change, their health behaviors. As such, mHealth interventions among middle-aged adults have spanned many different populations and contexts. That said, more research needs to be invested in workplace interventions, given the fact that many middle-aged adults have careers. Nonetheless, building healthy PA habits in middle-aged adulthood can help mitigate some of the health consequences present in old age.

Older adults (65+ years old)

As healthcare has improved, life expectancy has increased and contributed to a greater number of older adults still present in the population. In detail, if this cohort's growth continues at the current rate, by 2050 the Centers for Disease Control and Prevention (2013) projects the number of older adults to be 89 million. Notably, the high prevalence of overweight and obesity in older adults is a key factor in the high prevalence of chronic diseases (e.g., diabetes, cardiovascular disease, etc.), with 92% of older adults having at least one chronic disease and 77% having two or more (National Council on Aging, 2015). As a result, functional limitations are frequently observed among older adults which can include limitations in the ability to get dressed, walk from room to room, get up out of a chair, or drive, among other activities (An & Shi, 2015).

Little to no research on the use of mHealth interventions in the promotion of PA had been completed at the time of the writing of this book. The main reason for the lack of studies is likely a result of the fact that older adults represent a segment of the population least likely to own a mobile device capable of running an app. In fact, recent data found only 27% of individuals ≥65 years and older owned a smartphone, with fewer expected to own other mobile devices (e.g., tablets; Pew Research Center, 2015). That said, studies have indicated the elderly to have the lowest PA levels of any age cohort (Sun, Norman, & While, 2013). As such, more effort might be made among older adult populations to implement mHealth interventions.

What is clear from the preceding review of mHealth literature is the fact that mobile devices, most notably smartphones, are currently being used among a diverse array of populations and settings to promote PA and healthier behaviors. That said, few large-scale, methodologically rigorous studies have been conducted among the literature, with no study completed among older adults. The aforementioned limitations will need to be addressed if mHealth apps are to prove effective and be adopted by health professionals and PA specialists.

Application of mHealth apps in various contexts

As discussed in the introduction of this chapter, mobile devices such as smartphones and tablets are ever present in our lives. From the mobile devices we own personally, to mobile devices placed in hospitals, retailers, and numerous other settings (Figure 6.2), these devices are quickly becoming the manner by which we organize our lives and interact with the world. In the healthcare field, we have already seen the diversity present among the environments in which mHealth apps are being used to promote PA. While only a small amount of research is available on the use of mHealth in healthcare to increase PA participation, we have discussed mHealth interventions in weight loss and diabetes treatments as well as the treatment of cardio-obstructive pulmonary disease and psychiatric conditions. Indeed, the use of mHealth apps in the healthcare field—with special attention paid to barriers and future research directions of mHealth

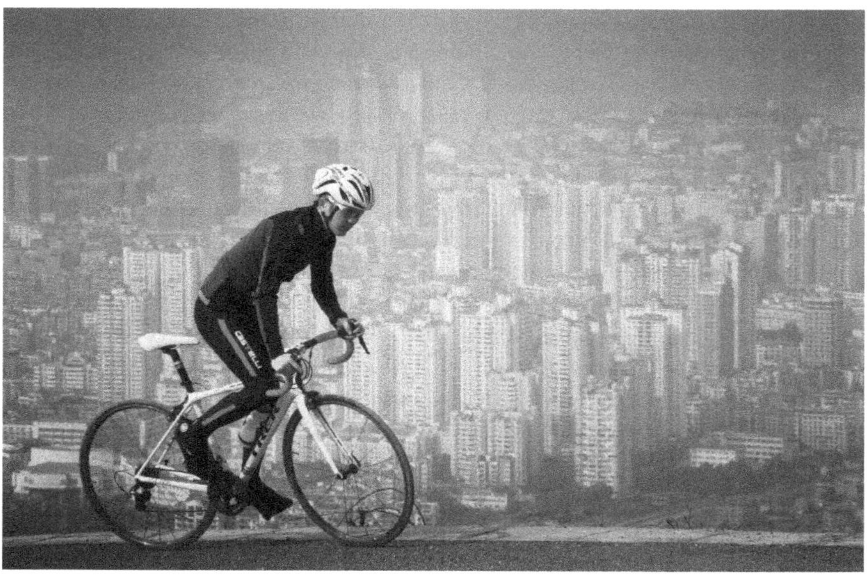

Figure 6.2 GPS tracking in biking.

Source: pixabay.com.

app use in this environment—will be the topic of the next section of the chapter. Moreover, we have highlighted the use of mHealth app interventions in free-living conditions such as college environments and in the workplace. Yet, there remains one environment where, despite the potentially major impact mHealth apps might have on PA promotion, little study of these apps has taken place: schools. As a result, a call has been made to promote healthy behaviors among children at younger ages to mitigate the poor health outcomes (i.e., chronic diseases) in adulthood arising due to childhood and adolescent overweight/obesity (Reilly & Kelly, 2011). Given the fact that the majority of children attend school, this environment is a prime location for PA and health promotion among youth.

As younger children are seldom mobile device owners, the paucity of literature to date on the use of mHealth apps for PA promotion has typically been among populations of adolescents. For example, a pair of randomized controlled trials by Lubans et al. (2014) and Smith et al. (2014), successfully increased PA and reduced screen-time using a theory-driven multi-component, app-based intervention, ATLAS. In fact, at the time of the writing, the aforementioned trial's success has resulted in a new ATLAS 2.0 protocol—a trial just getting underway (Lubans et al., 2016). Similar positive results have been seen in other mHealth studies implemented in a school-based environment (Watterson, 2012). Unfortunately, this represents the available high-quality literature on school-based mHealth interventions to promote PA—with younger children understudied. As youth represents a critical period during which to develop lifelong health habits, it is worthwhile outlining potential future research directions for school-based mHealth PA interventions among younger children.

As younger children are unlikely to own a mobile device, mHealth app-based PA interventions need to be implemented at the class level within schools, not the individual level. This puts the responsibility for such interventions on school administrators and teachers. Indeed, research reports that approximately 40% of teachers currently use mobile device apps within the classroom or physical education settings (Kervin, Verenikina, Jones, & Beath, 2013). In physical education settings, apps such as IronKids and Short Sequence: Kids Yoga Journey have been forwarded as potential facilitators of children's motor skill development and excitement with regard to greater PA participation (Martin, Ameluxen-Coleman, & Heinrichs, 2015). Specifically, mHealth apps like the two previously mentioned, were developed to aid physical educators in engaging all children within a class in greater PA participation. Yet, no known study has implemented these apps in a physical education setting. Further, given the fact many classroom teachers are currently using apps to aid teaching their children, why not use an mHealth app to teach these subjects while also getting children moving? For instance, a math teacher might use an app that helps children learn to add and subtract. Say a child was asked to add 4+7. Upon giving the answer, 11, the app might then ask all children within the class to do 11 jumping jacks, with answers to further questions tasking the children with completion of other exercises. This approach to teaching will not only promote greater PA, but might also have benefits to children's behavior. That said, a concerted effort needs to be made on the part of researchers to show school administrators, teachers, and physical educators the effectiveness of this type of intervention—not only with regard to engaging children in greater PA, but also showcase the benefits these types of activity breaks might have on classroom conduct.

As a final note, augmented reality apps also show promise for children's PA promotion in free-living settings. Indeed, the release of the popular Pokémon Go came on the heels of other augmented reality games such as Zombies, Run! Within days of its release, Pokémon Go was getting millions of children out the door, engaging in PA, and socializing with others—often walking and/or biking with friends to the nearest Pokéstop where the newest Pokémon were likely to be located. While no empirical research has yet been completed on Pokémon Go, researchers have posited that it might be worth examining exactly how much Pokémon Go is increasing PA levels (Baranowski, 2016). Studies of this type are particularly suited for children, given this populations' low PA levels and the need to prevent chronic disease progression in later life resulting from high levels of overweight/obesity during youth (Ogden et al., 2014).

Youth are our future. Schools are a prime venue to promote PA, health and wellness among youth. The fact that mHealth app-based interventions in children's PA and health promotion are understudied—especially given the current generation of youth's interest in technology—is a testament to the need for more push by researchers to change the current policies and regulations that continue to limit schools' focus on physical education/activity and, therefore, children's overall health and wellness. Moreover, researchers need to capitalize on gaming trends such as that currently seen for the augmented reality game Pokémon Go to increase children's free-living PA as well. Failure to use the amazing technology we have to ensure children possess the skills to become "lifelong movers" is a travesty and will only result in higher healthcare costs and lower quality of life for all involved.

Application of mHealth apps in the healthcare field

Imagine a world where treatments for diseases or adverse health conditions was more convenient and focused largely on proactively treating these diseases/conditions prior to their onset. Imagine a world where the focus of healthcare was not only to educate the patient about their disease/condition, but to empower the patient with the knowledge necessary to manage their long-term health and wellness. Imagine a world where access to a wellness team ready to help with any health malady an individual might be experiencing was right at your fingertips. While this description of healthcare might sound futuristic, the environment described is already here. Indeed, the present-day switch from reactive healthcare (i.e., treating diseases/conditions after onset) to proactive/preventive healthcare (i.e., treating diseases/conditions prior to onset) is placing mHealth apps as a major player in the current healthcare revolution.

In the previous section of this chapter, several examples were discussed regarding the effectiveness of mHealth app use in the healthcare field to promote

PA. Specifically, the paucity of literature to date has observed mHealth app-based PA interventions to be effective in the management/treatment of diabetes and/or weight loss (Arsand et al., 2010; Stuckey et al., 2011; Thomas & Wing, 2013), cardio-obstructive pulmonary disease (Verwey et al., 2014), and acute psychiatric conditions (Glynn et al., 2014)—with other mHealth app study protocols showing major promise in healthcare (Maddison et al., 2014). Yet, despite mHealth apps' initial demonstration of their ability to improve clinical outcomes through PA promotion, the preceding examples only represent literature discussing mHealth app-based interventions for PA promotion. As such, it is important to note other ways in which mHealth apps are being used in healthcare. This is best accomplished by discussing why mHealth apps are beneficial within an evolving healthcare field, with further discussion of barriers to mHealth app use in healthcare and how future research might overcome these barriers.

In discussing why mHealth apps will be advantageous in the future of healthcare, one cannot ignore the concept of "systems medicine" (Flores, Glusman, Brogaard, Price, & Hood, 2013; Hood, Balling, & Auffray, 2012). While a fuller explanation of "systems medicine" will be provided in the next section, a brief definition of systems medicine is provided here. Broadly, systems medicine takes a multi-faceted approach to patient treatment by considering multiple aspects of an individual's wellness—from the individual's genetics at the micro-level up to the environment in which the individual lives at the macro-level. Through the examination of each level of an individual's health, researchers can then surmise factors (and interactions between factors) that contribute to disease progression or attenuation. For example, health professionals could mandate various blood, physiological, and psychological testing for patients, after which all results could be uploaded to a secure online portal containing the patient's entire personal health history. Abnormal results from these tests could then be flagged for physician review, with the patient recommended for treatment and provided aid during this treatment by a dedicated wellness team. Notably, given present-day technology and the gradual shift to a systems-based approach to medicine, the majority of the patient's treatment could occur without the patient having to travel into the clinic. In order to employ this type of healthcare approach, however, a medium by which patients and healthcare professionals (e.g., physicians and wellness teams) to communicate is needed. Resulting from this need, mHealth apps have shown promise and continue to be at the forefront of the discussion on systems medicine.

Aside from being used to promote PA, West (2012) states that mHealth apps are being implemented in the systems medicine structure to increase patient medication adherence, ensure healthcare access to those living in rural areas, help patients effectively manage and improve chronic diseases, and enhance the efficiency of treatment delivery. This research also indicated that the use of mobile devices in the treatment and management of disease improved physicians' response times for medical test results, the error rate for patient discharge and medication prescription, and physician record keeping practices, among other aspects of healthcare. Furthermore, continued implementation and use of mHealth are projected to save the United States approximately $200 billion in healthcare costs by 2036, with projected mHealth revenue for the year 2017 projected to be $23 billion (West, 2012). However, with the plethora of benefits to the integration of mHealth apps in healthcare, what are some of the barriers to the widespread adoption of mobile devices in the field? Further, what future research/policy directions would prove most useful in reducing these barriers?

Confidentiality remains the largest barrier to the adoption of mHealth in healthcare. In a 2-year study of randomly selected U.S. adults, Richardson and Ancker (2015) found that while an increasing majority of individuals believed the use of a smartphone to share health data and communicate with physicians would improve healthcare quality, a significant concern regarding the privacy and security of the data was still present. As such, mHealth app developers need to ensure the data that would be shared with these mobile device apps was secure and at least as impenetrable as current electronic medical databases. Research proving the enhanced security of these apps would then have to be used to inform policies regarding the use of mHealth apps for medical record keeping and healthcare delivery. That said, it will be important for patients to decide upon the trade-off between keeping the health information collected via mHealth apps exceedingly private or giving up some right to this health information—providing some potentially identifiable health data to researchers and physicians. This large amount of data can then be analyzed via Big Data analysis techniques (see next section) to improve individual and population-level health policies and practice (Kvedar, 2015). Moreover, given the functional limitations often presenting among older adults (An & Shi, 2015)—at times, limiting this age cohort's ability to transport themselves to a health clinic—enhancing the security and confidentiality of mHealth might aid in increasing the popularity of mHealth app use among older adults as a result of not needing to physically go to a treatment facility. In turn, health professionals implementing interventions among older adults might be able to increase treatment adherence leading to potentially more effective treatment outcomes.

Another barrier to mHealth adoption in healthcare is access to mobile devices in developing countries. Indeed, in countries like Africa which are ravaged by deadly diseases, mHealth has seen the lowest adoption rates (West, 2012). As has been discussed, mHealth has been used to provide quality healthcare access to individuals living in rural areas. Therefore, more funding needs to be allocated to research examining the effectiveness of mHealth app use on individuals' health outcomes in countries where the rates of deadly disease are high and mHealth adoption is low. A final major barrier to mHealth adoption in healthcare applies not to the patient, but to the physicians. According to West (2012), even among the already established mHealth systems, physicians are rarely paid for the time they spend training to use mHealth apps or the time these physicians spend proving feedback to patients via the apps. Simply put, mHealth adoption will not increase if the doctors are not properly compensated for the time they are investing handling patient health inquiries via mHealth apps. Like patient confidentiality, policies and regulations pertaining to the compensation of physicians for the care they provide using mHealth apps within a systems medicine healthcare structure need to be more thoroughly considered.

While it is clear that mHealth apps have found a place within the healthcare field—most notably to help increase individuals' self-regulation of health behaviors—more can be done to fully adopt the extraordinary power of mHealth apps within this field. As such, it is imperative that a greater number of large-scale and methodologically rigorous studies be completed, showing how to securely provide access to quality healthcare via mHealth apps to individuals in developed and developing countries. Doing so will provide evidence that can later be used to show key stakeholders within the healthcare community the usefulness of mobile devices in the treatment and prevention of disease—improving mHealth policies and increasing adoption of this type of healthcare delivery method.

Use of mHealth apps in Big Data analysis

With the proliferation of mobile devices, it is not surprising to note that mobile device apps are gaining more attention in Big Data analysis. Big Data analysis refers to "large volumes of high velocity, complex, and variable data that require advanced techniques and technologies to enable the capture, storage, distribution, management, and analysis of the information" (TechAmerica Foundation's Federal Big Data Commission, 2012, p. 10). In simpler terms, our society is incredibly technologically advanced and capable of producing and storing large amounts of data in text, audio, and visual formats—seen on sites such as Facebook and YouTube. However, in some ways, the production and storage of data have outpaced society's ability to analyze this data and form meaningful conclusions regarding the relationships between ourselves and the environment. This ability to discern the relationships between ourselves and the environment around us has major implications for our health. Specifically, evaluation of this individual-environment relationship could be used in the healthcare system to inform health behavior decisions and facilitate new innovations which might improve our ability to prevent and/or manage disease and improve quality of life.

The use of mHealth in Big Data analysis is scarce, with little to no research available. That said, mHealth has great potential to facilitate Big Data analysis within the framework of systems health (Flores et al., 2013; Hood et al., 2012)—the concept alluded to in the previous section of this chapter. As stated, systems health is an integrated approach to healthcare which considers all levels of an individual's wellness—from the individual's genetic make-up to cells to organ structure/function to the environment within which this individual lives. Considering each bodily process, and how the environment interacts with each process, allows for an examination of the factors which might contribute most to disease (or the absence of disease). Once information regarding these individual-environment interactions is available, interventions can then be developed to attenuate disease progression or even prevent disease prior to onset.

As outlined by Hood et al. (2012), the end goal of systems health would be to create a "P4 Medicine" structure which posits that healthcare would be: (1) predictive (i.e., information will be available on an individual's health indices—allowing for prediction of an individual's risk for certain diseases or conditions); (2) preventive (i.e., provision of information regarding an individual's risk for certain diseases or conditions would facilitate lifestyle modifications to prevent certain maladies before onset); (3) personalized (i.e., lifestyle modifications in the prevention/treatment of diseases and conditions would be personalized to the individual—potentially leading to improved patient adherence and better treatment outcomes); and (4) participatory (i.e., individuals will be able to take an active and well-educated approach to the prevention or management of diseases/conditions). Nonetheless, the preceding health structure will require a medium by which patients/clients can provide information regarding their health habits (e.g., sleep, exercise, nutrition, etc.) and/or disease progression. Similarly, health professionals would need a medium by which to disseminate information regarding lifestyle modifications to promote proper health practices and/or directives for disease management in a cost-effective and accurate manner. This is where mHealth shows promise.

Through mHealth apps, a patient's communication with their physician can be facilitated within this P4 Medicine structure. For example, a male patient may visit his physician for a battery of health tests, such as blood assays as well as cardiorespiratory, strength, body composition, and neurological tests. Results from these tests could then be uploaded to a secure server and made available to both physician and patient via a P4 mobile device app, with results indicating disease or an adverse health condition flagged for physician's review. Perhaps in this example, the patient's tests revealed that he is 30 pounds overweight and has mild type II diabetes. Once this patient's results are reviewed by a physician, an appointment could be set up explaining treatment options. For cases mirroring our current patient's diagnosis, these appointments might take place via the P4 mobile device app in a manner similar to Microsoft's Skype or Apple's Facetime—reducing burden on both the physician and patient. Regardless of the meeting's format, the physician would then refer our patient to a wellness team who specialize in weight loss. This wellness team would hold an initial in-person meeting to explain what lifestyle modifications would be necessary to ensure weight loss and prevention of further diabetes symptoms. For instance, the wellness team might inform our patient that he must start taking Metformin, a diabetes medication, in addition to starting a structured exercise program.

In order to ensure our patient's adherence to his new program, the wellness team would send our patient daily reminders to take his Metformin as well as provide him with a 5-day exercise program each week. However, in contrast to current medical practice, this treatment would not take place at a clinic, nor would the treatment be explained only once to our patient, after which no further contact would be made. Instead, the wellness team would increase our patient's probability of adhering to treatment via the P4 mobile device app. Explicitly, daily reminders to take Metformin and a detailed outline of the exercise program would be placed on the P4 mobile device app. Further, the medication reminders and exercise program would be personalized to our patient's preferred daily time to take medication and to our patient's preferred exercise activities, respectively. As part of the P4 medicine structure, this personalization of our patient's program would improve our patient's long-term motivation to engage in the lifestyle changes needed to improve health. Finally, congruent with the P4 Medicine structure, the P4 mobile device app would be optimized to ensure communication between the wellness team and our patient. The app would not only ensure that our patient has the ability to interact via a secure messaging system with the wellness team, but the app would also allow the patient to chart his exercise, diet, and sleep, with reminders to do so sent to the patient's mobile device. In this manner, our patient can ask the team questions and/or receive timely feedback regarding his progression through the program—feedback which may make the difference between successful and unsuccessful treatment outcomes. Data from thousands of patients treated in the same manner as our patient could then be analyzed via Big Data analysis to further streamline treatment procedures and improve treatment outcomes.

Although a brief example of the role mHealth could play in Big Data analysis and how Big Data analysis might be used in the context of the healthcare field, the technology infrastructure and buy-in from key stakeholders (i.e., healthcare systems, private hospitals/clinics, etc.) remain a barrier. Indeed, new methods of analysis need to be made available to examine the relationships between an individual's health and their environment as, currently, the majority of the data available in the world of Big Data is unstructured in the form of text, videos, and pictures—not always in the numerical, spreadsheet-based format which has traditionally allowed for the analysis of large volumes of data (Gandomi & Haider, 2015). While it appears the day when systems medicine and the P4 Medicine structure are commonplace is drawing nearer, we are not quite there yet. Until then, however, mHealth has continued potential to help individuals self-regulate health behaviors and modify these behaviors in a manner more congruent with good health and be conducive to the Big Data analysis infrastructure.

Application of mHealth apps

Previous sections of this chapter have made clear the versatility of mHealth apps in the promotion of PA and health. From community, home, school and clinical settings and among diverse populations, mHealth apps offer a convenient way in which individuals can self-regulate their PA behavior, which—through incremental changes in these behaviors—aids in improving health. However, despite the promise of mHealth apps in the promotion of PA, successful PA interventions depend on more than the app itself. Indeed, it is often other factors, such as the theoretical backing of the intervention, the intervention's design and quality, and the app-related functionality that determine whether or not the mHealth intervention is effective.

To begin, PA interventions must have a theoretical backing. Theory allows researchers and practitioners to develop and implement an intervention which has a greater likelihood of being effective. Notably, however, the mere presence of a theory does not increase the probability of an intervention's success. As Brug, Oenema, and Ferreira (2005) state, theory has an *indirect* effect on the behavior change process. Instead, using theory to develop and implement a PA intervention allows interventionists to leverage determinants known to be closely associated with behavior change. For example, motivation has long been known to highly correlate with PA behavior. As such, a researcher might use Social Cognitive Theory to guide the construction of an mHealth app-based intervention to more effectively promote increased competence and subsequent PA self-efficacy, after which PA stands a greater chance of increasing. It is in this manner that the theory's indirect effect on an intervention's success can be seen. As such, theory allows researchers and practitioners to more effectively discern the mechanisms which lead to an intervention's success (or lack thereof), to better articulate these findings to interested individuals/parties, and to develop more effective interventions thereafter.

Once theory is in place, interventionists must then take care of ensuring intervention fidelity—a factor which is not mutually exclusive from the use of theory in an intervention. Borrelli (2011) states intervention fidelity to be "the ongoing assessment, monitoring, and enhancement of the reliability and internal validity" of an intervention (p. S52), after which she outlined five distinct domains related to this study design principle. These domains are (1) intervention design; (2) provider training; (3) intervention delivery; (4) intervention receipt; and (5) intervention enactment. Looking at each of these domains in relation to our Social Cognitive Theory example will allow for a better understanding of the importance of intervention fidelity in the implementation of an effective intervention.

To begin, intervention design allows an intervention to be constructed which more readily conforms to the intervention's chosen theory. Further, time spent ensuring the use of an appropriate intervention design will also help interventionists better investigate links between study variables—confident that the changes seen as a result of the intervention were not due to variables outside the study. As such, our interventionists would start by deciding upon what type of intervention design would be best for discerning whether a mobile device app is effective in increasing an individual's mastery (i.e., competency) to perform strength exercises, with the objective being to facilitate increased self-efficacy and PA. In this accord, our interventionists might decide to implement a randomized controlled trial where the experimental group uses a mHealth app containing video demonstrations of strength exercises in addition to an 8-week strength training program these individuals can follow. The comparison group would receive identical information, but via a paper-and-pencil packet. This would allow researchers to determine the effectiveness of an app-delivered program versus that of a traditional paper-and-pencil program in relation to the variables comprising Social Cognitive Theory that these researchers are using to frame their study.

The next two domains of intervention fidelity, provider training and intervention delivery, often go hand in hand. It is imperative that, following the selection of the intervention design, interventionists develop a standardized and highly detailed plan by which to train the providers responsible for intervention delivery—training that considers everything from the qualifications/characteristics of the individuals hired to deliver the intervention to how and where these individuals will be trained. Moreover, a detailed provider training plan will result in more consistent intervention delivery (i.e., the third intervention fidelity domain) as less variation/error will be present between providers, and more reliable adherence to the intervention's theoretical framework will be observed—increasing the likelihood of a successful intervention. Having decided upon the intervention's design, our interventionists would then go about the process of hiring and training providers to deliver the intervention, with the focus being to standardize the intervention's delivery as much as possible. As such, our interventionists would first develop a detailed plan to hire and train providers. In detail, our interventionists might desire to hire individuals with experience implementing theory-backed interventions and/or those with experience using mHealth apps to promote PA behavior change. Our interventionists would then train the individuals hired to deliver the intervention. This training would include instruction on how the providers will demonstrate use of the mobile device app (the experimental group) or the paper-and-pencil packet (the comparison group), how providers will engage in role playing scenarios to ensure individuals' understanding of the intervention, and the length of each training session to ensure equal contact time with both groups, among other plans. This plan would ensure that no matter which provider is informing an experimental or comparison group member of the different components of the intervention, the intervention's delivery is consistent.

The final two domains related to intervention fidelity shift the focus from the intervention's development and implementation as it relates to the intervention's personnel to the individuals participating in the intervention. Intervention receipt assesses whether or not the individual participating in the intervention understands the intervention's different components and can demonstrate the skills and knowledge related to the recommendations learned during the treatment. Providers can ensure intervention receipt through pre-post tests and even role-playing scenarios during the intervention sessions, wherein the provider is continually giving the individual feedback on each intervention participant's acquisition of the skills and knowledge related to the intervention. To ensure intervention receipt, our interventionists might seek to engage individuals in a role-playing scenario prior to the intervention wherein the provider can solicit feedback on the individual's demonstration of strength exercise form and knowledge of what major muscles each exercise targets. Notably, this role-playing scenario would be conducted for both the experimental group (i.e., using the mobile device app) and the comparison group (i.e., using the paper-and-pencil packet)—further ensuring that any differences in competency, self-efficacy, and PA between groups at the intervention's end are attributable to differences in content delivery between groups and not factors outside of the study.

Finally, intervention enactment evaluates an individual's use of the skills and knowledge they gained from intervention participation in the real world. Indeed, while pre-post tests or role playing scenarios may indicate an individual to have the skills and knowledge necessary to participate in an intervention, s/he still might not adhere to the intervention when asked to do so in the real-world. Our interventionists could measure intervention enactment simply by monitoring the average number of times the experimental group uses the mobile device app while completing the same observation on the comparison group's use of their paper-and-pencil packet. Aside from theory and study design, more practical matters also have to be kept in mind when developing and implementing a mobile app-based intervention. Chief among these considerations is the app's functionality.

To ensure intervention participants will use the mobile device app being used, a user-centered design process is suggested—an approach researchers have used to increase the usability of mobile device apps (Kirwan, Duncan, Vandelanotte, & Mummery, 2013; van der Weegen et al., 2013). Kirwan et al. (2013) make clear the importance of paying attention to many different aspects of the app design if researchers and clinicians want to develop an app that will be used regularly by participants and/or patients. These aspects include, but are not limited to: interface design, feedback, navigation, and terminology. While a number of subfunctions come under the four aforementioned aspects of app design, these researchers denote the importance of user input regarding these aspects of app design. These researchers go on to provide a general blueprint of effective user-centered app design to improve later usability of the app during an intervention and in real-world scenarios. Specifically, Kirwan et al. (2012) state that the following steps are needed during the app design process: (1) investigate the most popular commercially available health-related apps, noting features (e.g., color, layout, navigation structure, app feedback, etc.) that most appeal to individuals using the said apps; (2) develop and test an app "in house" among the design team to ensure the interface is ready to be trialed by participants; (3) field test the app with participants and ask for their thoughts—via self-reported questionnaires, interviews, etc.—regarding the app's functionality and issues or "bugs" which need modification; and (4) refine the app based on participant feedback, after which the apps can be used as part of an intervention and, possibly, put on the market. Development of an app in this manner greatly increases the probability that an individual participating in an intervention or consumers downloading the app will use the app regularly—potentially increasing the effectiveness of the app. Notably, increasing the regularity with which participants will use an app might also be promoted by providing tailored feedback to participants via the mHealth app. Unfortunately, tailoring of mHealth intervention protocol to individual participants has seldom occurred when using mHealth apps to promote PA/fitness—this is in contrast to recent literature tailoring feedback regarding healthy eating behavior to participants reporting their dietary intake via mHealth apps (Allen, Stephens, Dennison Himmelfarb, Stewart, & Hauck, 2013; Martin et al., 2015). Finally, attention to detail during app design will also allow for closer adherence to the theoretical underpinnings of the intervention which bodes well for the intervention's effectiveness.

That said, not all researchers or clinicians will want—or have the funds necessary—to develop their own app and, instead, might use a free, commercially available app. If this is the case, these researchers/clinicians would be wise to ensure that the mobile device app they want to use is compatible with the theoretical framework of the intervention. If the app is not able to promote the constructs within the intervention's guiding theory, the intervention stands a much lower likelihood of success. Nonetheless, the functionality of the mobile device app implemented is closely related to future intervention success and warrants as great a degree of attention as the selection of an intervention's guiding theory and the development of an intervention's fidelity measures.

Overall, effective mHealth app interventions, with the aim of promoting PA, are predicated upon three interrelated factors. First, effective mobile device app interventions need a strong theoretical framework on which the intervention can be developed. Theory allows for more effective intervention development and more accurate interpretations of the intervention's results. Second, to ensure that the intervention properly uses the selected theory, detailed intervention fidelity measures must be put in place by the research team. Proper intervention fidelity measures ensure smaller variation and error between providers with regard to intervention implementation—increasing the ability of researchers and clinicians to attribute intervention results to the different methodology used to implement the intervention, with little influence of outside factors. Finally, research teams developing their own app must consider the app's functionality. In doing so, interventionists can ensure the app is used with more regularity while still adhering to the theory backing the intervention. If interventionists decide not to develop their own app, opting instead to use a free, commercially available app, close attention needs to be paid to how well the app promotes the constructs related to the intervention's theory. Being mindful of the preceding information during the development and application of a mHealth app-based PA intervention should increase the likelihood of positive intervention outcomes.

Practical implications

The public health landscape is changing rapidly with increasingly powerful technology available at our fingertips. With the advent of smartphones and, later, tablets, mHealth apps represent an efficacious manner by which to promote increased PA participation and improved health at the population level, given mobile devices' widespread use among nearly all ages, races/ethnicities, and socioeconomic status. Further, not only do mHealth apps represent an effective manner by which to promote PA, implementation of these apps into fields such as healthcare promises to increase the efficiency with which treatments/interventions are delivered. However, barriers remain with regard to the widespread integration of mHealth apps into PA interventions in any setting. Among the biggest barriers reviewed were the privacy of individuals' health information, the disparity in access to live-saving mHealth apps present in lower-income countries fighting to manage and treat deadly diseases, and policy/regulatory practices that may not always compensate healthcare professionals for time spent providing care to patients/clients via an mHealth app-based medium. Finally, as we gaze into the future, the validity and reliability of mHealth apps, as well as apps associated with newer, more fashionable health wearable devices (e.g., necklaces, belts, and upscale smartwatches; Charara, 2016) capable of tracking PA and physiological variables, must be evaluated further.

Researchers and clinicians must work together to overcome these barriers through the development of improved mHealth app privacy mechanisms, the allocation of funding to research aimed at developing a methodology by which to implement mHealth app-based interventions in lower-income countries, and through the refining of current policies and regulations regarding the compensation of healthcare professionals for their provision of care by way of mHealth apps. Failure to improve upon the promising initial work on the use of mHealth apps in the promotion of PA and other health behaviors will not only limit the adoption of this novel form of healthcare, but will impede the provision of healthcare access to those individuals who might need it the most (e.g., those living in rural areas and lower-income countries).

References

Allen, J., Stephens, J., Dennison Himmelfarb, C., Stewart, K., & Hauck, S. (2013). Randomized controlled pilot study testing use of smartphone technology for obesity treatment. *Journal of Obesity*, 151597.

An, R., & Shi, Y. (2015). Body weight status and onset of functional limitations in U.S. middle-aged and older adults. *Disability and Health Journal, 8*, 336–344.

Arsand, E., Tatara, N., Ostengen, G., & Hartvigsen, G. (2010). Mobile phone-based self-management tools for type 2 diabetes: The few touch application. *Journal of Diabetes Science and Technology, 4*(2), 328–336.

Bandura, A. (1991). Social cognitive theory of self-regulation. *Organizational Behavior and Human Decision Processes, 50*(2), 248–287.

Baranowski, T. (2016). Pokémon Go, go, go, gone? *Games for Health Journal, 5*(5), 1–2.

Borrelli, B. (2011). The assessment, monitoring, and enhancement of treatment fidelity in public health clinical trials. *Jounral of Public Health Dentistry, 71*, S52–S63.

Brug, J., Oenema, A., & Ferreira, I. (2005). Theory, evidence, and intervention mapping to improve behavior, nutrition, and physical activity interventions *International Journal of Behavioral Nutrition and Physical Activity, 2*(2).

Carter, M., Burley, V., Nykjaer, C., & Cade, J. (2013). Adherence to a smartphone application for weight loss compared to website and paper diary: Pilot randomized controlled trial. *Journal of Medical Internet Research, 15*(4), e32.

Centers for Disease Control and Prevention. (2013). *The state of aging and health in America 2013.* Retrieved from www.cdc.gov/features/agingandhealth/state_of_aging_and_health_in_america_2013.pdf.

Charara, S. (2016). Fashion tech: 20 wearables that are more chic than geek. Retrieved from www.wareable.com/fashion/wearable-tech-fashion-style.

Direito, A., Jiang, Y., Whittaker, R., & Maddison, R. (2015). Apps for improving fitness and increasing physical activity among young people: The AIMFIT pragmatic randomized controlled trial. *Journal of Medical Internet Research, 17*(8), e210. doi:10.2196/jmir.4568.

Field, A., Coakley, E., Must, A., Spadano, J., Laird, N., Dietz, W., … Colditz, G. (2001). Impact of overweight on the risk of developing common chronic diseases during a 10-year period. *Archives of Internal Medicine, 161*, 1581–1586.

Flores, M., Glusman, G., Brogaard, K., Price, N., & Hood, L. (2013). P4 medicine: How systems medicine will transform the healthcare sector and society. *Personalized Medicine, 10*(6), 565–576.

Fukuoka, Y., Vittinghoff, E., Jong, S., & Haskell, W. (2010). Innovation to motivation-pilot study of a mobile phone intervention to increase physical activity among sedentary women. *Preventive Medicine, 51*, 287–289.

Gandomi, A., & Haider, M. (2015). Beyond the hype: Big Data concepts, methods, and analytics. *International Journal of Information Management, 35*, 137–144.

Gasser, R., Brodbeck, D., Degen, M., Luthiger, J., Wyss, R., & Reichlin, S. (2006). Persuasiveness of a mobile lifestyle coaching application using social facilitation. *Persuasive Technology, 3962*, 27–38.

Glynn, L., Hayes, P., Casey, M., Glynn, F., Alvarez-Iglesias, A., Newell, J., … Murphy, A. (2014). Effectiveness of a smartphone application to promote physical activity in primary care: The SMART MOVE randomised controlled trial. *British Journal of General Practice*, e384–e391.

Hallal, P., Andersen, L., Bull, F., Guthold, R., Haskell, W., & Ekelund, U. (2012). Global physical activity levels: Surveillance progress, pitfalls, and prospects. *The Lancet, 380*(9838), 247–257.

Harries, T., Eslambolchilar, P., Stride, C., Rettie, R., & Walton, S. (2013). Walking in the wild: Using an always-on smartphone application to increase physical activity. *Human-Computer Interaction, 8120*, 19–36.

Hebden, L., Cook, A., van der Ploeg, H., & Allman-Farinelli, M. (2012). Development of smartphone applications for nutrition and physical activity behavior change. *Journal of Medical Internet Research: Research Protocols, 1*(2), e9.

Hebden, L., Cook, A., van der Ploeg, H., King, L., Bauman, A., & Allman-Farinelli, M. (2014). A mobile health intervention for weight management among young adults: A pilot randomised controlled trial. *Journal of Human Nutrition and Dietetics, 27*, 322–332.

Hood, L., Balling, R., & Auffray, C. (2012). Revolutioning medicine in the 21st century through systems approaches. *Biotechnology Journal, 7*, 992–1001.

Intercontinental Marketing Services Institute for Health Informatics. (2015). *Patient adoption of mHealth*. Retrieved from www.imshealth.com/en/thought-leadership/ims-institute/reports/patient-adoption-of-mhealth.

Kervin, L., Verenikina, I., Jones, P., & Beath, O. (2013). Investigating synergies between literacy, technology and classroom practice. *Australian Journal of Language and Literacy, 36*(3), 135–147.

Kirwan, M., Duncan, M., Vandelanotte, C., & Mummery, W. (2012). Using smartphone technology to monitor physical activity in the 10,000 steps program: A matched case-control trial. *Journal of Medical Internet Research, 14*(2), e55.

Kirwan, M., Duncan, M., Vandelanotte, C., & Mummery, W. (2013). Design, development, and formative evaluation of a smartphone application for recording and monitoring physical activity levels: The 10,000 steps "iStepLog". *Health Education & Behavior, 40*(2), 140–151.

Kvedar, J. (2015). The privacy trade-offs. In *The internet of healthy things*. Boston, MA: Partners HealthCare Connected Health.

Lubans, D., Smith, J., Peralta, L., Plotnikoff, R., Okely, A., Salmon, J., … Morgan, P. (2016). A school-based intervention incorporating smartphone technology to improve health-related fitness among adolescents: Rationale and study protocol for the NEAT and ATLAS 2.0 cluster randomised controlled trial and dissemination study. *BMJ Open, 6*, 6.

Lubans, D., Smith, J., Skinner, G., & Morgan, P. (2014). Development and implementation of a smartphone application to promote physical activity and reduce screen-time in adolescent boys. *Frontiers in Public Health, 2*.

Maddison, R., Rawstorn, J., Rolleston, A., Whittaker, R., Stewart, R., Benatar, J., … Gant, N. (2014). The remote exercise monitoring trial for exercise-based cardiac rehabilitation (REMOTE-CR): A randomised controlled trial protocol. *BMC Public Health, 14*(1236).

Martin, C., Miller, A., Thomas, D., Champagn, C., Han, H., & Church, T. (2015). Efficacy of SmartLoss, a smartphone-based weight loss intervention: Results from a randomized controlled trial. *Obesity, 23*, 935–942.

Martin, N., Ameluxen-Coleman, E., & Heinrichs, D. (2015). Innovative ways to use modern technology to enhance, rather than hinder, physical activity among youth. *Journal of Physical Education, Recreation & Dance, 86*(4), 46–53.

Mattila, E., Lappalainen, R., Parkka, J., Salminen, J., & Korhonen, I. (2010). Use of a mobile phone diary for observing weight management and related behaviours. *Jounral of Telemedicine and Telecare, 16*, 260–264.

National Council on Aging. (2015). *Healthy aging facts*. Retrieved from www.ncoa.org/news/resources-for-reporters/get-the-facts/healthy-aging-facts/.

Ogden, C., Carroll, M., Kit, B., & Flegal, K. (2014). Prevalence of childhood and adult obesity in the United States, 2011–2012. *Journal of the American Medical Association, 311*(8), 806–814.

Patten, M. (2014). The role of theory in research. In M. Patten (Ed.), *Understanding research methods: An overview of the essentials* (9th ed., pp. 27–29). Glendale, CA: Pyrczak Publishing.

Pew Research Center. (2015). *The smartphone difference*. Retrieved from www.pewinternet.org/2015/04/01/us-smartphone-use-in-2015/.

Reilly, J., & Kelly, J. (2011). Long-term impact of overweight and obesity in childhood and adolescence on morbidity and premature mortality in adulthood: Systematic review. *International Journal of Obesity, 35*, 891–898.

Richardson, J., & Ancker, J. (2015). *Public health perspectives of mobile phones' effects on healthcare quality and medical data security and privacy: A 2-year nationwide survey*. Paper presented at the AMIA Annual Conference Proceedings, 2015.

Sarwar, M., & Soomro, T. (2013). Impact of smartphones on society. *European Journal of Scientific Research, 98*(2), 216–226.

Smith, J., Morgan, P., Plotnikoff, R., Dally, K., Salmon, J., Okely, A., … Lubans, D. (2014). Smart-phone obesity prevention trial for adolescent boys in low-income communities: The ATLAS RCT. *Pediatrics, 134*(3), e723-e731.

Statista. (2016). *Number of apps available in leading apps stores as of July 2015*. Retrieved from www.statista.com/statistics/276623/number-of-apps-available-in-leading-app-stores/.

Stuckey, M., Russell-Minda, E., Read, E., Munoz, C., Shoemaker, K., Kleinstiver, P., & Petrella, R. (2011). Diabetes and technology for increased activity (DaTA) study: Results of a remote monitoring intervention for prevention of metabolic syndrome. *Journal of Diabetes Science and Technology, 5*(4), 928–935.

Sun, F., Norman, I., & While, A. (2013). Physical activity in older people: A systematic review. *BMC Public Health, 13*(449).

TechAmerica Foundation's Federal Big Data Commission. (2012). *Demystifying Big Data: A practical guide to transforming the business of government.* Retrieved from www-304.ibm.com/industries/publicsector/fileserve?contentid=239170.

Thomas, J., & Wing, R. (2013). Health-E-Call, a smartphone-assisted behavioral obesity treatment: Pilot study. *JMIR Mhealth Uhealth, 1*(1), e3.

Toscos, T., Faber, A., Connelly, K., & Upoma, A. (2008). *Encouraging physical activity in teens: Can technology help reduce barriers to physical activity in adolescent girls?* Paper presented at the 2008 Second International Conference on Pervasive Computing Technologies for Healthcare, Tampere, Finland.

Troiano, R., Berrigan, D., Dodd, K., Masse, L., Tilert, T., & McDowell, M. (2008). Physical activity in the United States measured by accelerometer. *Medicine and Science in Sport and Exercise, 40*(1), 181–188.

Tsai, C., Lee, G., Raab, F., Norman, G., Sohn, T., Griswold, W., & Patrick, K. (2007). Usability and feasibility of PmEB: A mobile phone application for monitoring real time caloric balance. *Mobile Networks and Applications, 12*, 173–184.

U.S. Department of Health and Human Services. (2008). *2008 Physical Activity Guidelines for Americans* Retrieved from https://health.gov/paguidelines/pdf/paguide.pdf.

van der Weegen, S., Verwey, R., Spreeuwenberg, M., Tange, H., van der Weijden, T., & de Witte, L. (2013). The development of a mobile monitoring and feedback tool to stimulate physical activity of people with a chronic disease in primary care: A user-centered design. *Journal of Medical Internet Research, 1*(2).

Verwey, R., van der Weegen, S., Spreeuwenberg, M., Tange, H., van der Weijden, T., & de Witte, L. (2014). A pilot study of a tool to stimulate physical activity in patients with COPD or type 2 diabetes in primary care. *Journal of Telemedicine and Telecare, 20*(1), 29–34.

Watterson, T. (2012). Changes in attitudes and behaviors toward physical activity, nutrition, and social support for middle school students using the AFIT app as a supplement to instruction in a physical education class. PhD thesis, University of South Florida.

West, D. (2012). How mobile devices are transforming healthcare. *Issues in Technology Innovation, 18*(1), 1–11.

Wyatt, S., Winters, K., & Dubbert, P. (2006). Overweight and obesity: Prevalence, consequences, and causes of a growing public health problem. *The American Journal of the Medical Sciences, 331*(4), 166–174.

7 Global positioning systems and geographic information systems and physical activity

Zachary Pope and Zan Gao

Up to this point in the book, several novel ways in which emerging technologies are being used to promote physical activity (PA)—each with the aim of reducing sedentary behavior and preventing the development of chronic diseases. Indeed, many of the previously reviewed technologies have literature dating from the turn of the twenty-first century to the present day—indicating the use of these complex technologies to promote PA is at the cutting-edge. One of the most sophisticated modern technologies to be used in PA and health promotion is Global Positioning Systems (GPS) and Geographic Information Systems (GIS)—two related technologies that, while only recently popularized for health and fitness, are older than many other technologies reviewed in this book.

Originally developed and used by the military in the late 1970s, GPS was finally made available for civilian use in 2000 (Maddison & Mhurchu, 2009). Since being made available for civilian use, numerous GPS devices have been developed to allow individuals to track all types of movement and activity. Moreover, GPS PA data have more recently been analyzed in relation to the built environment using GIS (Kirtland et al., 2003). In brief, GIS software allows for PA data captured by GPS to be analyzed in relation to the locations where these activities took place and, thus, facilitating researchers' ability to discern relationships between locations and features of the built environment (e.g., sidewalk construction, land use, and trail systems) which may facilitate or inhibit PA participation (Troped et al., 2001). While a fuller explanation of GIS and associated techniques is beyond the scope of this chapter, the reader is directed to other sources which devote themselves to simply and fully explaining this technology (National Geographic Society, 2016). Nonetheless, the combination of GPS/GIS is among the most promising technologies available to advocate for changes to the built environment which may better promote PA participation in addition to facilitating the development, implementation, and assessment of PA interventions.

Throughout this chapter the reader will be provided an in-depth look into how GPS/GIS is currently being used to promote PA and health. Specifically, the chapter will first focus attention on the use of this technology in different populations after which the discussion will switch to an examination of the literature regarding GPS/GIS in the assessment of different intensities and types of PA, as well as the limitations of GPS/GIS use in different contexts. Following a discussion of the preceding topics, the emphasis of the chapter will switch to the use of GPS/GIS in healthcare with a further discussion of how health professionals might develop an effective PA interventions using this technology. Finally, the chapter will close with a brief review of the practical implications of the topics discussed.

GPS/GIS and health promotion in various populations

Many readers may personally use a GPS device for the purpose of tracking activities such as walking, running, biking, and hiking (Figure 7.1), among other activities. Indeed, it is during the aforementioned situations where it was most common to see GPS in use (i.e., sport-related performance tracking and assessment) a decade ago. However, noteworthy is the fact that GPS and, now, GIS, are presently being more frequently used by non-athlete populations. Specifically, these technologies have been used in two broad segments of the population: (1) PA and health promotion during PA interventions and environmental audits among the general population; and (2) sport-related performance tracking and assessment among athletes. As the focus of this book is on PA and health promotion, we will first discuss the extant GPS/GIS literature on this topic among the general population before turning to the latter topic regarding sport-related performance tracking and assessment. Emphasis will be placed on the

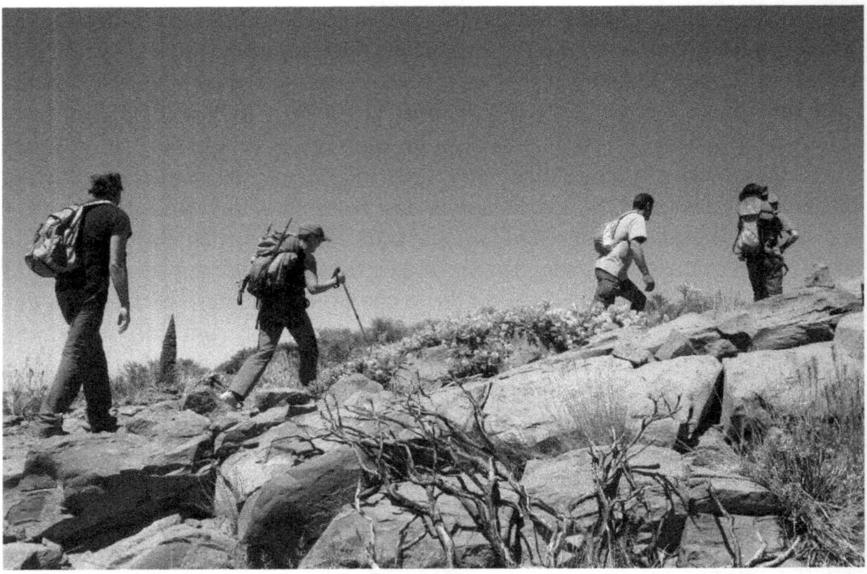

Figure 7.1 Application of a GPS-embedded physical activity app in hiking.

Source: pixabay.com.

discussion of the populations in which these GPS/GIS studies took place and the findings of the literature.

Use of GPS/GIS in the general population

The use of GPS/GIS in PA and health promotion is still seen less frequently than that of other wearable technologies which may or may not have GPS embedded in them (e.g., health wearables such as the Fitbit, Jawbone, etc.). That said, the present literature has looked first to prove the validity and reliability of GPS/GIS technologies after which the effectiveness of these technologies in the promotion of PA and health has been investigated. In a population of 20 older adults, Webber and Porter (2009) examined the feasibility of tracking the mobility patterns of this population. As is common to GPS research due to GPS's poorer ability to discern PA type or track PA well indoors, these older adults were fitted with one GPS watch and two accelerometers. Findings indicated that while the older adults had no difficulty using the GPS watches and did not perceive these watches to be bothersome, the data obtained from these devices was significantly impacted by the amount of time the participants spent indoors—highlighting further the inability of GPS to accurately track indoor movement. In a similar study, Oliver Badland, Mavoa, Duncan, and Duncan (2010) investigated the feasibility of combining GPS, GIS, and accelerometry to assess transportation-related PA, indicating that out of 259 potential trips which could have been analyzed using the GPS data collected, only 29 were analyzed as other trips had issues related to the GPS devices such as signal loss, device failure, lost devices, and unworn devices. Notably, to reduce measurement error, a more recent study developed and validated a model mathematic equation allowing researchers to use GPS and accelerometry data to accurately predict PA intensity and duration, as well as energy expenditure during controlled and free-living conditions (Nguyen, Lecoultre, Sunami, & Schutz, 2013). However, widespread use of this model has yet to be seen.

As a more sophisticated GPS has been developed in the last several years, however, a small body of literature has shifted concentration from the validity and reliability of GPS/GIS to these technologies' capability to promote individuals' PA participation. In fact, the majority of the literature to date has focused not on interventions *per se*, but on the assessment of PA patterns, in addition to the built environment, and how the promotion of PA might be achieved in these environments through later behavioral interventions or initiatives which seek to modify the built environment to be more conducive to PA participation. Moreover, much of the research to date has focused on youth populations. For example, several large-scale projects have been initiated using GPS/GIS, in combination with accelerometry, to examine and facilitate youth PA promotion by investigating the locations in which youth PA takes place.

The UK-based Personal and Environmental Associations with Children's Health (PEACH) project (Wheeler, Cooper, Page, & Jago, 2010) is one such large-scale study which gathered GPS/GIS data from 1307 10-year-old and

11-year-old children, finding children spent an average 13% of after-school time outdoors, with further findings indicating that outdoor time contributed to 30% of children's daily PA participation and 35% of their daily MVPA. Similar results were seen in the Teen Environment and Neighborhood (TEAN) study, with Carlson et al. (2016) indicating the highest proportion of adolescent PA (42%) to occur at school, with approximately 19% and 21% of PA occurring at home or near home/school, respectively. These findings mirrored that of a smaller, earlier study indicating the majority of adolescent participation in PA takes place near or at school/home (Maddison et al., 2010). As a result, it is clear that increasing PA among youth must consider the impact of the built environment on PA behavior.

Despite the fact that the built environment plays a role in influencing youth PA behavior, modifying the built environment through reconstruction is challenging. As such, recent studies have focused on educating youth regarding approaches in which they can use their current built environment to engage in more PA. The 6-month Children's Use of the Built Environment (CUBE) study among youth aged 10–16-years-old used GPS/GIS, along with accelerometry, to observe moderate-to-vigorous PA (MVPA) in different locations of their environment. Following baseline measurement, the intervention youth and their parents met with researchers who counseled the youth on how to use their most frequently traversed built environments (data provided by GIS analysis of each child's GPS data) to increase PA (Oreskovic, Goodman, Park, Robinson, & Winickoff, 2015; Oreskovic, Winickoff, Perrin, Robinson, & Goodman, 2016). Control group youth received standard information regarding PA participation and healthier living. Researchers found that, on average, the intervention youth receiving counseling had just over 9 more minutes of daily MVPA than controls at post-intervention. Similarly, researchers in New Zealand used GPS/GIS to discern if playground upgrades resulted in greater PA (PA) among 5–10-year-olds, observing significant higher PA over time as a result of these upgrades (Quigg, Reeder, Gray, Waters, & Holt, 2013). Findings from the preceding studies indicate the usefulness of examining the built environment when investigating how to best intervene and increase children's PA levels.

The built environment has also been the largest area of inquiry among adults in the general population. Among the earliest studies in this line of research was a pilot study by Rodriguez, Brown and Troped (2005) during which GPS/GIS was used to investigate the location of MVPA in 35 adults, finding 46% of MVPA occurred within the participant's neighborhood—congruent with the later results of Troped and associates (2010). Notably, both studies found environmental variables such as land use, housing unit/population density, intersection density, and vegetation index had an effect on PA. Nonetheless, GPS/GIS research among adults has also found that as much as 60% of PA occurs further than 800 meters from individuals' homes (Hillsdon, Coombes, Griew, & Jones, 2015)—necessitating the investigation of PA participation in other locations within communities solely built to promote PA participation.

Indeed, other studies have investigated how the provision of biking/running trails and parks within a community can influence PA. Troped et al. (2001) used GPS/GIS to assess the biking/running trail use of 413 adults, observing significantly decreased trail use the farther the participant lived from the trail, when the study participants were older, and when the study participant was female. Interestingly, recent multi-site research using GPS/GIS to assess adult use of 31 parks in five U.S. states found that adults who visit a park at least once weekly had significantly higher MVPA compared to adults who did not visit a park (Evenson, Wen, Hiller, & Cohen, 2013). Finally, GPS/GIS data have even shown that the implementation of public transit can promote greater PA among adults in the surrounding community, and this does not necessarily displace other active forms of transportation such as walking or biking (Miller et al., 2015).

While the aforementioned studies are not meant to be exhaustive, they are representative of the high-quality literature available regarding the use of GPS/GIS to aid in the promotion of PA and health among the general population. What should be clear in the discussion above is the usefulness of GPS/GIS in studying the influence of the built environment on the PA participation of youth and adults. Specifically, information gleaned from studies using GPS/GIS to study the PA patterns of youth and adults can be used to advocate for modifications and policy changes governing community land use, in addition to aiding in the development, implementation, and assessment of PA interventions.

For instance, modifications could be made to a local park (e.g., updated playground equipment) or community governing bodies could implement policies which designate certain areas of land to be only for recreational use—all changes which would increase the likelihood of greater PA participation. Moreover, it might be worth examining how new augmented reality games such as Pokémon Go—which use GPS-enabled devices to display on the screensof these devices a virtual world overlaid onto real-world environments (Figure 7.2)—might be used to increase PA at the population level. Indeed, researchers have postulated the possibility of using games such as Pokémon Go to increase PA at the population level (Baranowski, 2016).

Finally, with 64% of adults currently owning a smartphone (Pew Research Center, 2015), it would be advantageous for researchers to use GPS-enabled smartphones in future studies, given the breadth of contextual information these devices might provide regarding PA environments. For example, Hirsch and colleagues (2014) described how researchers might use commercially available GPS-enabled smartphone apps (e.g., MapMyFitness) to track where PA occurs in a given environment (e.g., an urban environment) and what type of PA is most likely to occur at a given location. Indeed, participants of a study could send the GPS coordinates of locations where PA is impeded due to broken sidewalks or poorly maintained trails to researchers interested in how to modify the built environment to promote PA. These coordinates could then be used to promote changes to the built environment at the government level. Overall, it is clear the promise of GPS/GIS in PA and health promotion remains great, with the use of GPS/GIS for health promotion among the general population continuing to grow.

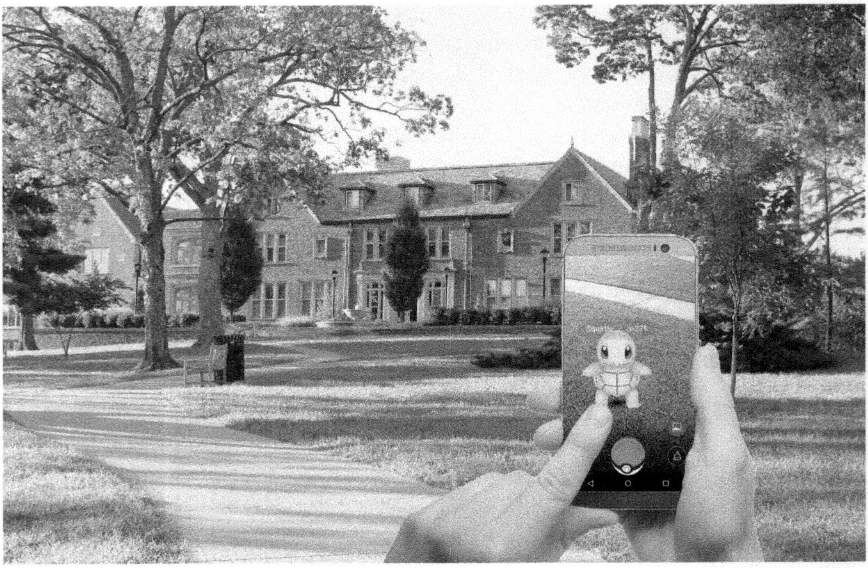

Figure 7.2 Pokémon Go app outdoors.
Source: pixabay.com.

That said, sport-related performance has also been another area of research wherein GPS and/or GIS have been used.

Sport-related performance tracking and assessment among athletes

Although sport-related performance tracking and assessment are not the main focus of this book, it is noteworthy to briefly discuss the use of GPS and/or GIS during sport participation, given the breadth of literature available on this topic. Moreover, participation in recreational sports throughout the lifespan has been shown to lead to better health outcomes in late life among recreationally active individuals in the general population (Hirvensalo & Lintunen, 2011). As such, the development of accurate sport-related performance tracking and assessment tools, such as GPS/GIS, is paramount if recreationally active individuals are going to make informed choices about the sport activities they participate in. Notably, little use of GIS is seen in studies of sport performance as researchers typically assess the competitor's performance on the field of play and do not try to discern barriers in the built environment inhibiting gameplay.

Both team and individual sports have been of interest to researchers using GPS to track and assess sport performance. MacLeod Morris, Nevill, and Sunderland (2009) investigated the validity of an advanced GPS system, the Spi Elite™, as worn by nine recreational trained field hockey players during a circuit requiring the athletes to run and change direction. Findings indicated that the GPS system was highly accurate, with GPS-recorded distance off by an average of only three meters for the pre-measured course and average GPS speed measurements being identical to that provided by the timing gates. However, Johnston et al. (2012) conducted a similar study, suggesting that while GPS was accurate in tracking distance covered and peak speed, the error associated with these measures increased as athlete velocity increased. The results of the Johnston et al. (2012) study are congruent with earlier findings by Coutts and Duffield (2010) and Jennings and colleagues (2010), which found distance and peak velocity measures become less reliable as athlete training intensity increased.

The use of GPS in the assessment of PA patterns among professional sports has also been investigated to better inform athlete training practices. Two studies have used GPS to examine between-position differences in gameplay intensity as measured by parameters such as overall time in light, moderate, and vigorous exercise; distance traveled during the game; and average/peak velocities (Kempton, Sullivan, Bilsborough, Cordy, & Coutts, 2015; Macutkiewicz & Sunderland, 2011). Findings indicated that, generally, high-speed running, distance covered, and player load varied by position and was higher during and was often higher late in the season. Data from studies like the preceding two investigations can be used to better inform trainers and coaches of the volume of activity each player is engaging in—allowing the trainers and coaches to manipulate training practices to optimize performance/recovery and reduce likelihood of injury. Notably, optimizing performance/recovery and reducing injury hae been the focus of a growing body of GPS literature in recent years which has examined athlete training load and volume (Figure 7.3) (Malone et al., 2015; Nielsen et al., 2013; Smith, Moran, & Foley, 2013).

The aforementioned literature, however, is limite in that few studies have investigated recreationally active athletes or sports in which recreationally active athletes are likely to participate—again, a drawback given sport participation continued throughout the lifespan can result in better health long-term health outcomes (Hirvensalo & Lintunen, 2011). Geocaching, a sport which functions much like a real-world treasure hunting game, requires participants with GPS-enabled devices to walk, bike, hike, and climb their way to a specific location denoted by GPS coordinates (Groundspeak, 2016). Upon reaching the GPS coordinates, the players find containers (termed "geocaches" or "caches") at which point they are able to take and keep the contents of the cache. Per the rules of geocaching, however, players must log their find within the cache logbook and leave within the cache an item of at least the same value as the item they took (Groundspeak, 2016). While some scholars have stated geocaching to be a twenty-first-century form of outdoor hide-and-seek (Schlatter & Hurd, 2005), scarce literature is available which has tested the effectiveness of a geocaching program in the promotion of PA. Indeed, while researchers have posited that geocaching might be a sport capable of increasing PA across adults, children, and families, concerns about the safety of geocaching have likely inhibited the implementation of geocaching-based PA interventions (Flett, Moore, Pfeiffer,

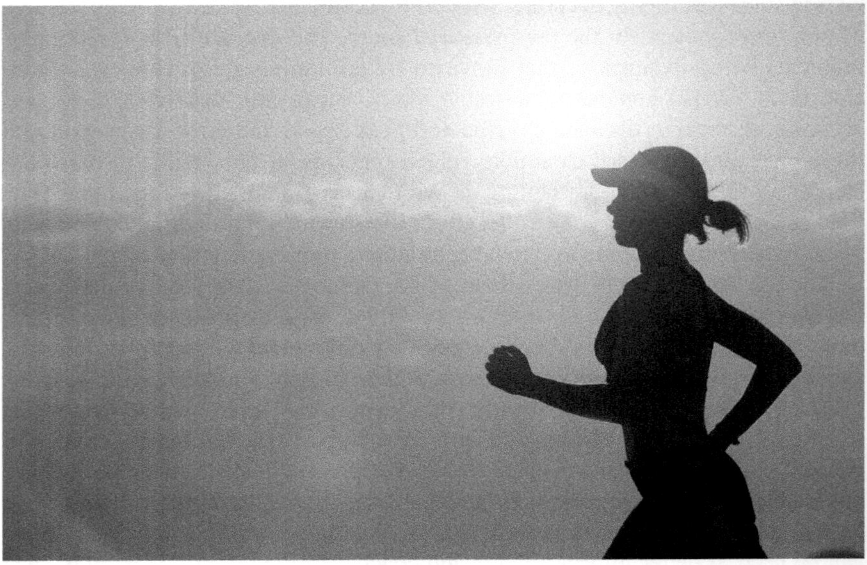

Figure 7.3 Tracking physical activity with a mobile phone app.
Source: pixabay.com.

Belonga, & Navarre, 2010). Therefore, future research might consider how to minimize safety concerns (e.g., the need to, at times, travel to obscure locations to reach a geocache) before implementing a geocaching-based PA intervention.

As can be seen, GPS and GIS demonstrate great utility among both the general population for PA and health promotion and populations of professional and some recreational athletes for sport performance tracking and assessment. However, some issues remain. For instance, how do studies decrease the signal loss common when using GPS? Further, despite GPS devices' ability to track the speed and distance of PA, how do researchers improve the ability of GPS to track PA intensity and type so that further GPS studies do not have to rely on the concurrent use of GPS and accelerometer devices to track PA? Finally, how might researchers better integrate GPS devices into the natural behaviors of individuals? Presently this integration is difficult as it might interfere with certain activities. For example, it would be difficult to wear a GPS device during a football game. In subsequent sections of this chapter, these questions will be addressed.

GPS/GIS and different intensity levels and types of PA

As stated in the previous section of this chapter, it is common to have participants in GPS and GIS studies wear accelerometers in addition to the GPS devices provided by the research teams. While some of the rationale behind wearing accelerometers arises due to the fact GPS devices have difficulty accessing and keeping a signal when tracking PA indoors, wearing accelerometers also addresses the limitation of GPS devices to assess PA intensity and type.

With regard to PA intensity, previous studies have indicated that, as PA intensity increases, the error associated with measurements made by GPS also increases (Coutts & Duffield, 2010; Jennings et al., 2010; Johnston et al., 2012). While some researchers are developing mathematical models to help correct for error in measures of PA intensity made by GPS (Nguyen et al., 2013), widespread use of these models has not taken place. Inaccurate measures of PA intensity have major implications when designing and implementing PA interventions. Specifically, if inaccurate GPS measures of PA intensity lead to the design and implementation of a PA intervention that is too intense, intervention participants may lose motivation to participate in PA—decreasing the effectiveness of the intervention and the ability to expand the intervention to the larger population.

The assessment of PA type is also an important consideration as it pertains to the limitations of GPS. Maddison and Mhurchu (2009) stated that, while GPS is able to provide good information on the distance, velocity, and location of PA participation, the inability of GPS to provide data which can help differentiate different activities done at the same velocity—for example, slow walking versus slow biking—the usefulness of this technology in PA tracking and assessment is limited. Unfortunately, few investigations into increasing GPS devices' capability to accurately assess PA type have been completed, with studies having this objective finding the use of accelerometers is still necessary for the most valid discernment of PA type (Troped et al., 2008). Unfortunately, the necessity of wearing both a GPS device and an accelerometer increases participant burden and subsequently reduces intervention compliance—both outcomes which, again, limit the researchers' ability to generalize the findings of these investigations to subsequent large-scale intervention development and implementation.

Given the previously described limitations of GPS in the measurement of PA intensity and type, future studies must look at ways in which to improve the capability of GPS devices to provide these measurements concurrently and in a manner that does not result in high participant burden—meaning GPS and accelerometry need to be integrated in a single device. However, of the most recent studies seeking to measure both PA intensity and type concurrently and accurately, it was found that one GPS device and two accelerometer are still needed for the most accurate measurements (Nguyen et al., 2013). Furthermore, while integration of GPS and accelerometry into one device has taken place with the proliferation of smartphones, the validity and reliability of these devices in the systematic tracking and assessment of PA intensity and type—not to mention the ability of smartphones to accurately track PA distance, velocity, and location—remain to be seen. Moreover, while vests and clothing are available which integrate GPS and accelerometry—such as the Catapult vest (Catapult, 2016; www.catapultsports.com) and the Hexoskin Biometric Shirt (Hexoskin,

2016; www.hexoskin.com)—these articles of clothing may still be uncomfortable and burdensome for participants to wear.

It is suggested, therefore, that researchers and companies engage in greater collaboration to develop products that have the capability to provide accurate GPS and accelerometer data concurrently and meet the style and comfort preferences of users interested in technology of this type. Nonetheless, researchers and health professionals should still strive to integrate GPS into the tracking and assessment of PA intensity among the general population as well as among athletes—particularly recreational athletes. Indeed, despite the limitations of GPS in the assessment of PA intensity and type, this technology is still powerful and has the ability to impact public health policy and initiatives—promoting health at both the individual and population levels.

Application of GPS/GIS in different contexts

As has been addressed in the previous two sections of this chapter, GPS and GIS are used across a diverse array of populations to assess a number of activities. As a result of the aforementioned diversity, these technologies are used in numerous contexts. Broadly, the contexts could be reduced to two main environments: (1) PA and health promotion in relation to the built environment; and (2) sport-related performance tracking and assessment on various fields of sport play. While much of the literature within these categories has been touched upon, it is important to note where improvements to the use of GPS and/or GIS can be made within each context to offer greater benefit to clients and consumers who benefit from the data these two related technologies provide.

Within the context of PA and health promotion, we have discussed the use of GPS/GIS to discern the relationship between an individual's built environment and their PA participation. Examining this relationship has become paramount, given the increasingly obesogenic environment of the present-day wherein technology continues to make our lives easier, with less need for PA (Jones, Bentham, Foster, Hillsdon, & Panter, 2007). That said, improvements to a couple major aspects of GPS/GIS studies for PA and health promotion are needed to overcome the aforementioned challenges.

First, despite the utility of GIS software in the analysis of participant GPS location data in relation to PA, the privacy of this software has been questioned for nearly a decade (Brownstein, Cassa, Kohane, & Mandl, 2006; Maddison & Mhurchu, 2009). It has been observed that reverse identification of participants' residencies is possible nearly 80% of the time using publication quality GIS maps (Brownstein et al., 2006). Not only does the possibility of discerning an individual's residence pose a danger to these individuals, the potential breach in confidentiality may deter individuals from future GPS/GIS study participation—limiting the investigation of the built environment's influence on PA and slowing advantageous PA-related modifications to the built environment. Fortunately, recent work has begun to investigate how researchers can "obfuscate," or mask, data points when analyzing GPS data with GIS software (Seidl, Jankowski, &

Tsou, 2016). This work is preliminary, however, and further research into the masking of participant GPS data without compromising researchers' ability to accurately analyze these data is needed.

While minor in relation to questions regarding privacy of GPS/GIS data, a second improvement with regard to the use of GPS/GIS data in studies on PA and health promotion concerns the need for participants to wear both a GPS device and an accelerometer. The previous section of this chapter offered a fuller discussion of why this concurrent measurement by two devices is necessary; namely, GPS devices have poor ability to discern PA intensity and type while also having limited use indoors due to signal loss. Although GPS and clothing companies are working to integrate GPS and accelerometry, the fact that two devices are necessary in GPS/GIS studies is noteworthy as it increases participant burden. Increased participant burden can lower compliance to the study protocol—negatively impacting study outcomes and the conclusions which can be drawn as a result of a given study (Matthews, Hagstromer, Pober, & Bowles, 2012). As stated previously, increased collaboration will be needed between researchers and companies to develop products that not only collect GPS and accelerometer data concurrently, but that also meet the style and comfort preferences of users (Figure 7.4).

Among professional and recreational athletes on the field of play, two major improvements to the use of GPS could also be made. To begin with, as addressed

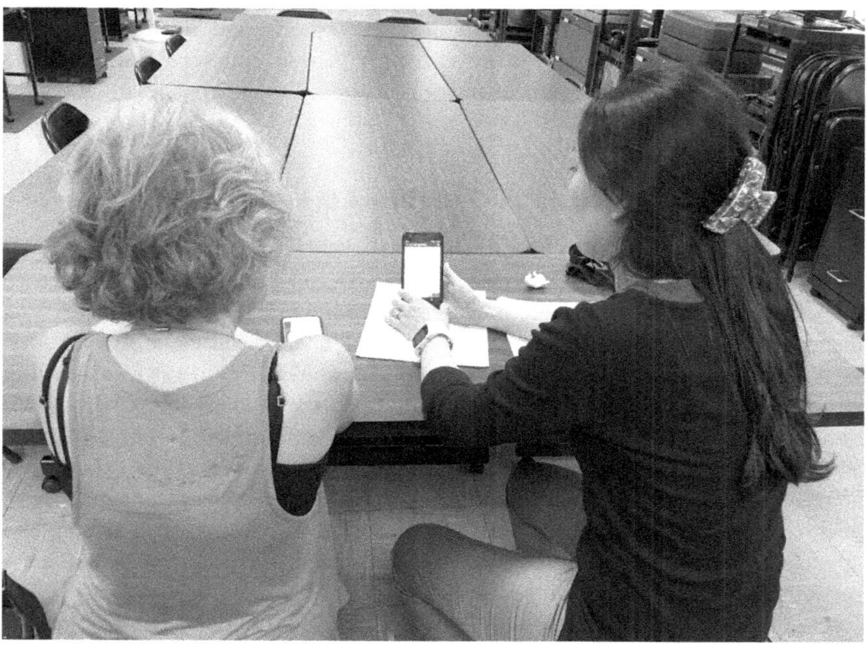

Figure 7.4 A researcher teaching a patient to use a smartphone physical activity app.
Source: Photo by Zan Gao.

above, GPS has demonstrated higher error as athlete velocity increases (Coutts & Duffield, 2010; Jennings et al., 2010; Johnston et al., 2012). Training load is also of serious concern to athletes and trainers, given the fact that too high or too low a training load can have a negative impact on player performance (Manzi, Bovenzi, Impellizzeri, Carminati, & Castagna, 2013). Therefore, research into the development of more-sensitive GPS devices—which might also be integrated with accelerometry—is necessary to ensure the most accurate tracking and assessment of athlete performance, with an additional objective being to reduce injury. Second, if GPS is going to be fully employed in a wide variety of sports, the devices need to be minimally intrusive. While GPS-enabled devices such as the Catapult (Catapult, 2016) are available, often the devices are still too large and temperamental to be used in sports where large amounts of contact are to be expected (e.g., football). Researchers might look further at how to integrate small GPS units into currently available biometric clothing lines, such as the Hexoskin Biometric Shirt (Hexoskin, 2016), as this type of integration would be less intrusive to the overall performance of the athletes wearing the technology.

Despite the need for improvements in GPS in different contexts, GPS data is still changing the way in which researchers/health professionals improve the ability of the general population to participate in PA, in addition to aiding coaches/trainers to prepare their athletes to compete at the highest level of sport. Given the fast pace at which technology continues to advance, it is likely that many of the major improvements desired within the context of PA and health promotion as well as sport-related performance tracking and assessment will be partially or fully solved in the next decade. These solutions will facilitate improved health and performance among community members and athletic populations, respectively.

Application of GPS/GIS in the healthcare field

The use of GPS/GIS in healthcare differs slightly from that seen using other forms of technology. Specifically, while GPS/GIS can and has been implemented in clinical settings, the literature is scarce. Indeed, while these technologies lend themselves well to the assessment of PA among healthy individuals in addition to athletes and other recreationally active populations, GPS/GIS is less useful in clinical populations where treatment often takes place indoors—making acquisition of the satellite signal needed for GPS devices difficult and inhibiting further analysis via GIS techniques. Given these limitations, as well as the extant literature reviewed previously, it might be stated that GPS/GIS is of greatest use in healthcare in the public health field—particularly as it pertains to assessing and advocating for changes in the built environment which would better facilitate PA participation by individuals in poorer health.

One way in which to harness the power of GPS/GIS among clinical populations is to use this technology to complete environmental assessments of the individuals for a set period of time, after which the individuals can be brought back to the health clinic and counseled on how to take advantage of the environment around them to increase PA. For example, a male named John who is currently 40 pounds overweight and in the early stages of type 2 diabetes could be provided a GPS device by a wellness team at the weight management clinic where he is currently enrolled. The wellness team would then request that John wear the GPS device over the course of the next month. Following a month of GPS wear, John would then bring the GPS device back to the weight management clinic, at which point the wellness team would use GIS software to analyze the GPS data and create maps of the locations where John engages in the greatest amount of PA. An appointment could then be set up with John, when these maps would be provided to him. Using these maps, the wellness team could highlight locations within the environment which John interacts with or frequently passes, where greater PA participation is possible (e.g., nearby walking paths, parks, fitness facilities, etc.). John could then set goals with the wellness team regarding increasing his PA participation (e.g., setting a goal to use the walking path near his house at least three times per week). Periodic calls by wellness team personnel could then be made to John, assessing his adherence to his goals and discussing any new barriers to PA which have arisen since his previous meeting with the wellness team.

While the preceding example is hypothetical in nature, the same design has been used among overweight youth 10–16 years of age within the CUBE study—implemented via an outpatient community health clinic. Specifically, Oreskovic et al. (2016) asked youth to wear GPS devices during three different time periods over the course of one month, before taking part in a counseling session reviewing their GPS data and how to use the built environment they most frequently traversed to increase PA. At the study's end, researchers observed daily MVPA to be approximately 9 minutes higher among the intervention group compared to controls. Although the usefulness of GPS/GIS for healthcare delivery was first addressed nearly a decade ago (see Hanjagi, Srihari, & Rayamane, 2007), a study in healthcare akin to that of the CUBE study has yet to take place among adults. Thus, more attention needs to be paid to this line of investigation as findings regarding the built environment from GPS data may have wide implications as these pertain to advocating for public policy changes, affecting how communities use land and the provision of recreational facilities by these same communities. These same policy changes could also complement healthcare delivery approaches which seek to use the built environment to increase PA participation and promote health—akin to John's example above. In this manner, we can change a normally obesogenic built environment into a place where the unique aspects of the built environment can be a catalyst for improved PA and health.

Finally, crowdsourcing might also be an innovative way in which healthcare can use GPS/GIS to improve health at the population level. Briefly, crowdsourcing references large numbers of public citizens being given the opportunity to complete tasks for companies, organizations, or institutions, ranging from the categorization of galaxies in space to solving complex engineering problems (Ranard et al., 2014). Within the healthcare field, crowdsourcing has been used in the surveillance and monitoring of malaria symptoms in India (Chunara et al., 2012) in addition to being used for data processing purposes to identify blood smears containing malaria-infected parasites (Mavandadi et al., 2012). GPS has also been used for crowdsourcing within the healthcare field to allow users equipped with a smartphone application to document—using GPS coordinates—where they or others were experiencing flu-like symptoms as well as constructing maps of automated external defibrillators around a city. Indeed, given the high smartphone ownership among individuals in developed countries (Pew Research Center, 2015), use of GPS-enabled smartphones via a crowdsourcing manner akin to the two examples just mentioned might go a long way to improving population health. For instance, smartphones could be used by patients enrolled in a health management program to send GPS coordinates of places in their environment that are impeding their PA. This information could then be used by researchers and health professionals to advocate for changes in the built environment to promote population-level increases in PA participation—much like the strategy mentioned in the first section of this chapter. Nonetheless, with a concerted effort by researchers and health professionals, GPS/GIS could have major benefits in the healthcare field via public health policy.

Use of GPS/GIS in developing effective PA interventions

GPS/GIS are different from other emerging technologies in that GPS/GIS technologies are typically used to inform subsequent interventions or describe PA patterns and are not typically the medium by which researchers and health professionals intervene. Nonetheless, when using GPS/GIS to complement the PA intervention development, implementation, and development process, a few different considerations must be made to ensure an effective PA intervention.

As is recommended for all interventions, a theoretical backing in studies looking to use GPS/GIS to develop, implement, and assess an intervention is necessary. Theory allows for leveraging the indirect effects of certain determinants of PA engagement (e.g., self-efficacy, motivation, etc.) while also facilitating external and accurate interpretations of study findings (Patten, 2014). With regard to GPS/GIS, theoretical foundations are paramount in discerning how these two emerging technologies may best benefit the PA intervention.

Second, effective use of GPS/GIS in PA and health promotion studies needs to consider intervention fidelity. While a fuller description of intervention fidelity is available in Chapter 6, the term refers to how researchers go about protecting the reliability and internal validity of their study (Borrelli, 2011). In studies using GPS/GIS to track and assess PA levels of participants, the greatest threat to intervention fidelity is signal loss and, as a related metric, participant adherence. One review found that out of 17 studies reporting the amount of GPS data loss, data loss rates were 2.5%–92% (Krenn et al., 2011). Therefore, researchers must provide thorough information to participants regarding GPS device wear which outlines, among many possible instructions, the proper wear location, the required amount of wear time per day, the GPS syncing procedures to allow sufficient satellite signal/reduction of signal loss, and the charging procedures given often limited battery life of GPS devices. Further, researchers should periodically check up on the participants to ensure adherence to these procedures. These fidelity measures will ensure low loss of GPS data—often stated to be the largest limitation of PA research using GPS devices (Krenn et al., 2011)—and facilitate subsequent analysis of this GPS data via GIS software.

Finally, like most new research fields, future studies must increase the representativeness of the study participants as it pertains to the demographics of the general population (Krenn et al., 2011). This will allow for the findings of said studies to be more effective in influencing the design and implementation of PA interventions across a wide array of populations in the academic and healthcare fields. Not only will this increased representativeness come in the form of more diverse race/ethnicity make-up of studies using GPS/GIS, it must also arise from a more evenly distributed age make-up of these studies. As was evident in the first section of this chapter, a great deal of research has been done on children, adults, and athletes, but far less research is available regarding middle-aged and older adults and their activity patterns. Investigating middle-aged and older adults' PA patterns—and ways the built environment might be modified to promote PA participation in these older populations—is paramount, given the fact that functional limitations brought about by decreased PA and increased disease commonly observed with aging are currently a public health concern (An & Shi, 2015).

Practical implications of GPS/GIS use in promoting health

Aside from the considerations that future research must take into account when using GPS/GIS to design, implement, and assess PA interventions to ensure these technologies' limitations do not bias results and/or limit the use/generalization of the data gathered, GPS/GIS holds major promise. In particular, these two related technologies have a bright future related to examining the relationships between individuals' PA patterns and objects within the built environment. Indeed, through the examination of the built environment via this technology, researchers can advocate for changes at the city, state, and national government levels, influencing policies regarding the assignment of land use while also integrating this technology further into healthcare—teaching clinical populations how to use the built environment around them to increase PA levels.

That said, over the next decade, researchers and industry members must work together: (1) to integrate GPS and accelerometry into single devices which appeal to and reduce the burden of study participants, in addition to being capable of providing PA type and intensity information—with the capability of these devices to also measure physiological variables, such as heart rate and energy expenditure also needed; (2) to develop GPS/accelerometry devices which can be worn by athletes in all types of professional and recreational sports, to effectively manage training load to improve performance and reduce injury; and (3) to learn how to effectively mask the maps published using GIS software to protect study participant confidentiality and facilitate further desire by community members to participate in studies of this type. Nonetheless, GPS/GIS promises to play a major role in the future of PA and health promotion. Indeed, as GPS/GIS has demonstrated tremendous growth and use in the technologies' first 15 years of civilian use, it will be amazing to see where another 15 years of improvements will take this technology.

References

An, R., & Shi, Y. (2015). Body weight status and onset of functional limitations in U.S. middle-aged and older adults. *Disability and Health Journal, 8*, 336–344.

Baranowski, T. (2016). Pokémon Go, go, go, gone? *Games for Health Journal, 5*(5), 1–2.

Borrelli, B. (2011). The assessment, monitoring, and enhancement of treatment fidelity in public health clinical trials. *Jounral of Public Health Denistry, 71*, S52–S63.

Brownstein, J., Cassa, C., Kohane, I., & Mandl, K. (2006). An unsupervised classification method for inferring original case locations from low-resolution disease maps. *International Journal of Health Geographics, 5*(56).

Carlson, J., Schipperijn, J., Kerr, J., Saelens, B., Natarajan, L., Frank, L., … Sallis, J. (2016). Locations of physical activity as assessed by GPS in young adolescents. *Pediatrics, 137*(1).

Catapult. (2016). Catapult. Retrieved from www.catapultsports.com/

Chunara, R., Chhaya, V., Bane, S., Mekaru, S., Chan, E., Freifeld, C., & Brownstein, J. (2012). Online reporting for malaria surveillance using micro-monetary incentives, in urban India, 2010–2011. *Malaria Journal, 11*, 43.

Coutts, A., & Duffield, R. (2010). Validity and reliability of GPS devices for measuring movement demands of team sports. *Jounral of Science and Medicine in Sport, 13*, 133–135.

Evenson, K., Wen, F., Hiller, A., & Cohen, D. (2013). Assessing the contribution of parks to physical activity using global positioning system and accelerometry. *Medicine and Science in Sport and Exercise, 45*(10), 1981–1987.

Flett, M., Moore, R., Pfeiffer, K., Belonga, J., & Navarre, J. (2010). Connecting children and family with nature-based physical activity. *American Journal of Health Education, 41*(5), 292–300.

Groundspeak. (2016). *Geocaching 101*. Retrieved from www.geocaching.com/guide/

Hallal, P., Andersen, L., Bull, F., Guthold, R., Haskell, W., & Ekelund, U. (2012). Global physical activity levels: Surveillance progress, pitfalls, and prospects. *The Lancet, 380*(9838), 247–257.

Hanjagi, A., Srihari, P., & Rayamane, A. (2007). A public health care information system using GIS and GPS: A case study of Shiggaon. In *GIS for Health and the Environment*. Berlin: Springer.

Hexoskin. (2016). *Hexoskin wearable body metrics*. Retrieved from www.hexoskin.com/

Hillsdon, M., Coombes, E., Griew, P., & Jones, A. (2015). An assessment of the relevance of the home neighbourhood for understanding environmental influences on physical activity. *International Journal of Behavioral Nutrition and Physical Activity, 12*(100).

Hirsch, J. A., James, P., Robinson, J. R. M., Eastman, K. M., Conley, K. D., Evenson, K. R., & Laden, F. (2014). Using MapMyFitness to place physical activity into neighborhood context. *Frontiers in Public Health, 2*, 19. http://doi.org/10.3389/fpubh.2014.00019.

Hirvensalo, M., & Lintunen, T. (2011). Life-course perspective for physical activity and sports participation. *European Review for Aging and Physical Activity, 8*, 13–22.

Jennings, D., Cormack, S., Coutts, A., Boyd, L., & Aughey, R. (2010). The validity and reliability of GPS units for measuring distance in team sport specific running patterns. *International Journal of Sports Physiology and Performance, 5*, 328–341.

Johnston, R., Watsford, M., Pine, M., Spurrs, R., Murphy, A., & Pruyn, E. (2012). The validity and reliability of 5-Hz global positioning system units to measure team sport movement demands. *Journal of Strength & Conditioning Research, 26*(3), 758–765.

Jones, A., Bentham, G., Foster, C., Hillsdon, M., & Panter, J. (2007). *Tackling obesities: Future choices – obesogenic environments – evidence review*. London: Government Office for Science.

Kempton, T., Sullivan, C., Bilsborough, J., Cordy, J., & Coutts, A. (2015). Match-to-match variation in physical activity and technical skill measures in professional Australian Football. *Journal of Science and Medicine in Sport, 18*, 109–113.

Kirtland, K., Porter, D., Addy, C., Neet, M., Williams, J., Sharpe, P., … Ainsworth, B. (2003). Environmental measures of physical activity support: Perception versus reality. *American Journal of Preventive Medicine, 24*(4), 323–331.

Krenn, P., Mag, D., Titze, S., Oja, P., Jones, A., & Ogilvie, D. (2011). Use of global positioning systems to study physical activity and the environment. *American Journal of Preventive Medicine, 41*(5), 508–515.

MacLeod, H., Morris, J., Nevill, A., & Sunderland, C. (2009). The validity of a non-differential global positioning system for assessing player movement patterns in field hockey. *Journal of Sports Sciences, 27*(2), 121–128.

Macutkiewicz, D., & Sunderland, C. (2011). The use of GPS to evaluate activity profiles of elite women hockey players during match-play. *Journal of Sports Sciences, 29*(9), 967–973.

Maddison, R., Jiang, Y., Hoorn, S., Exeter, D., Mhurchu, C., & Dorey, E. (2010). Describing patterns of physical activity in adolescents using global positioning systems and accelerometry. *Pediatric Exercise Science, 22*, 392–407.

Maddison, R., & Mhurchu, C. (2009). Global positioning system: A new opportunity in physical activity measurement. *International Journal of Behavioral Nutrition and Physical Activity, 6*(73). doi:10.1186/1479–5868–6-73.

Malone, J., Michele, R., Morgans, R., Burgess, D., Morton, J., & Drust, B. (2015). Seasonal training-load quantification in elite English Premier League soccer players. *International Journal of Sports Physiology and Performance, 10*, 489–497.

Manzi, V., Bovenzi, A., Impellizzeri, M., Carminati, I., & Castagna, C. (2013). Individual training-load and aerobic-fitness variables in Premiership soccer players during the precompetitive season. *Journal of Strength & Conditioning Research, 27*(3), 631–636.

Matthews, C., Hagstromer, M., Pober, D., & Bowles, H. (2012). Best practices for using physical activity monitors in population-based research. *Medicine and Science in Sport and Exercise, 44*(Suppl. 1), S68-S76.

Mavandadi, S., Dimitrov, S., Feng, S., Yu, F., Sikora, U., Yaglidere, O., … Ozcan, A. (2012). Distributed medical image analysis and diagnosis through crowd-sourced games: A malaria case study. *PloS One, 7*(5), e37245.

Miller, H., Tribby, C., Brown, B., Smith, K., Werner, C., Wolf, J., … Oliveira, M. (2015). Public transit generates new physical activity: Evidence from individual GPS and accelerometer data before and after light rail construction in a neighborhood of Salt Lake City, Utah, USA. *Health & Place, 36*, 8–17.

National Geographic Society. (2016). *GIS (geographic information system)*. In *Encyclopedia.* Retrieved from http://nationalgeographic.org/encyclopedia/geographic-information-system-gis/.

Nguyen, D., Lecoultre, V., Sunami, Y., & Schutz, Y. (2013). Assessment of physical activity and energy expenditure by GPS combined with accelerometry in real-life conditions. *Journal of Physical Activity and Health, 10*, 880–888.

Nielsen, R., Cederholm, P., Buist, I., Sorensen, H., Lind, M., & Rasmussen, S. (2013). Can GPS be used to detect deleterious progression in training volume among runners? *Journal of Strength & Conditioning Research, 27*(6), 1471–1478.

Oliver, M., Badland, H., Mavoa, S., Duncan, M., & Duncan, S. (2010). Combining GPS, GIS, and accelerometry: Methodological issues in the assessment of location and intensity of travel behaviors. *Journal of Physical Activity and Health, 7*, 102–108.

Oreskovic, N., Goodman, E., Park, E., Robinson, A., & Winickoff, J. (2015). Design and implementation of a physical activity intervention to enhance children's use of the built environment (the CUBE study). *Contemporary Clinical Trials, 40*, 172–179.

Oreskovic, N., Winickoff, J., Perrin, J., Robinson, A., & Goodman, E. (2016). A multimodal counseling-based adolescent physical activity intervention. *Journal of Adolescent Health*, In press.

Patten, M. (2014). The role of theory in research. In M. Patten (Ed.), *Understanding research methods: An overview of the essentials* (9th ed., pp. 27–29). Glendale, CA: Pyrczak Publishing.

Pew Research Center. (2015). *The smartphone difference*. Retrieved from www.pewinternet.org/2015/04/01/us-smartphone-use-in-2015/

Quigg, R., Reeder, A., Gray, A., Waters, D., & Holt, A. (2013). Using GPS units and accelerometers to evaluate the effect of playground upgrades on the amount of child physical activity. *Australian Parks and Leisure, 16*(1), 21–26.

Ranard, B., Ha, Y., Meisel, Z., Asch, D., Hill, S., Becker, L., … Merchant, R. (2014). Crowdsourcing: Harnessing the masses to advance health and medicine, a systematic review. *Journal of General Internal Medicine, 29*(1), 187–203.

Rodriguez, D., Brown, A., & Troped, P. (2005). Portable global positioning units to complement accelerometry-based physical activity monitors. *Medicine and Science in Sport and Exercise, 37*(11 (Suppl.)), S572–S581.

Schlatter, B., & Hurd, A. (2005). Geocaching: 21st-century hide-and-seek. *Journal of Physical Education, Recreation & Dance, 76*(7), 28–32.

Seidl, D., Jankowski, P., & Tsou, M.-H. (2016). Privacy and spatial pattern preservation in masked GPS trajectory data. *International Journal of Geographical Information Science, 30*(4), 785–800.

Smith, J., Moran, M., & Foley, J. (2013). Effect of GPS feedback on lactate threshold pacing in intercollegiate distance runners. *International Journal of Exercise Science, 6*(1), 74–80.

Troped, P., Oliveira, M., Matthews, C., Cromley, E., Melly, S., & Craig, B. (2008). Prediction of activity mode with global positioning system and accelerometer data. *Medicine and Science in Sport and Exercise, 40*(5), 972–978.

Troped, P., Saunders, R., Pate, R., Reininger, B., Ureda, J., & Thompson, S. (2001). Associations between self-reported and objective physical environmental factors and use of a community rail-trail. *Preventative Medicine, 32*, 191–200.

Troped, P., Wilson, J., Matthews, C., Cromley, E., & Melly, S. (2010). The built environment and location-based physical activity. *American Journal of Preventive Medicine, 38*(4), 429–438.

Webber, S., & Porter, M. (2009). Monitoring mobility in older adults using global positioning system (GPS) watches and accelerometers: A feasibility study. *Journal of Aging and Physical Activity, 17*, 455–467.

Wheeler, B., Cooper, A., Page, A., & Jago, R. (2010). Greenspace and children's physical activity: A GPS/GIS analysis of the PEACH project. *Preventative Medicine, 51*, 148–152.

8 Health wearable devices and physical activity promotion

Nan Zeng and Zan Gao

Nowadays, physical activity (PA) monitoring devices are increasingly popular, with commercially available wearable activity monitors and trackers—hereafter referred to as health wearables—representing a rapidly growing health-focused industry. Health wearables typically cost US$100–250 , making these devices relatively cheap compared to research-grade accelerometers (often ≥US$250). In fact, approximately 3.3 million health wearable devices were sold between April 2013 and March 2014 in the United States—representing a sales growth of over 500% as compared to the previous year (Danova, 2014). By 2018, almost 60 million health wearables will be in use worldwide (Sullivan, 2014). The popularity of such devices has risen as they are affordable, stylish, and useful.

Generally speaking, health wearables (e.g., fitness wristbands and sport watches) use sensors to help users automatically track and set PA-related goals (e.g., calories burned, step counts, distance traveled, etc.), sleep, diet, and other behaviors so as to optimize health (Almalki, Gray, & Sanchez, 2015). In early 2016, Samsung showcased an innovative technology called WELT, a smart wearable healthcare belt offering consumers a more discrete way of using smart sensor technology to monitor health. WELT is capable of recording the user's waist size, eating habits, step counts, and inactive time (e.g., sitting). A similar smart belt, introduced by Belty, contains integrated artificial intelligence to promote a healthy lifestyle. For example, while walking, Belty can increase your walking pace through rhythmic sounds. Currently, an interactive helmet, the Open Heart Helmet, is being developed by the Exertion Games Laboratory. This helmet provides a visual of real-time heart rate data—an effective approach for cyclists to monitor their PA intensity.

To facilitate tracking, many health wearables wirelessly connect to free mobile- and Internet-based applications which provide users immediate feedback and the ability to store long-term PA information (e.g., stairs climbed, heart rate, active time, etc., see Table 8.1 and Figure 8.1; Cadmus-Bertram, Marcus, Patterson, Parker, & Morey, 2015; Lyons, Lewis, Mayrsohn, & Rowland, 2014). The capability of health wearables to upload health statistics to mobile and Internet-based applications allows health wearables to promote self-regulation via the tracking of health metrics (e.g. steps taken, calories burned, etc.) in addition to facilitating social support among connected users of these applications—aiding

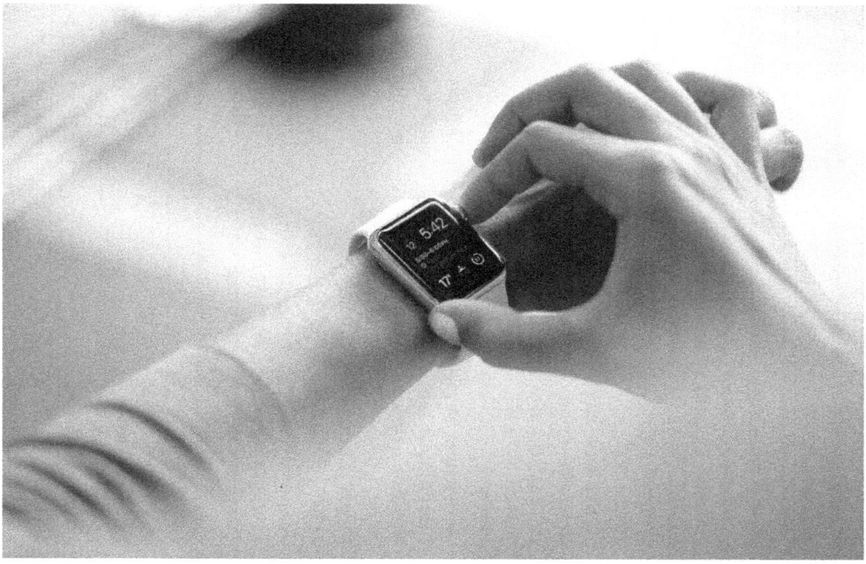

Figure 8.1 The use of a smart watch in tracking.
Source: pixabay.com.

wearers to achieve their fitness and health goals (Evenson, Goto, & Furberg, 2015; Lyons et al., 2014).

To date, health wearable devices have been widely employed to improve overall well-being in a variety of ways. Health wearable-based interventions (e.g., studies employing Fitbits, Apple Watches, Microsoft Bands, etc.) are used for self-evaluation, self-monitoring, self-reinforcement, and goal setting to increase PA with the aim of promoting health/wellness among various populations including children and adolescents, young adults, older adults, and patients (Cadmus-Bertram et al., 2015; Michie et al., 2011; Wang et al., 2015). These increasingly advanced devices enable the wearers to improve their health outcomes by constantly monitoring their bodily responses to PA, with most users believing health wearable technology has enhanced their lives (Michie et al., 2011). A national telephone survey conducted by the Pew Research Center's Internet and American Life Project in 2012 found that 69% of U.S. adults keep track of at least one health indicator such as weight, diet, PA participation, or disease symptoms for themselves, family members, or friends using journals, spreadsheets, and/or mobile devices. Notably, among those who tracked at least one health behavior or condition, 21% reported they used modern technology, such as health wearables, to track their health data. Finally, in a study by Fox and Duggan (2013), 46% of health wearable users indicated that the use of trackers had changed their overall approach to maintaining their health or the health

Table 8.1 Selected devices and descriptions

Device	*Model*	*Reference price*	*Display type/ compatibility*	*Activity type*	*Parameters measured*	*Other possible tracking*	*Battery life*
Fitbit	Surge	$249.99	Sports watch; built-in GPS; Windows, Mac, Android, iOS, Web	Running, hiking, weights, elliptical, spinning, workout, walking, circuit training	Active time, steps, heart rate, distance traveled, calories burned, floors climbed, heart rate zones	Sleep patterns, exercise history, historical stats, diet, weight, balance	About 5 days with continuous heart rate; 5 hours with GPS
Fitbit	Charge HR	$119.99	Wrist band; no GPS; Windows, Mac, Android, iOS, Web	Running, walking, outdoor bike, elliptical, sport, aerobic workout	Active time, steps, heart rate, distance traveled, calories burned, floors climbed	Sleep patterns, exercise history, historical stats	Up to 5 days
Apple	38 mm	$299	Sports watch; Mac, iOS	Outdoor/indoor run, walk, cycle, elliptical, rower, stair stepper, other	Active time, steps, heart rate, distance traveled, calories burned, floors climbed, heart rate zones	Sitting time, sleep patterns, exercise history, historical stats, diet, weight, balance	6.5 hours for workout, up to 18 hours for normal use
Jawbone	UP4	$149.99	Wrist band; Windows, Mac, Android, iOS, Web	Running, walking, weights, bike, elliptical, cardio, zumba, cross train, stationary	Active time, steps, heart rate, distance traveled, calories burned, pace, intensity	Sleep patterns, exercise history, historical stats, diet, weight	Up to 7 days
TomTom	Multi-Sport Cardio	$189.99	Sports watch; built-in GPS; Windows, Mac, Android, iOS, Web	Running, cycling, swimming, treadmill, freestyle	Active time, heart rate (workout only), distance traveled, calories burned, heart rate zones, speed/pace, elevation	None	Up to 8 hours (GPS+HR), up to 10 hours (GPS), up to 10 days for normal use

Microsoft Band	2	$174.99	Wrist band; built-in GPS; Windows, Mac, Android, iOS, Web	Running, biking, explore, golf, exercise, guided workouts	Active time, steps, heart rate, distance traveled, calories burned, floors climbed, heart rate zones	Sleep quality, exercise history, historical stats	Up to 48 hours
Garmin	Vivoactive	$169.99	Sports watch; Windows, Mac, Android, iOS, Web	Running, walking, swimming, cycling, lifting	Active time, steps, heart rate, distance traveled, calories burned, pace, elevation	Sleep quality, exercise history, historical stats	3 weeks of battery life with 10 hours of GPS tracking
Polar	M400	$179.95	Sports watch; built-in GPS; Windows, Mac, Android, iOS, Web	Running, crossfit, strength, cycling, other indoor/ outdoor	Active time, steps, heart rate, distance traveled, calories burned, heart rate zones, pace	Exercise history, historical stats	Up to 8 hours (GPS+HR), 24 days in time mode with daily activity monitoring
Mio	Fuse	$129	Sports watch; Android, iOS	Running, walking, cycling, hiking, biking	Active time, steps, heart rate, distance traveled, calories burned, heart rate zones, pace/speed	Sleep patterns, exercise history, historical stats	Up to 7 days with 1 hour of workout time per day
Misfit	Shine	$69.99	Wrist band; Android, iOS	Basketball, tennis, swim, soccer, cycling, running, walking, yoga, dancing	Steps, distance traveled, calories burned	Sleep patterns, exercise history, historical stats, diet, weight	Up to 6 months (uses coin cell battery)

of people for whom they provide care, and 34% declared that tracking activity has affected decisions about how to treat an illness or condition. Stated simply, health wearable devices have potential benefits for positive health behavior change. Therefore, it comes as no surprise that health wearable devices are a major wellness trend. This chapter will review the literature regarding health wearables in evaluating PA behavior as well as implementing PA plans. Furthermore, data collection, processing, and reporting will be discussed. Finally, evidence concerning the application of health wearables in PA and health promotion in various populations and settings will be presented.

Wearable devices in assessing and promoting PA

Current techniques to assess PA and sedentary behavior can be classified as direct observation, self-reported instruments, and motion sensors. Although direct observation is regarded as the gold standard in measuring PA behavior (Sirard & Pate, 2001), this technique may not be feasible in many situations because of expectancy bias, observation effect, and even participant privacy concerns (Liggett, Gray, Parnell, McGee, & McKenzie, 2012). Additionally, self-reported instruments have some weaknesses including measurement error and recall bias, failure to assess one or more dimensions of behavior, and inability to assess some activities (Prince et al., 2008). Moreover, some questionnaires are not recommended to be used with children 10 or 11 years of age or younger as children often lack the required cognitive skills needed to complete the questionnaires, leading to inaccurate reporting of PA behaviors (Sallis, 2010). Consequently, objective assessment tools such as health wearable devices with built-in motion sensors are increasingly being used to evaluate PA behaviors among various populations.

In recent years, using health wearables to evaluate PA has become increasingly accepted in observational and experimental research. Advances in the technology of health wearable devices provide professionals and researchers a variety of PA measurement options to assess multiple health-related outcomes. For instance, pairing devices with their associated mobile applications could help track physiological responses to PA such as heart rate, energy expenditure, and other health-related indicators like food consumption or sleep quality indices. Indeed, self-monitoring with health wearables permits individuals to evaluate and regulate their health behaviors and evaluate their progress toward individual wellness goals. In a recent study by Case et al. (2015), researchers gauged the accuracy of smartphone applications and wearable devices compared with direct observation of step counts. Eighteen healthy adults were required to walk on a treadmill set at 3.0 mph for 500 and 1500 steps while wearing the Flex (Fitbit), the UP24 (Jawbone), the Fuelband (Nike), and a Digi-Walker SW-200 pedometer (Yamax). Meanwhile, each participant carried an iPhone 5s (Apple) simultaneously running 3 iOS applications: Fitbit (Fitbit), Health Mate (Withings), and Moves (ProtoGeo Oy); and a Galaxy S4 (Samsung Electronics) running 1 Android application: Moves (ProtoGeo Oy). Overall, most smartphone applications and health wearable devices were accurate for tracking step counts. The findings may help reinforce individuals' trust in using smartphone applications and health wearable devices to track health behaviors since step counts are often used to derive other measures of PA, such as distance or calories burned.

Clinicians have also begun employing health wearables to measure patients' PA. For instance, Alharbi and associates (2016) conducted research involving 48 cardiac patients and family members who wore Fitbit-Flex and Actigraph simultaneously over four days to monitor daily step counts and minutes of moderate-to-vigorous PA (MVPA). Researchers found Fitbit-Flex had high sensitivity in classifying participants who achieved the recommended PA guidelines—seen as relatively accurate in assessing the achievement of PA recommendations and as useful for monitoring PA in cardiac patients.

It should also be noted that researchers are increasingly interested in the accuracy of using health wearables to track sleep. Baroni and colleagues (2015) utilized the Fitbit Flex to measure sleep parameters longitudinally in a sample of college students for one week at three time points—baseline, post-test, and 3-month follow-up. Unfortunately, the devices did not capture a significant amount of sleep data at baseline, only about 14% of the Fitbit Flexes recorded sleep six or seven nights, and nearly 35% failed to record any sleep data. Similarly, Lillehei, Halcón, Savik, and Reis (2015) reported an unacceptably high volume of missing data (86%) with the use of Fitbit One. As sleep is vital to health, improvements in health wearables' capability to track sleep quality need to be made.

In summary, using health wearable devices to evaluate PA behavior is possible as most health wearables are deemed valid and reliable in monitoring PA—despite these devices' sometimes insufficient ability to track other health metrics such as sleep. That said, some caution must be taken when using these devices for research purposes as some devices may slightly overestimate or underestimate PA behavior. Nonetheless, health wearables are capable of continuously monitoring free-living conditions and providing valuable PA data for all stakeholders to track PA levels.

As a result of their validity and reliability, health wearable devices may aid in the design and implementation of personal PA plans. Frequently, health wearables are used to motivate people to engage in more PA by viewing data and results captured in real time, after which structured PA plans can be developed. Specifically, once an individual has established long-term health goals, they may then consider the various features that different health wearables offer, which are most congruent with their goals. For example, if an individual sets a daily goal of 8000 steps, and only 7000 were achieved by 7:00 p.m., the user might want a health wearable on which they can set reminders for themselves to go for a walk or at least stand up after sitting for a long period. Aside from simply tracking data, the mobile and Internet-based applications associated with health wearable devices can also be used as an easy and practical way to increase PA participation by encouraging peer interaction and motivation through PA contests and games. For instance, the first person to reach a PA milestone (e.g., 10,000 daily steps) every day for one week will be awarded a certain prize via the application. In this manner, wearers can compete with and support friends, family, colleagues, and even strangers as they work toward a common PA goal and share their accomplishments—motivating one another to engage in greater PA. In fact, many mobile and Internet-based apps are specially designed to enable users to easily post PA outcomes such as exercise time, distance and calories on social media platforms like Facebook and Twitter.

Health wearable devices are also a convenient tool to improve overall well-being in the workplace—encouraging employees to plan and participate in PA at work, which can positively impact productivity (Brown, 2014). For example, health wearables can remind employees to go for a "walk meeting" to log extra steps or to plan to hit the gym for 30 minutes to avoid fatigue caused by spending most of the day sitting in front of the screen. In this situation, the health wearables make workplace wellness more efficient and practical for full-time employees by eliminating the need to track activity manually. Moreover, health wearables, used in conjunction with wellness challenge platforms, can bring employees together to increase PA engagement and boost morale by encouraging staff to support each other and make more connections on individual and team PA goals (Brown, 2014). For an international organization, these health wearable devices have the added benefit of engaging and connecting staff all over the world—helping a large number of individuals live more active, healthier lives.

As mentioned previously, selection of a health wearable is crucial. While some health wearables are more basic, measuring metrics such as step counts, calories burned, and distance traveled, others employ more advanced options, giving the user crucial feedback on training progress when assessing physiological variables such as heart rate and allowing logging of food (Figure 8.2). For instance, if an individual is hoping to qualify for a marathon, this individual may want to choose a health wearable that measures heart rate (e.g., Fitbit Surge and TomTom) allowing them to plan training runs to be completed within certain heart rate ranges. Conversely, an individual desiring to improve their golf skill should seek out health wearables capable of conducting golf swing analytics (e.g., Microsoft Band). Nonetheless, if an individual is simply striving to increase daily PA participation, a health wearable with only step counts and distance traveled will likely suffice (e.g., Misfit Xiaomi Band) (Havey, 2015).

Whatever the PA goal, however, health wearables offer numerous features—akin to those reviewed above—which can aid individuals in the development and implementation of a PA plan capable of aiding progress toward personal PA goals. In fact, research has demonstrated health wearable use is effective in motivating participants to implement exercise regimens and not simply as a device used to just set goals. Wearers suggested that they often relied on the data (e.g., checklists and exercise history) offered by health wearables to keep them motivated during training, and that reviewing the device's PA feedback engendered a sense of satisfaction and motivation (Baker & Mutrie, 2005). In this manner, health wearables reduce the day-to-day variation in PA participation and aid individuals in implementing plans to achieve long-term health goals. Moreover,

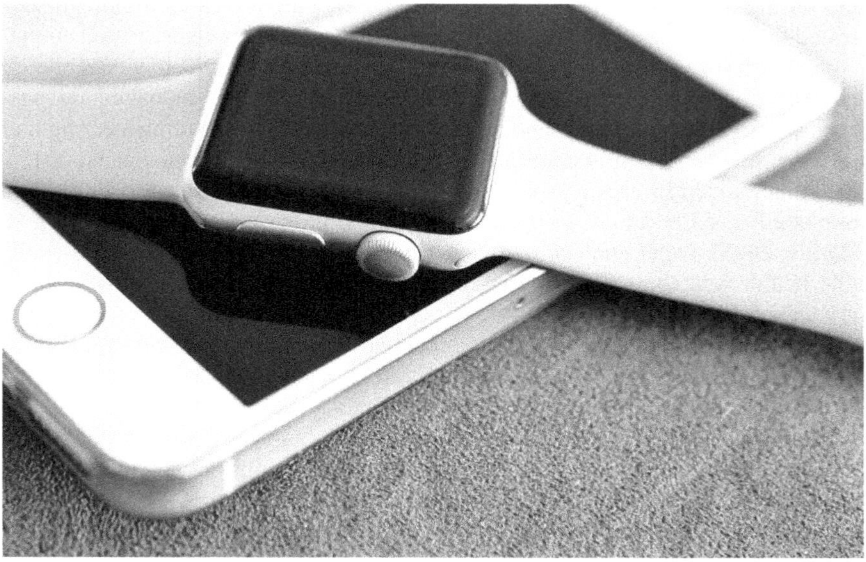

Figure 8.2 Synchronizing a smart watch with a smartphone.
Source: pixabay.com.

the mobile and Internet-based applications associated with health wearables allow for the tracking of sleep quantity and quality—promoting more restful sleep habits—and food logs to facilitate weight loss (Havey, 2015). Finally, statistics regarding PA, diet, and sleep can then be uploaded onto social media platforms where friends and family can support these healthy changes, thereby increasing the likelihood an individual will stay committed to their PA plan (Havey, 2015). Therefore, health wearables users should take advantage of these devices to help design and implement their PA plans.

Health wearable devices and different PA intensities

Generally, PA can be quantified according to intensity (how hard), duration (how long), frequency (how often), and type (e.g., walking, running, swimming, etc.) (Hills, Mokhtar, & Byrne, 2014). Presently, research-grade accelerometer-based activity monitors, such as the ActiGraph and Actical, are the most common devices used to objectively measure free-living PA and sedentary behavior among various populations. There is, however, a paucity of evidence regarding the accuracy and precision of commercially available health wearable devices (i.e., Fitbit, Jawbone Up, TomTom Sport Watch, etc.) in free-living settings, with most of these studies being conducted in highly controlled laboratory settings. For example, one study examined the accuracy of the Fitbit classic wireless activity tracker in assessing energy expenditure during a treadmill test and during a simulated free-living PA routine of nine activities. Findings suggested that, when worn on the hip, the Fitbit significantly underestimated energy expenditure for most activities, indicating the variability in this device's energy expenditure measurements may be problematic for weight management programs as accurate energy expenditure estimates are crucial for implementing and tracking the energy deficit necessary to promote weight loss (Sasaki et al., 2015). A similar underestimation was observed for step counts when the Fitbit was employed in older adults completing two walking trials (Phillips, Petroski, & Markis, 2015). Other studies involving a greater number of commercially available health wearables in both free-living and laboratory conditions have been conducted (Figure 8.3).

Ferguson and colleagues (2015) compared the performance of seven commercial health wearables (Fitbit One, Fitbit Zip, Jawbone Up, Misfit Shine, Nike Fuelband, Striiv Smart Pedometer, and Withings Pulse) and two research-grade accelerometers (BodyMedia SenseWear, and ActiGraph GT3X+) during 48 hours of free-living conditions. Findings indicated that most commercially available health wearables showed strong validity for step counts and sleep time measurements and moderate validity for energy expenditure measurements and time spent in MVPA. However, large differences were observed across devices,

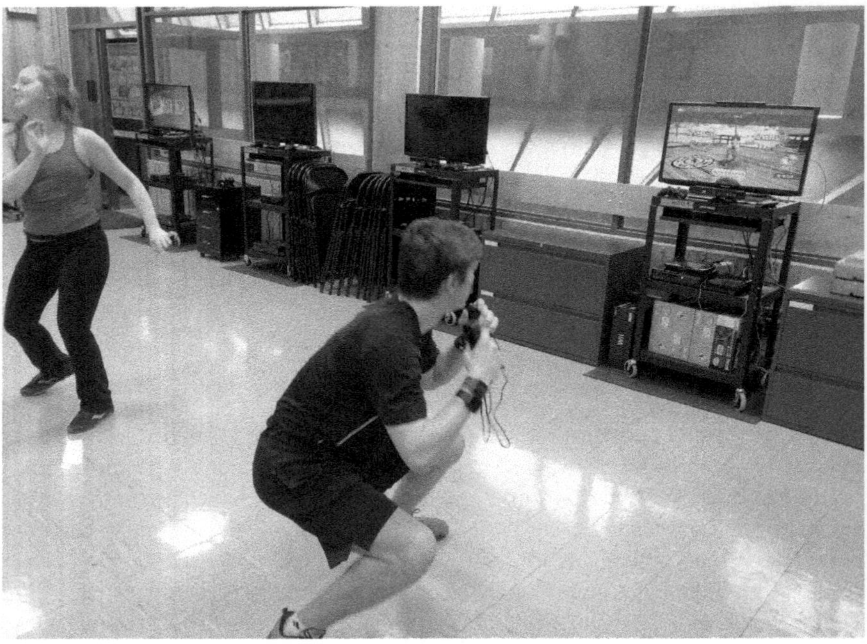

Figure 8.3 Testing smart watches.

Source: Photo by Zan Gao.

with the Fitbit One, Fitbit Zip, and Withings Pulse providing the most accurate intensity readings. Similar results were seen in an earlier study where the Body-Media Fit armband and the Fitbit Zip were observed to be promising tools in measuring energy expenditure (Lee, Kim, & Welk, 2014). Finally, the most recent study in the literature compared nine health wearable devices (ActiGraph GT3X+, activPAL, Fitbit One, GENEactiv, Jawbone Up, LUMOback, Nike Fuelband, Omron pedometer, and Z-Machine) for accuracy during a 24-hour activity measurement. The results showed the research-grade ActiGraph GT3X+ had the closest measurement for sleep and steps, while the most accurate measures of sedentary behavior, light-intensity PA, and MVPA were completed by the LUMOback, GENEactiv, and Fitbit One, respectively (Rosenberger, Buman, Haskell, McConnell, & Carstensen, 2016).

Currently, long-term activity measurement is only possible with research-grade devices, such as the ActiGraph GT3X+ and GT9X. Most of the commercially available health wearable devices are unable to measure the long-term performance of a wide array of health-related outcomes. As evidenced above, there is still a marked lack of measurement standards among commercial health wearable devices for PA measurements as measurement of these PA outcomes is highly varied among devices when tested outside the laboratory (Rosenberger et al., 2016). For instance, light PA is usually defined as 1.1–2.9 METs (i.e., walking less than three miles per hour, bicycling less than five miles per hour, performing light housework, etc.), but not all devices identify these activities as light PA. Indeed, time spent at different PA intensities is highly related to optimal health. Unfortunately, many health wearable devices were not designed with the explicit purpose of measuring PA intensity. Therefore, individuals choosing a health wearable device should consider the PA outcome measures of greatest importance to their health goals, while researchers and health professionals should give thought to the health outcome most important for the purposes of their intervention before selecting a health wearable to implement. Nonetheless, as rapid changes in health wearable technology continue to take place, evaluations of these devices' measurement with more robust criterion measures in free-living settings are warranted as future iterations of health wearables must demonstrate high accuracy and precision in order to be used to guide exercise and improve overall health.

Using wearable devices to collect data, process data, and interpret feedback

Health wearable devices are normally designed to be worn on the body. These devices are typically small and light, allowing users to wear them on the wrist as a wristband or watch (Barcena, Wueest, & Lau, 2014), although some health wearables can also be attached to sports equipment like running shoes, clothes, bikes, etc. Today, commercially available health wearables are equipped with a 3-axis accelerometer that enables movement tracking in every direction, orientation, and rotation. Furthermore, these health wearables usually contain gyroscopic sensors which are responsible for generating the data (Nield, 2016). By reading the real-time data from these sensors and then applying the data to process algorithms, the devices can recognize patterns and identify user's current PA type and intensity (Barcena et al., 2014). Simply put, health wearable devices measure motion, and then transform everyday activities into discrete data that can be stored, analyzed, and used to guide a process of PA behavior change and the promotion of improved health.

Typically, three steps are required when using health wearables to track PA. First, researchers collect PA data. This step requires participants to adhere to proper wear procedures which facilitate the tracking of acceleration and movement frequency, duration, intensity and patterns by health wearables which can then be used to discern PA outcomes, such as the number of flights of stairs climbed and the distance one has traveled during the day. Discerning the preceding outcomes requires the processing of data and represents the next step in the data collection process. Movement information which has been stored in raw form on the health wearable device can then be converted via mobile and Internet-based applications, which display the previously raw movement information using easily interpretable metrics, such as steps per day, calories burned, total active minutes, and sleep quality, among others. Notably, data analysis varies as different devices use different algorithms to calculate the gathered data in a precise and specialized way (Bogdanov, 2015). These differences necessitate once again that consumers and researchers/health professionals consider beforehand the type of PA information most important to them, so as to ensure that the health wearable provides this data. Finally, the third step in the data collection process concerns the interpretation by the user of PA data displayed on mobile/Internet-based apps. Through an examination of the data, individuals can read active versus sedentary time in order to facilitate modifications in their PA behavior, in addition to comparing current PA with previous statistics so as to derive motivation and examine progress toward their desired health goal (Barcena et al., 2014; Nield, 2016).

Today, the vast majority of health wearable devices only perform a data collection function—requiring a separate computing device to allow the user to access the data analysis functions. In order to perform the previously reviewed data interpretation functions, most current health wearable devices synchronize with mobile or Internet-based applications, giving users the ability to upload and interpret the data collected by the devices. Nevertheless, the ways the devices are synced with mobile and Internet-based apps are quite different. For example, Misfit Shine and Fitbit sync via Bluetooth, while health wearables like the Jawbone Up sync with a mobile device via an embedded mini jack to save the device's battery life.

Given the increasing use of health wearables in the collection, analysis, and interpretation of PA and related health metrics, developers of future health wearable devices need to focus on the design of devices which deliver higher precision and more valid data. Increasing the accuracy and validity of these devices is paramount as health wearable users and researchers have reached a point where the collection of PA data is not sufficient. Indeed, an increasing number of individuals want devices that not only can accurately track and interpret PA habits in real time, but which can also provide moment-by-moment feedback that will help users modify their poor health habits and improve their good habits—in order to optimize health and wellbeing.

Application of wearable devices in developing PA interventions

Over the last five years, health wearable technology has fast become a popular accessory. Rapid developments in technology have encouraged the use of health wearable devices (i.e., fitness bands and sport watches) in PA research and have offered new opportunities for promoting healthy lifestyles across diverse populations. Nowadays, commercially available health wearables have become popular devices for objectively assessing PA. These devices typically provide PA feedback to users through the devices' monitor displays or mobile and Internet-based applications to aid in motivating users to increase their PA. That is, these devices offer numerous features (e.g., goal setting, tracking activity over time, reminders and prompts, and social connections) to promote greater PA participation and make being physically active more fun (Beebe & Harris, 2012). Health wearables such as Polar, Fitbit, and Jawbone, among others, are marketed to individuals trying to improve their health and physical fitness. These health wearables promise greater convenience in connecting to social networks, often via mobile device-based applications, and can be effective among various populations as an intervention tool. Therefore, health wearables are of interest for use in scalable PA interventions, as these devices represent a novel and appealing approach to health promotion.

Despite the novelty of health wearable technology, these devices are beginning to be used frequently as a PA intervention tool among various populations. For example, Thorndike et al. (2014) designed a randomized controlled trial (RCT) using Fitbit to promote PA among 104 medical residents. Phase 1 was a 6-week RCT, with participants assigned to an intervention group receiving a traditional Fitbit with an external display or a control group given a Fitbit without an external display. Phase 2 was a 6-week non-randomized trial immediately following Phase 1 during which all participants wore traditional Fitbits. During both phases, median steps/day, blood pressure, high-density lipoprotein (HDL) cholesterol, and proportion of days participants wore the health wearable were measured. Findings indicated that, although the health wearable intervention did not have a major impact on PA or health outcomes, the high implementation rates by physicians and the modest changes in steps, blood pressure, and HDL among patients suggested that more intensive wellness programs using health wearables might have potential in promoting healthier lifestyles among clinical populations. Similarly, a RCT by Thompson et al. (2014) examined whether offering a health wearable capable of providing feedback regarding PA via an external display, while concurrently using Go4Life wellness education material for PA counseling, could promote health among 49 sedentary and overweight older adults. Researchers observed no significant change among intervention participants for PA, weight loss, glucose, lipids, blood pressure, or body fat, indicating alternative approaches to exercise counseling may be warranted for older adults to improve health. In addition, health wearable interventions have also taken place among women and overweight/obese adults.

Cadmus-Bertram et al. (2015) evaluated the feasibility and preliminary efficacy of integrating the Fitbit and its associated Internet-based app into a PA intervention for 51 post-menopausal women. Findings indicated the intervention group (Fitbit and Internet-based-based self-monitoring intervention) to have significantly increased MVPA and steps minutes/week compared to non-significant increases in the control group (only received a standard pedometer). Additionally, the Fitbit was well accepted in this sample of women and associated with increased PA at post-intervention. In a 6-week RCT among African American college women, Melton and colleagues (2016) examined the effectiveness of the Jawbone UP platform to promote PA and sleep quality versus a comparison group using the MyFitnessPal smartphone application. Interestingly, at the 8-week follow-up, the intervention group experienced a significantly greater decrease in step counts versus the comparison group, with neither group demonstrating any significant changes in sleep quality at the 6-week post-test or 8-week follow-up. Findings indicated that among African American female college students, there is no evidence to suggest health wearables were effective at improving PA participation or sleep quality—necessitating further study to discern whether gender or cultural differences act as mediating factors. Finally, Wang and colleagues (2015) assessed the utility of the Fitbit and short message service (SMS) text-messaging prompts to increase PA in overweight and obese adults. Sixty-seven participants were randomized to an intervention group receiving a Fitbit One in addition to three daily SMS-based PA prompts or to a comparison group receiving only the use of the Fitbit One. Findings showed the intervention group to have significantly higher steps per day (1266 steps), minutes/week of MVPA (17.8 minutes), and total PA per week (38.3 minutes), with the only significant increase among the comparison group being a 4.3 minutes/week increase in MVPA at the 6-week follow-up. Study findings suggested that Fitbit One was able to promote a small increase in MVPA.

Overall, the market for health wearable devices continues to grow in popularity, and the potential for using these devices to promote health is great (Figure 8.4). Indeed, health wearable devices provide opportunities to overcome limitations of self-reported PA and may lead to more effective behavior change (Hickey & Freedson, 2016). Although evidence regarding the effectiveness of health wearable devices in developing effective PA interventions is inconclusive, studies have demonstrated that these devices do hold great potential in improving PA and promoting healthier lifestyles in a diverse array of populations. While some preliminary work has been conducted using commercially available health wearable devices, more studies are warranted to better understand the possible effects of these devices when used for developing efficacious PA interventions in the near future.

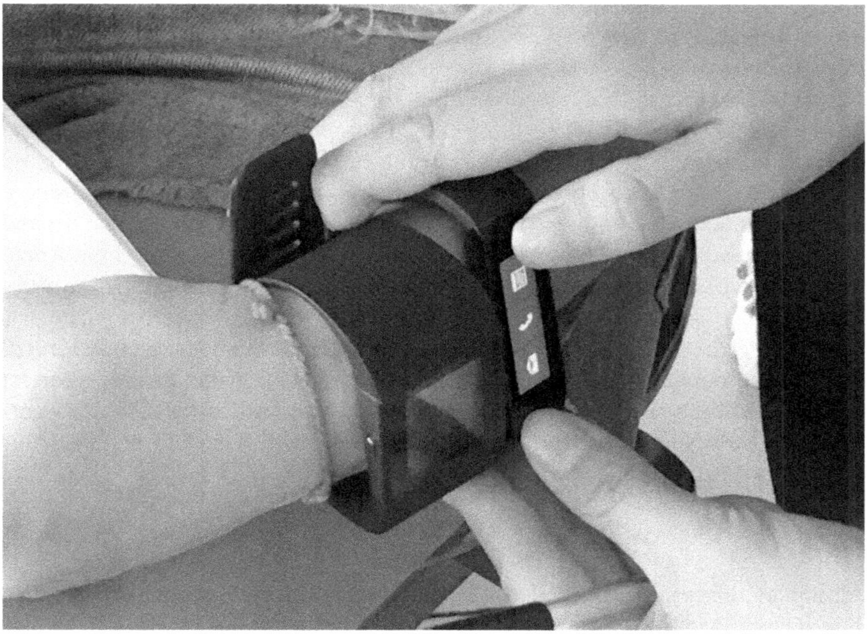

Figure 8.4 Validation of smart watches.
Source: Photo by Zan Gao.

Practical implications

To date, health wearables play a significant role in health promotion. These devices offer individuals the ability to track and modify their health-related outcomes, such as PA and sleep patterns, as well as guide researchers and health professionals in the design and implementation of health promotion interventions seeking to promote PA behavior change. Nevertheless, using health wearables to effectively promote health behavior change is currently facing challenges which must be considered in future studies. To begin with, there is a paucity of evidence regarding the accuracy and precision of health wearables in free-living conditions. Although research-grade accelerometers (e.g., ActiGraph and Actical) have been well investigated in tracking PA and step counts during free-living conditions, commercially available health wearables (e.g., fitness wristbands and sport watches) capable of tracking metrics such as step counts, energy expenditure, heart rate, or sleep quality, among others, have not been well validated (Powell, Landman, & Bates, 2014). It is important to note that recently ActiGraph has produced a watch called ActiGraph Link that has an app function on mobile devices, which is convenient for research and daily use. Second, convincing an individual who has never previously considered participating in health or fitness activities to use a health wearable to track and assess their progress toward health goals is a challenge. Indeed, despite the initial novelty of health wearables to new users, the attrition rate for use may be high. According to one survey (N=6223), at least one-third of owners who purchased a health wearable abandon their devices within 4 to 6 months (Ledger & McCaffrey, 2014). Notably, the individuals most likely to stop using these devices are those who are in poorer health but who need health behavior change the most. Finally, a wearable device must be affordable, so that an individual is able to purchase and use the device to implement a PA plan that is meant to achieve the desired health outcome. However, some devices, such as the Fitbit Surge and the Apple Watch, can cost hundreds of dollars. This is a notable challenge as the individuals most likely to benefit from using these devices to self-regulate PA behavior for the purposes of improving health are most likely to be underserved, low-income populations (Patel, Asch, & Volpp, 2015). In the coming years, a concerted effort needs to be made to overcome these limitations if health wearables are truly able to achieve their full potential with regard to helping individuals live healthier and more active lives.

References

Alharbi, M., Bauman, A., Neubeck, L., & Gallagher, R. (2016). Validation of Fitbit-Flex as a measure of free-living physical activity in a community-based phase III cardiac rehabilitation population. *European Journal of Preventive Cardiology, 23*(14), 476–485.

Almalki, M., Gray, K., & Sanchez, F. M. (2015). The use of self-quantification systems for personal health information: Big Data management activities and prospects. *Health Information Science and Systems, 3*(1), 1–11.

Baker, G., & Mutrie, N. (2005). *Are pedometers useful motivational tools for increasing walking in sedentary adults?* Paper presented at Walk21-VI "Everyday Walking Culture." The 6th International Conference on Walking in the 21st Century, September 22–23, 2005, Zurich, Switzerland.

Barcena, M. B., Wueest, C., & Lau, H. (2014). *How safe is your quantified self?* Mountain View, CA: Symantec.

Baroni, A., Bruzzese, J. M., Di Bartolo, C. A., & Shatkin, J. P. (2015). Fitbit Flex: An unreliable device for longitudinal sleep measures in a non-clinical population. *Sleep Breath, 20*(2), 853–854.

Beebe, L. H., & Harris, R. F. (2012). Using pedometers to document physical activity in patients with schizophrenia spectrum disorders: A feasibility study. *Journal of Psychosocial Nursing and Mental Health Services, 50*(2), 44–49.

Bogdanov, V. (2015). *How wearables work: Fitness bracelets and activity trackers.* Retrieved from http://intersog.com/blog/tech-tips/how-wearables-work-fitness-bands-and-activity-trackers/.

Brown, J. (2014). *How can wearables improve overall wellbeing?* Retrieved from www.shapeup.com/how-can-wearables-improve-overall-wellbeing/.

Cadmus-Bertram, L. A., Marcus, B. H., Patterson, R. E., Parker, B. A., & Morey, B. L. (2015). Randomized trial of a Fitbit-based physical activity intervention for women. *American Journal of Preventive Medicine, 49*(3), 414–418.

Case, M. A., Burwick, H. A., Volpp, K. G., & Patel, M. S. (2015). Accuracy of smartphone applications and wearable devices for tracking physical activity data. *The Journal of the American Medical Association, 313*(6), 625–626.

Danova, T. (2014). Just 3.3 million fitness trackers were sold in the US in the past year. *Business Insider*. Retrieved from www.businessinsider.com/33-million-fitness-.

Evenson, K. R., Goto, M. M., & Furberg, R. D. (2015). Systematic review of the validity and reliability of consumer-wearable activity trackers. *International Journal of Behavioral Nutrition and Physical Activity, 12*(1), 1–22.

Ferguson, T., Rowlands, A. V., Olds, T., & Maher, C. (2015). The validity of consumer-level, activity monitors in healthy adults worn in free-living conditions: A cross-sectional study. *International Journal of Behavioral Nutrition and Physical Activity, 12*(1), 1–9.

Fox, S., & Duggan, M. (2013). *Tracking for health*. Pew Research Center, Pew Internet and American Life Project. Retrieved from www.pewinternet.org/2013/01/28/tracking-for-health/.

Havey, M. L. (2015). The athlete's guide to tracking. Retrieved from https://blog.underarmour.com/devices/activity-trackers/the-athletes-guide-to-tracking/.

Hickey, A. M., & Freedson, P. S. (2016). Utility of consumer physical activity trackers as an intervention tool in cardiovascular disease prevention and treatment. *Progress in Cardiovascular Diseases, 58*(6), 613–619.

Hills, A. P., Mokhtar, N., & Byrne, N. M. (2014). Assessment of physical activity and energy expenditure: An overview of objective measures. *Frontiers in Nutrition, 1*, 1–16.

Ledger, D., & McCaffrey, D. (2014). *How the science of human behavior change offers the secret to long-term engagement*. Retrieved from http://endeavourpartners.net/assets/Wearables-and-the-Science-of-Human-Behavior-Change-EP4.pdf.

Lee, J. M., Kim, Y., & Welk, G. J. (2014). Validity of consumer-based physical activity monitors. *Medicine & Science in Sports & Exercise, 46*(9), 1840–1848.

Liggett, L., Gray, A., Parnell, W., McGee, R., & McKenzie, Y. (2012). Validation and reliability of the New Lifestyles NL-1000 accelerometer in New Zealand preschoolers. *Journal of Physical Activity and Health, 9*(1), 295–300.

Lillehei, A. S., Halcón, L. L., Savik, K., & Reis, R. (2015). Effect of inhaled lavender and sleep hygiene on self-reported sleep issues: A randomized controlled trial. *The Journal of Alternative and Complementary Medicine, 21*(7), 430–438.

Lyons, E. J., Lewis, Z. H., Mayrsohn, B. G., & Rowland, J. L. (2014). Behavior change techniques implemented in electronic lifestyle activity monitors: A systematic content analysis. *Journal of Medical Internet Research, 16*(8), e192.

Melton, B. F., Buman, M. P., Vogel, R. L., Harris, B. S., & Bigham, L. E. (2016). Wearable devices to improve physical activity and sleep: A randomized controlled trial of college-aged African American women. *Journal of Black Studies*, published online before print June 8, 2016.

Michie, S., Ashford, S., Sniehotta, F. F., Dombrowski, S. U., Bishop, A., & French, D. P. (2011). A refined taxonomy of behaviour change techniques to help people change their physical activity and healthy eating behaviours: The CALO-RE taxonomy. *Psychology & Health, 26*(11), 1479–1498.

Moore, L. V., Harris, C. D., Carlson, S. A., Kruger, J., & Fulton, J. E. (2012). Trends in no leisure-time physical activity—United States, 1988–2010. *Research Quarterly for Exercise and Sport, 83*(4), 587–591.

Nield, D. (2016). *How it works: We explain how your fitness tracker measures your daily steps*. Retrieved from www.wareable.com/fitness-trackers/how-your-fitness-tracker-works-1449.

Patel, M. S., Asch, D. A., & Volpp, K. G. (2015). Wearable devices as facilitators, not drivers, of health behavior change. *The Journal of the American Medical Association, 313*(5), 459–460.

Phillips, L. J., Petroski, G. F., & Markis, N. E. (2015). A comparison of accelerometer accuracy in older adults. *Research in Gerontological Nursing, 8*(5), 213–219.

Powell, A. C., Landman, A. B., & Bates, D. W. (2014). In search of a few good apps. *Jama, 311*(18), 1851–1852.

Prince, S. A., Adamo, K. B., Hamel, M. E., Hardt, J., Gorber, S. C., & Tremblay, M. (2008). A comparison of direct versus self-report measures for assessing physical activity in adults: A systematic review. *International Journal of Behavioral Nutrition and Physical Activity, 5*(1), 1.

Rosenberger, M. E., Buman, M. P., Haskell, W. L., McConnell, M. V., & Carstensen, L. L. (2016). Twenty-four hours of sleep, sedentary behavior, and physical activity with nine wearable devices. *Medicine and Science in Sports and Exercise, 48*(3), 457–465.

Sallis, J. F. (2010). Measuring physical activity: Practical approaches for program evaluation in Native American communities. *Journal of Public Health Management and Practice, 16*(5), 404–410.

Sasaki, J. E., Hickey, A., Mavilia, M., Tedesco, J., John, D., Kozey Keadle, S., & Freedson, P. S. (2015). Validation of the Fitbit wireless activity tracker for prediction of energy expenditure. *Journal of Physical Activity and Health, 12*(2), 149–154.

Sirard, J. R., & Pate, R. R. (2001). Physical activity assessment in children and adolescents. *Sports Medicine, 31*(6), 439–454.

Sullivan, M. (2014). *Fitness tracker sales will triple by 2018, then smartwatches take over (report)*. Retrieved from http://venturebeat.com/2014/11/25/fitness-tracker-sales-will-triple-by-2018-then-smartwatches-take-over-report/.

Thompson, W. G., Kuhle, C. L., Koepp, G. A., McCrady-Spitzer, S. K., & Levine, J. A. (2014). "Go4Life" exercise counseling, accelerometer feedback, and activity levels in older people. *Archives of Gerontology and Geriatrics, 58*(3), 314–319.

Thorndike, A. N., Mills, S., Sonnenberg, L., Palakshappa, D., Gao, T., Pau, C. T., & Regan, S. (2014). Activity monitor intervention to promote physical activity of physicians-in-training: Randomized controlled trial. *PloS One, 9*(6), e100251.

Wang, J. B., Cadmus-Bertram, L. A., Natarajan, L., White, M. M., Madanat, H., Nichols, J. F., … & Pierce, J. P. (2015). Wearable sensor/device (Fitbit One) and SMS text-messaging prompts to increase physical activity in overweight and obese adults: A randomized controlled trial. *Telemedicine and e-Health, 21*(10), 782–792.

9 Active video games and physical activity promotion

Zan Gao, Nan Zeng, and Zachary Pope

Sedentary video games have become an increasingly integral part of individuals' lifestyles since their advent in 1972. Presently, nearly three billion hours are spent playing video games by various populations worldwide every week. In the United States, the number of video game players who play at least one hour per day (via consoles and computers) reached a stunning 183 million. Traditionally, video games have been blamed for individuals' sedentary lifestyles, which contribute to extremely high rates of overweight/obesity and associated chronic diseases including diabetes and cardiovascular diseases (Gao & Chen, 2014; Gao, Huang, Liu, & Xiong, 2012).

Despite the negative impact that sedentary video games have on healthy behavior, active video games (AVGs) have great potential to promote physically active lifestyles (Barnett, Cerin, & Baranowski, 2011; Gao, Chen, Pasco, & Pope, 2015). Briefly, AVGs (a.k.a., exergaming) refer to video games that are also a form of exercise. Indeed, the fast growth of AVGs (e.g., Dance Dance Revolution [DDR], Wii Sports/Fit, and Xbox Sports) has led to the development of new interactive exercise strategies, which in turn have had a great impact on field-based physical activity (PA) interventions (Gao et al., 2012; Gao, 2012; Guy, Ratzki-Leewing, & Gwadry-Sridhar, 2011). These games generally capitalize on individuals' interest in computer and video interactions with gaming console-specific PA equipment to promote increased PA and decreased sedentary time (Mears & Hansen, 2009; Primack et al., 2012).

Recently, some AVGs such as DDR, Wii Just Dance, and Kinect Sports have been implemented outside of home and laboratory settings, and are beginning to find their way into schools and community centers as a potential solution to curbing physical inactivity and obesity (Gao et al., 2015). As AVGs have been and continue to be used by many individuals, particularly children and adolescents, it is of critical importance to synthesize research findings derived from laboratory-based and field-based contexts, with the goal of providing meaningful practical implications and recommendations for health professionals and PA specialists. In response, this chapter provides an overview of AVGs and health promotion in various populations (Figure 9.1), followed by a review of the effect AVGs have on PA and health-related outcomes. Additionally, the implementation and effectiveness of AVGs in different contexts, the application of AVGs in

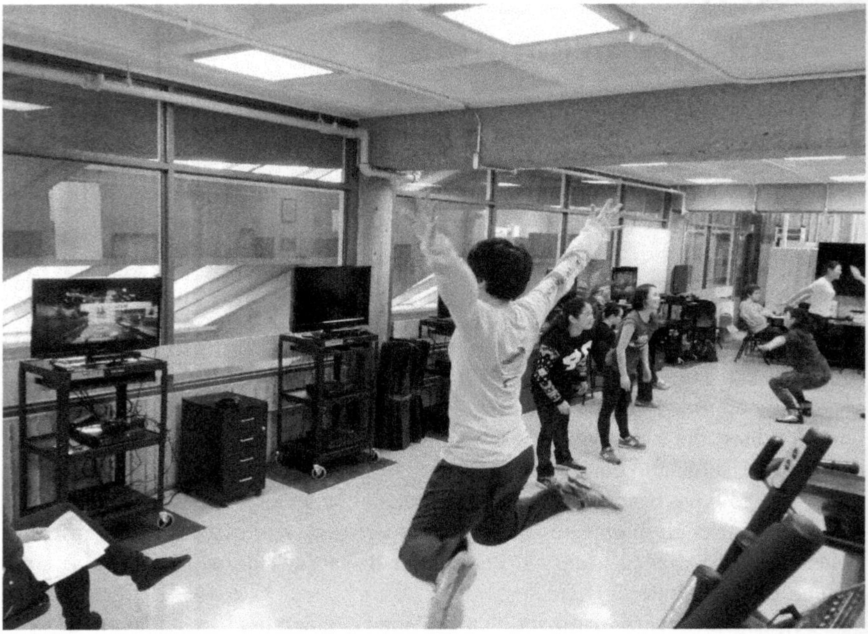

Figure 9.1 Elite athletes playing active video games.
Source: Photo by Zan Gao.

the healthcare field, and the emerging relationship of AVGs and augmented reality video games will be discussed. Finally, the chapter will conclude with practical implications of applying AVGs in interventions promoting PA and health.

Active video games and health promotion in various populations

Regular PA participation makes a significant contribution to healthy body weight among children and adolescents, a satisfactory quality of life in the general adult population, and the maintenance of physical functioning among older adults. Currently, AVGs have emerged as an innovative approach in promoting PA and health. Presently, numerous empirical studies and reviews have completed investigations regarding the effects of AVGs among children and adolescents, adults, and older adults.

Normal weight populations

Children and adolescents

The increasing childhood obesity rate has become a public health concern in the United States. Regular PA participation helps prevent and reduce childhood obesity (McManus & Mellecker, 2012). Hence, AVGs may be used to encourage children and adolescents to develop a physically active lifestyle (Baranowski, 2013; Gao & Podlog, 2012). As a result, AVGs have been implemented in laboratories, homes, schools, and community centers as an innovative solution to promote health and fight obesity among children and adolescents. Indeed, studying the efficacy and effectiveness of AVGs in this youth populations has become a popular research topic over the past decade (Christison & Khan, 2012; Daley, 2009; Gao, 2012). Evidence from these studies proves that AVGs can generate some health benefits among children and adolescents. To date, research studies conducted in laboratory-based settings have documented the positive effects of AVGs on acute energy expenditure (Bailey & McInnis, 2011; Daley, 2009; Foley & Maddison, 2010). For example, it was found that energy expenditure values of DDR were equivalent to 7.0 METs—an intensity classified as a moderate-to-vigorous-intensity level of PA. By contrast, other studies conducted in field-based settings appear to have diverse research results, with some supporting the benefits of AVGs and others indicating no benefit (Baranowski et al., 2012; Gao, Podlog, & Huang, 2013; Graves, Ridgers, & Stratton, 2008; Maddison, Mhurchu, Jull, Prapavessis, & Rodgers, 2007).

Healthy adults and old adults

Although most AVG studies have focused on children and adolescents, a number of research studies targeting adult populations have also been conducted to evaluate the physical, psychological, and cognitive effects of AVGs. Evidence from these studies has provend that AVGs can result in some health benefits (e.g., improving physical fitness, weight loss, and enjoyment) among healthy adults and older adults (Franco, Jacobs, Inzerillo, & Kluzik, 2012; Rendon et al., 2012, Toulotte, Toursel, & Olivier, 2012). To date, the majority of AVG studies in adults were conducted in laboratory-based settings, which observed positive effects of AVGs on outcomes such as energy expenditure, maximal oxygen consumption, heart rate and timed up and go compared to resting values. Additionally, it has been evident that the effects of AVGs on heart rate, maximal oxygen consumption, and energy expenditure were similar to those of traditional PA (Pope, Lee, Li, & Gao, 2016; Zeng, Lee, Pope, Li, & Gao, 2016). Details of such effects of the extant literature will be fully addressed in the following section.

Obese populations

The worldwide prevalence of obesity has increased dramatically over the past 30 years. Given the fact that AVGs have become an increasingly popular activity in which both children and adults can participate, it is necessary to provide an overview of the current evidence regarding the effects of AVGs on health-related outcomes among overweight or obese individuals, with the ultimate goal of offering meaningful practical implications for future research. Overall, evidence concerning the effects of AVGs on physiological and physical indicators is mixed, as some studies have indicated positive results while others have suggested otherwise (e.g., Goldfield et al., 2012; Staiano et al., 2016). Among the positive findings, evidence suggests that AVGs have the potential to attenuate weight gain for overweight or obese youth as AVGs can help children and adolescents be more physically active (Figure 9.2). Further, it has been observed that AVGs can improve children's skill-related fitness and lead to increases in trunk and spine bone mass density among overweight and obese girls. Among the general obese populations, AVGs have demonstrated positive effects on psychological outcomes such as self-efficacy, body image, perceived scholastic competence, and social competence. As was the case for the discussion of healthy populations, details regarding the study of the efficacy and effectiveness of AVGs among obese populations will be illustrated in a lat*er section of this chapter.

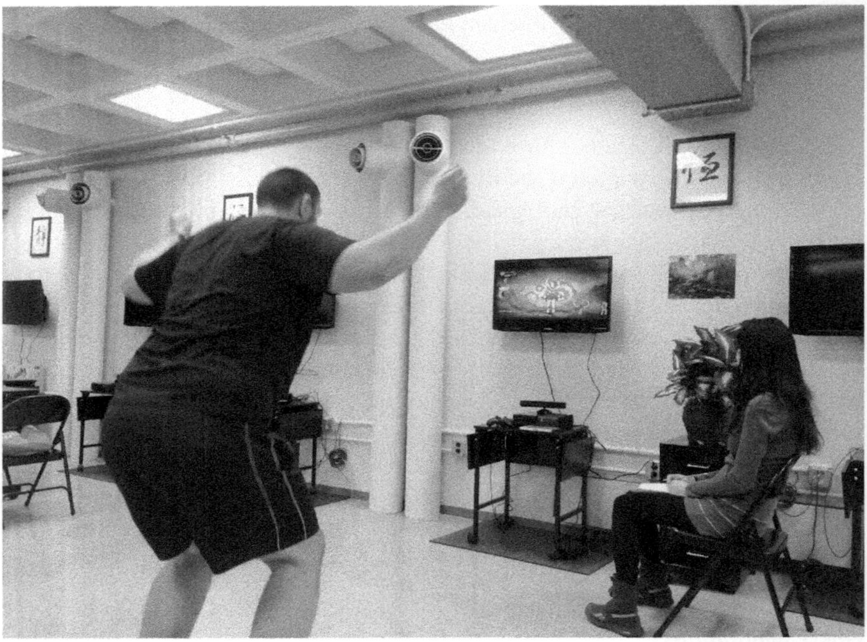

Figure 9.2 Young adults playing active video games.

Source: Photo by Zan Gao.

Effects of active video games on PA and health-related outcomes

Normal weight populations

To determine the effectiveness of AVG on individuals' health-related outcomes, randomized controlled trials and control trials were consulted first when examining the literature. Generally, the intervention dose varied considerably across studies. Explicitly, the intervention duration ranged from 6–52 weeks, with the majority of studies less than 30 weeks in duration. Moreover, the duration of each AVG session ranged from 10–50 minutes, and the frequency varied from 1–5 sessions per week. Notably, given the nature of the AVGs, most empirical studies were conducted with children and adolescents. However, findings of AVG studies with adults were also reviewed.

Physiological and physical effects

Examining the physiological and metabolic effects of AVGs has been the focus of most laboratory-based research (Bailey & McInnis, 2011; Daley, 2009; Foley & Maddison, 2010). Overall, the majority of AVGs have been reported to increase individuals' exercise intensity to a point equivalent to light-to-moderate-intensity PA, as measured by heart rate, oxygen consumption, and rate of perceived exertion in children/adolescents and young adults (Graves et al., 2008; Maddison et al., 2007). Despite these findings, the effects of AVGs varied greatly, due to the nature of different AVGs (Biddiss & Irwin, 2010). Indeed, some AVGs are designed to be more physically demanding than others. For instance, games that actively engage the lower body have higher energy costs due to the involvement of larger muscle mass when compared to games that only engage the upper body (Biddiss & Irwin, 2010). The preceding fact is none too surprising as research shows that only one-third of the 68 Wii Sports and Wii Fit Plus games are capable of promoting moderate-intensity PA. Therefore, the AVGs requiring the use of more muscle mass (e.g., DDR, Wii boxing, Xbox Just Dance) should be encouraged for use in interventions with health promotion objectives.

The effects of home-based AVG intervention on physiological/physical outcomes have yielded mixed findings. Some researchers suggested that AVG interventions had significantly positive effects on individuals' health-related outcomes, such as cardiovascular fitness, body composition, and PA participation. For example, Bethea and colleagues (2012) reported children's cardiovascular fitness was enhanced and maintained after a 30-week DDR intervention. Other researchers asserted that the AVG treatment effects on PA, body mass index (BMI) and body fat favored the AVG (e.g., Eyetoy, Kinect Sport) intervention group over control children (Ni Mhurchu et al., 2008). Working with healthy elderly, Rendon et al. (2012) found that participants in Wii Fit and exercise group had greater improvements in functional balance compared to the control group after an 8-week program. The same was true for Toulotte et al.'s (2012) study, when comparing Wii Fit or Wii Fit plus exercise to a control condition in a 20-week intervention among healthy elderly. However, several studies have reported that AVG interventions have no effect on children's body composition (e.g., BMI, body fat percentage) and PA levels (Baranowski et al., 2012; Madsen, Yen, Wlasiuk, Newman, & Lustig, 2007). For instance, Baranowski et al. (2012) found no differences in accelerometer-determined PA levels between AVG intervention children and sedentary video game control children (Figure 9.3). Franco et al. (2012) also failed to find differences between Wii Fit or Wii Fit plus exercise and control conditions on balance in a short-duration intervention (i.e., 3 weeks).

It is plausible that intervention fidelity may have caused the inconsistency of the findings across studies. Even with a randomized controlled trial design, intervention fidelity may still be a concern. For example, Baranowski et al.'s (2012) study had two major limitations: (1) no instructions or prescriptions on how to be physically active were offered for children; and (2) no home visits and phone calls were performed to ensure the intervention fidelity. These strategies are crucial and need to be used in home-based AVG studies as well as other population-based PA interventions. Hence, the implementation of standardized intervention fidelity procedures across studies presents an important challenge for AVG researchers in the future.

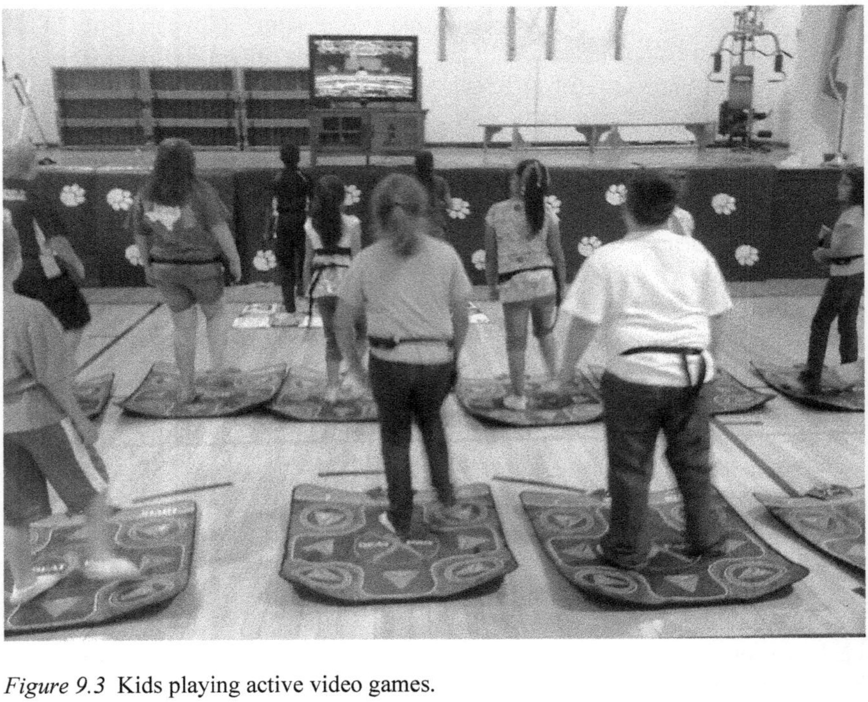

Figure 9.3 Kids playing active video games.

Source: Photo by Zan Gao.

Additionally, the relatively low effectiveness of AVGs used in a non-structured or self-directed manners (e.g., in home settings) for PA promotion among children may result from low self-regulation in children. Explicitly, children are not as adept as adults in the regulation of their thoughts and behaviors while playing AVGs. Indeed, children are not capable of contemplating the purpose of AVGs, how much time to allocate to game play, and what benefits they could acquire from the AVG experiences. Instead, children may be attracted and engaged simply by the appealing features of the games (Figure 9.4). Thus, devising strategies that could make self-directed use of AVGs more successful is a challenge.

Evidence of the effectiveness of school-based AVG interventions are also inconclusive, with the majority of research indicating significantly positive effects (Gao, Hannan, Xiang, Stodden, & Valdez, 2013; Gao et al., 2012; Gao & Xiang, 2014; Sheehan & Katz, 2013) while a few other studies reported the opposite (Gao, Hannon, Newton, & Huang, 2011; Gao, 2012). Specifically, two studies reported that children engaged in significantly more minutes of PA and had improved balance development as a result of AVG play than they did in the traditional physical education programs (Fogel, Miltenberger, Graves, & Koehler, 2010; Sheehan & Katz, 2013). Three other intervention studies also reported positive trends, indicating that AVG interventions significantly improved children's cardiorespiratory fitness and PA over time (Gao, Hannan, Xiang, et al., 2013; Gao et al., 2012; Gao & Xiang, 2014). Conversely, however,

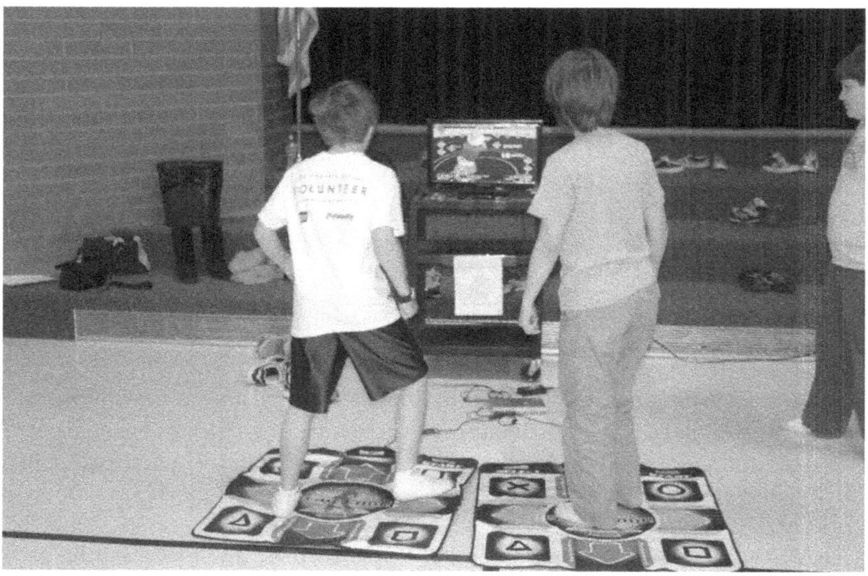

Figure 9.4 Kids playing active video games.

Source: Photo by Zan Gao.

one study found that an AVG intervention performed worse at increasing PA participation and energy expenditure versus a comparison group (Duncan & Staples, 2010).

Finally, evidence suggests playing AVGs does not result in as much PA as traditional sports. Whittman (2010) reported AVGs resulted in greater increased PA levels in children compared to two traditional after-school activities. However, Gao et al. (2011) found adolescents had significantly higher percentages of time in moderate-to-vigorous PA in fitness and football when compared to a DDR unit during physical education classes. Two other studies carried out among elementary school children demonstrated that children's in-class PA levels during the AVG unit were significantly lower than during the fitness or aerobic dance units in physical education classes (Gao, Zhang, & Stodden, 2013; Sun, 2012). Lastly, Miller and colleagues (2013) suggested children's energy expenditure was significantly greater during physical education compared to AVG classes. It is possible the contradictory findings may be attributable to the nature of AVGs (e.g., some games are more active than others), the research design, the target population, instruments, and other confounding factors (e.g., the fidelity of the physical education or AVG programs, familiarity with AVGs). Thus, caution is advised when evaluating these mixed research findings.

While not all AVGs are physically demanding enough to result in health benefits, it is widely acknowledged that AVGs can be a viable replacement for many mundane sedentary behaviors like sedentary video games. Pate (2008) argued that, unlike the 1950s when kids would go out to play if bored, today's societies are enriched by convenient technologies such as video games, the Internet, cellphones, and television. These technologies have enabled people to live a sedentary lifestyle since a young age. Therefore, AVGs, with their exercise utility, are believed to be a substitute for less active forms of entertainment (i.e., computer games), but not as a standalone replacement for traditional PA. Indeed, as AVGs are beginning to be seen with greater frequency in homes, studies have reported AVGs to be naturally replacing individuals' sedentary screen time (Maloney et al., 2008). That said, care must be taken to ensure AVGs do not draw kids away from the traditional physical activities that they already participate in.

Psychosocial effects

The most appealing aspect of AVGs lie in their entertaining or motivating features. It is well documented that many AVGs, besides their requirement of physical exertion, are perceived as enjoyable by players (Bailey & McInnis, 2011). Such perceptions are critical to engage individuals' participation in AVGs and, more importantly, sustain their continued participation in these games. Thus far, there have been only a handful of studies which have examined individuals' psychosocial outcomes. The majority of these studies seem to suggest that, generally, individuals enjoy playing AVGs (Gao, 2012; Sun, 2013). Gao (2012) reported that adolescents were intrinsically motivated to play DDR. Further, when provided with the opportunity to play DDR and other AVGs, children and adolescents were more interested and self-efficacious for these activities compared to conventional physical education classes learning fitness exercises or aerobic dance (Gao et al., 2013; Sun, 2012). Indeed, using a longitudinal study design, Gao and colleagues reported that an AVG intervention exerted a positive effect on children's self-reported social support and self-efficacy over time (Gao et al., 2012). Furthermore, working with college students, researchers (Pope et al., 2016; Zeng et al., 2016) suggested that exergaming may also increase perceived enjoyment and intrinsic motivation in this population compared to treadmill exercise which may improve exercise adherence. Undoubtedly, as an attractive form of modern technology, AVGs challenge or complement conventional physical education classes in giving children enjoyable and psychosocially beneficial experiences (Figure 9.5). As such, AVGs have potential as a technological tool in education as well as in public health promotion.

Although AVGs are appealing to most game players, it remains questionable whether this effect is sustainable for the institution implementing the AVG program (e.g., schools) or whether the AVG program results in long-term PA adherence as only one study reported positive results over time (Gao et al., 2012). Unfortunately, two other studies reported that elementary school children's situational interest in AVGs declined significantly between the beginning

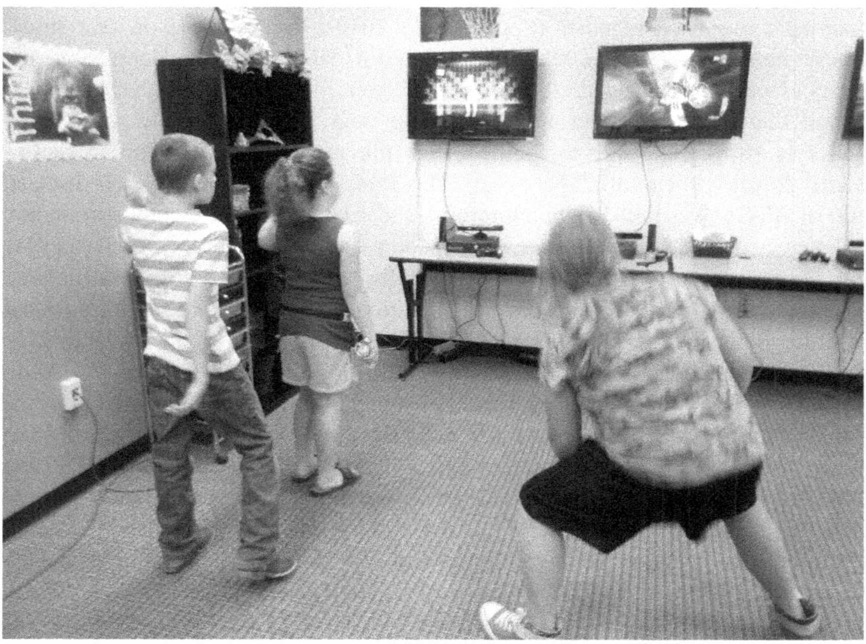

Figure 9.5 Kids playing active video games.

Source: Photo by Zan Gao.

and end of instruction (Sun, 2012, 2013). These results suggest that AVGs may have strong motivational power at the beginning of their use, but it is premature to claim they will help children develop a physically active and healthy lifestyle in the long term.

In fact, the sustainability of AVG use is a primary concern for the field-based PA interventions. Several studies illustrated that children's enthusiasm toward AVGs waned over time (Duncan & Staples, 2010; Sun, 2012, 2013). As a result, some researchers have suggested that AVG play exerts only acute effects and is not a sustainable activity to promote children's long-term PA participation (Duncan & Staples, 2010). Unfortunately, this perspective has not taken into account confounding factors such as study design problems, measurement issues, and other methodological concerns associated with previous studies. Indeed, most AVG studies were not randomized controlled trials and often lacked rigorous control of confounding factors. Specifically, previous studies have pinpointed a number of confounding factors (e.g., game types, game experience, age, and gender) associated with AVG studies that limit the strength of evidence.

Engaging in AVGs could bring about other psychosocial benefits. Specifically, playing AVGs can significantly influence children's PA attitudes, subjective norms (i.e., perceived social pressure from significant others), intention, and strenuous exercise behavior (Maddison et al., 2007). AVGs provide opportunities for social support among children and teachers who were involved in the gaming experience together (Fogel et al., 2010). For example, in one study, researchers (Paw et al., 2008) implemented a dance AVG and compared the level of participation in the game between two different social groups. It was found that the multiplayer group (playing with peers) played approximately twice as many minutes as the home group (playing alone), with dropout significantly lower in the multiplayer group. This study points out that the self-directed use of AVGs over time might compromise the success of AVG intervention and subsequent PA behavior. Hence, it is recommended to promote structured play by setting up multiple AVG stations in the same setting. With a structured program, players rotate from one AVG station to another station with minimal waiting time. In this manner, all players would have the opportunity to play AVGs simultaneously, with the continuous ability to play different AVG activities during the program. Players can also configure the game in workout mode prior to the PA session to maximize exercise time while minimizing transition time. This can be accomplished through some game consoles such as DDR and Xbox One. To enhance the maintenance of long-term AVG participation it might also be suggested to involve family and friends. As mentioned earlier, AVGs can promote social support among children and their peers (Fogel et al., 2010; Gao et al., 2012; Paw et al., 2008). It is, therefore, desirable to get their family members (parents and sibling) and friends involved in the AVG interventions. Additionally, once children are confident in their AVG skills, launching a tournament may be a fun way for them to demonstrate their psychomotor skills. For example, players usually compete for higher scores or number of perfect moves in DDR; and compete directly with other players in-person or online when playing Wii or Kinect. In fact, AVGs like iDance have networking capabilities, allowing the establishment of an online social group for gaming play. Therefore, it is recommended that, in future research, professionals help children build a global social network of AVG players, which facilitate children's shared experiences and socialization as they connect with new friends who share similar interests (Figure 9.6).

Finally, successful AVG implementation is contingent on the appropriate instruction and training of players—an aspect of AVG implementation researchers have neglected in field-based settings. That is, health professionals should teach and guide individuals as they learn to play AVGs as opposed to just "rolling out the ball" and letting them play. Indeed, AVGs do not define the learning objectives and contents for players. Rather, health professionals must first decide what they want players to learn and accomplish through AVGs, with failure to do so resulting in marginal effects of AVGs. Decisions on the progression of skills, behavioral maintenance, and the learning environment should be carefully designed, arranged, and monitored. Health professionals should have the faith to manipulate AVG activities and the learning environment in a way to maximize individuals' perceptions of enjoyment, self-efficacy, and motor skill development. Taken together, if professionals carefully plan and provide opportunities for all

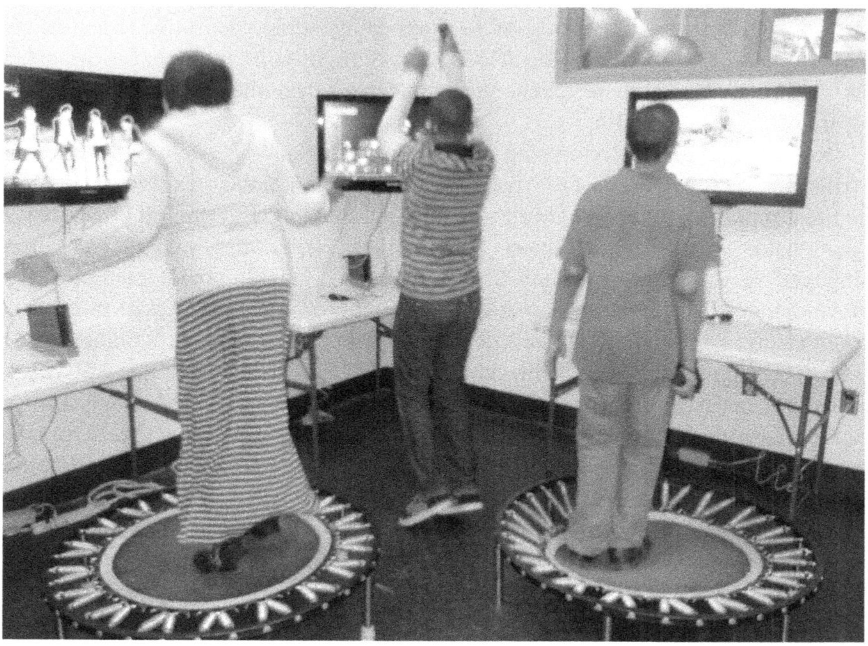

Figure 9.6 Kids playing active video games.

Source: Photo by Zan Gao.

individuals' engagement and quality learning, implementing motivating and sustainable AVGs is feasible in homes, schools, and community centers.

Effects on movement skill outcomes

Recently, AVGs have been considered an innovative approach to facilitate development of fundamental motor skills, which include locomotor skills (e.g., running, hopping, jumping, and walking), object control skills (e.g., kicking, striking, throwing, and catching), and body management skills (e.g., static/dynamic balancing, landing, and twisting and turning) (Gallahue, Ozmun, & Goodway, 2012).

Thus far, only one study has examined the effect of AVGs on locomotor skills. Interestingly, this study was part of a large study examining children's PA during AVGs. Specifically, the researchers (Barnett, Hinkley, Okely, Hesketh, & Salmon, 2012) investigated whether preschool children who reported playing the Nintendo Wii and PlayStation Eye Toy AVGs had higher movement skills than those who reported engaging in non-interactive electronic games (PlayStation and X-box) for 6 weeks. They found no significant group differences on locomotor skills. In fact, it was not possible to ascertain whether playing AVGs could facilitate locomotor skill development since some participants might have had low levels of locomotor skills prior to the study. Moreover, the small sample size of the study indicates the findings of the study should be interpreted with caution. Given the limitations of the preceding study, definitive conclusions cannot be ascertained regarding AVGs' ability to promote improved locomotion skills. As such, future research must concentrate on the ability of AVGs to promote locomotor skills.

Research evidence concerning the effectiveness of AVGs on object control skills is mixed, with half of the available literature indicating positive effects and the rest reporting otherwise. More specifically, two studies (Barnett et al., 2012; Vernadakis, Papastergiou, Zetou, & Antoniou, 2015) suggested that children engaged in AVG interventions had significantly greater object control skills development than those in non-AVG or specific object control skill programs. Conversely, two studies (Barnett, Ridgers, Reynolds, Hanna, & Salmon, 2015; Johnson, Ridgers, Hulteen, Mellecker, & Barnett, 2015) indicated that AVGs did not significantly improve intervention players' perceived or actual object control skills over time as compared to the control group. Notably, however, these two investigations (Barnett et al., 2015; Johnson et al., 2015) let children randomly play with designated AVGs with no gameplay instructions given, whereas the other study employed an experienced motor skill instructor at each AVG intervention session, who taught children how to perform the required movements (Vernadakis et al., 2015). Lack of instruction in the former two studies may have led to the biased result and the appearance of AVGs as having no potential to develop an individual's motor skills, while one may assume skill acquisition in the Vernadakis et al. (2015) study was attributable to the instructor as opposed to AVG itself. Further, we speculate that intervention dose may play a big role in the differences. Indeed, Vernadakis et al. (2015) conducted an 8-week intervention (twice a week, 30 minutes per session) with a total amount of 480 minutes of AVG-based program implementation. Yet, the intervention length in the other randomized controlled trials (Barnett et al., 2015; Johnson et al., 2015) were 278 minutes and 300 minutes, respectively. The lower dose of the AVG interventions in the latter two studies may not have been sufficient to trigger motor skill improvement. Finally, the nature of AVGs (i.e., Wii vs. Kinect) may result in different amounts of bodily engagement.

The effectiveness of AVGs on body management of individuals with physical disabilities (e.g., Developmental Coordination Disorder, Autism Spectrum Disorder (ASD), and balance problems) is promising (Hilton, et al. , 2014; Hammond, Jones, Hill, Green, & Male, 2014; Jelsma, Geuze, Mombarg, & Smits-Engelsman, 2014; Salem, Gropack, Coffin, & Godwin, 2012). However, studies investigating non-disabled children and adults are still warranted. Generally, studies among non-disabled populations reported that engaging in AVGs could improve balance (Gioftsidou et al., 2013; Vernadakis, Gioftsidou, Antoniou, Ioannidis, & Giannousi, 2012) and postural stability (Sheehan & Katz, 2012;, 2013) among children and college students. The preceding findings were congruent with findings that indicated AVGs were effective in improving overall balance capabilities in older adults (Bateni, 2012; Orsega-Smith, Davis, Slavish, & Gimbutas, 2012; Van Diest, Lamoth, Stegenga, Verkerke, & Postema, 2013). Additionally, the benefits of AVGs on flexibility (McCarthy, Brazil, Greene, Rendell, & Rohr, 2013), coordination, reaction time, speed and agility (Van Biljon & Longhurst, 2012) were also reported. In another qualitative study (Barnett, Ridgers, Hanna, & Salmon, 2014), children indicated that they would consider AVGs a learning tool in developing movement skills because they thought skill acquisition through AVG to be highly transferable. In this way, AVGs might be used as a method by which to promote motor control and overall physical functioning.

Obese populations

Physiological and physical effects

Among the AVG studies in obese populations, seven examined whether AVGs affected individuals' physiological outcomes. Three randomized controlled trials suggested AVGs had no effect on certain physiological outcomes. Specifically, Staiano et al. (2016) found no significant changes in cardiovascular risk factors including blood pressure, cholesterol, triglycerides, glucose and insulin, but did observe significant increases in trunk and spine bone mineral density post-intervention in overweight and obese girls. Adamo et al. (2010) also reported no significant differences in peak heart rate, peak workload, time to exhaustion, and blood assay after an AVG intervention, suggesting AVGs may not help obese children improve cardiorespiratory fitness. Additionally, Maddison et al. (2011) indicated that obese individuals' cardiovascular fitness improved after AVG play but differences were not significant between the intervention and control groups. In contrast, Goldfield and associates (2012) indicated aerobic fitness such as peak heart rate and rate of perceived exertion significantly increased after a 10-week AVG-based intervention. In addition, researchers reported absolute energy expenditure was significantly higher, but maximal heart rate lower, in obese children compared to their lean counterparts during AVG play (Chaput et al., 2015). Lastly, one quasi-experiment study (Penko & Barkley, 2010) suggested obese individuals' average heart rate and VO_2 were significantly greater in Nintendo Wii intervention than during treadmill walking and traditional sedentary video game play, partially due to the greater mass of the children/individuals, while another study found no improvements in any physiological outcomes such as heart rate, rate of perceived exertion, VO_2, and METs (Marti, Alvarez-Pitti, Provinciale, Lison, & Rivera, 2015).

Several studies examined the effects of AVG play on obese populations' adiposity levels. Five randomized controlled trials supported that AVG interventions had a positive effect on BMI, body composition, or body fat percentage (Christison & Khan, 2012; Maddison et al., 2011; Staiano, Abraham, & Calvert, 2013; Staiano et al., 2016; Trost, Sundal, Foster, Lent, & Vojta, 2014). Conversely, three randomized controlled trials failed to report positive effects of AVGs on adiposity (Adamo et al., 2010; Goldfield et al., 2012; Wagener, Fedele, Mignogna, Hester, & Gillaspy, 2012). For example, Wagener et al. (2012) suggested no significant improvement in BMI after a 10-week (three times a week) DDR intervention.

As a final note, the effects of AVGs on overweight and/or obese individuals' habitual PA and fitness are promising. One randomized controlled trial indicated AVG intervention children to have significantly increased moderate-to-vigorous PA post-intervention (Trost et al., 2014). Another randomized controlled trial found greater increased daily time spent playing AVGs, indicating AVG play may increase children's PA (Maddison et al., 2011) (Figure 9.7). Lastly, one control trial revealed children in an AVG group showed significantly improved fitness including coordination, reaction time, and speed and agility after a 6-week AVG-based intervention (Van Biljon & Longhurst, 2012).

Psychosocial effects

The psychological effects of AVG on overweight or obese individuals are very similar to those normal weight populations. Specifically, Staiano et al. (2013) reported that cooperative AVG players significantly increased in self-efficacy, and both cooperative and competitive AVG groups exhibited more peer support compared to a control group after a 20-week AVG intervention. Wagener et al. (2012) stated participants in a dance-based AVG condition had significantly increased perceived competence to exercise regularly, with Goldfield et al. (2012) suggesting significant pre-post improvements for body image, perceived scholastic competence, and social competence after an AVG-based intervention. The preceding two studies are in contrast with the findings of one quasi-experimental study which

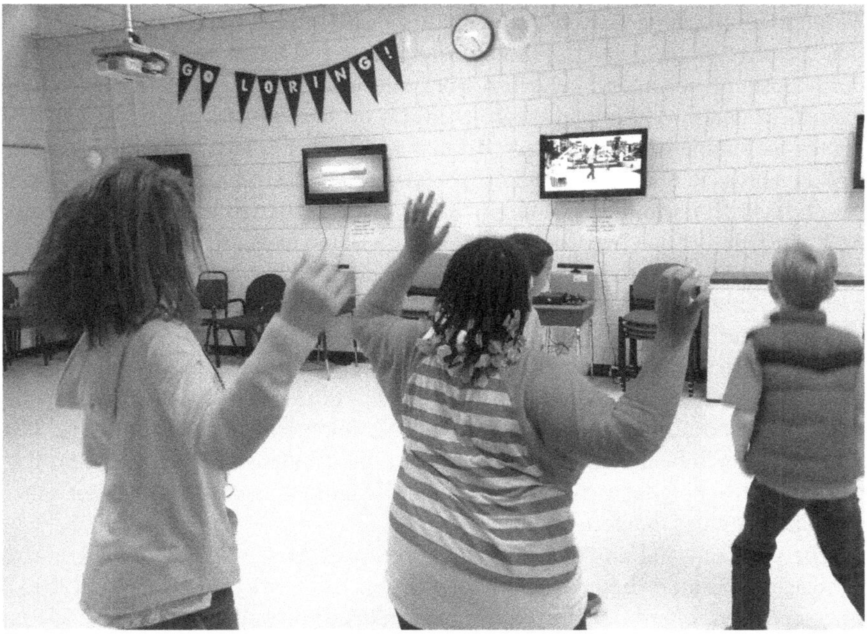

Figure 9.7 Kids playing an active video game.
Source: Photo by Zan Gao.

indicated improvements in global self-worth, but not in scholastic competence, social acceptance, athletic competence, and physical appearance among obese population (Christison & Khan, 2012). Finally, a recent study suggested obese children scored significantly higher in expectations and satisfaction, but not in self-efficacy and perceived exertion, during an AVG intervention (Marti et al., 2015).

In summary, we conclude that some AVGs can be considered a strategic tool for promoting a physically active and healthy lifestyle, and may be useful in attenuating and reversing the obesity epidemic; as well as in improving psychological well-being among obese populations.

Application of active video games in different contexts

AVGs are often deemed as home entertainment, and are popular and available to younger generations. As such, one might expect, more AVG studies have been completed in home-based settings. However, based upon the extant literature, laboratories seem to be the most common context to test AVGs' efficacy and validity, whereas schools appear to be a popular field-based venue to use AVG for PA and health promotion. Overall, more than two-thirds of the AVG intervention studies were conducted in laboratories and schools.

Laboratory-based contexts

Based upon the large number of laboratory-based studies on AVGs, it is known that the physiological and psychological responses induced by AVGs are higher than those of sedentary behaviors like sitting, resting, and sedentary video games. In detail, AVGs had positive effects on individuals' physiological outcomes as compared to sedentary behaviors. These findings suggested playing AVGs increased energy expenditure, heart rate, METs, VO_2 max, and PA from rest, which is in accordance with previous reviews (Barnett et al., 2011; Biddiss & Irwin, 2010; Foley & Maddison, 2010; LeBlanc et al., 2013). Findings also favored AVGs over sedentary behaviors for rate of perceived exertion and enjoyment. Given that many people spend a large amount of time in sedentary behaviors on a daily basis, the findings represent an optimistic message for public health. Explicitly, the findings suggest that AVGs can be used to replace individuals' sedentary behaviors, such as screen time, while maintaining game enjoyment and attractiveness over time. It is important to note, however, this finding needs to be taken with caution in that the challenge facing health professionals is to encourage players to replace sedentary behaviors, but not other physical activities or sports, with AVGs.

The physiological and psychological responses induced by AVGs were also similar to laboratory-based traditional exercises. According to Gao et al. (2015), in comparison to traditional exercise, heart rate considerably favored the AVGs, while all other variables were similar for both exercise modalities. Importantly, laboratory-based exercises can be further categorized into different types of exercise: walking (e.g.,1–2.6 km/hr), brisk walking (e.g., 4.2 km/hr), fast walking (e.g., 5.7 km/hr), running, and biking. Indeed, findings demonstrated that AVGs' effect size margin over that of laboratory-based traditional exercises declined as the exercise intensity increased from slow-paced walking to biking and to running (Gao et al., 2015). That said, enjoyment favored AVGs versus laboratory-based exercises—an encouraging finding given that AVG gameplay produces not only the equivalent magnitude of effect as light-to-moderate-intensity PA, but is also fun and enjoyable for players (Figure 9.8). The increases the likelihood of long-term PA adherence.

Field-based context

In home-based settings, two studies indicated that AVG interventions were more effective than control/comparison groups in increasing energy expenditure, PA, and METs (Murphy et al., 2009; Ni Mhurchu et al., 2008). However, three home-based randomized controlled trials found no significant differences for PA, BMI and weight loss, between the intervention and control/comparison groups (Baranowski et al., 2012; Maloney et al., 2008; Ni Mhurchu et al., 2008). Finally, one randomized controlled trial indicated mixed results in that AVG intervention children had greater increased self-reported PA, but not objectively measured PA, compared to control children (Maloney, Stempel, Wood, Patraitis, & Beaudoin, 2012).

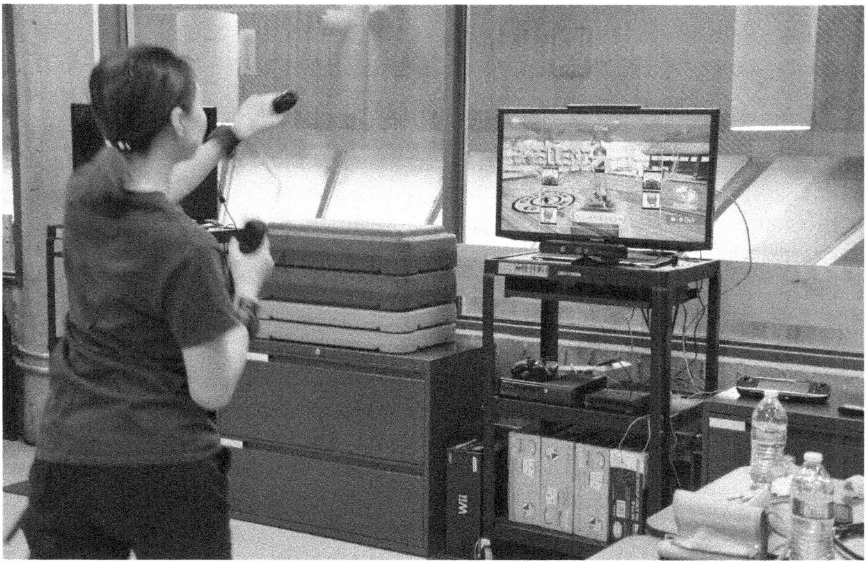

Figure 9.8 Elite athletes playing active video games.

Source: Photo by Zan Gao.

In school settings, two randomized controlled trials and two control trials found AVG interventions were more effective than control/comparison groups in promoting a variety of health-related outcomes, including PA, cardiorespiratory fitness, and weight loss (Gao & Xiang, 2014; Sheehan & Katz, 2013; Staiano, Abraham, & Calvert, 2013). Furthermore, three control trials suggested that AVG interventions had positive effects on some outcomes (e.g., PA, self-efficacy, enjoy/liking, intrinsic motivation) but no significant effects on other outcomes (e.g., outcome expectancy) as compared to control/comparison groups (Gao, Hannan, Xiang, et al., 2013; Gao et al., 2012; Lwin & Malik, 2014). Conversely, one control trial revealed that an AVG intervention was worse than a comparison group at influencing PA participation and energy expenditure (Duncan & Staples, 2010). When comparing the effectiveness of AVGs with traditional sports or PA, one study (Whittman, 2010) indicated AVGs were better while four studies (Gao et al., 2011; Gao, Zhang, & Stodden, 2013; Miller et al., 2013; Sun, 2012) suggested otherwise. Finally, within other field-based settings, one randomized controlled trial (Wagener, Fedele, Mignogna, Hester, & Gillaspy, 2012) indicated positive effects of an AVG intervention compared to control while two other studies found no differences between the groups (Bethea, Berry, Maloney, & Sikich, 2012; Paw et al., 2008).

The aforementioned findings appear inconclusive with regard to physiological and physical outcomes suggesting more research studies utilizing AVGs in field-based contexts are warranted and encouraged. Psychologically, however, AVGs produced improved self-efficacy, enjoyment/liking, and attitudes as compared to tradition field-based PA programs—a result in line with many empirical studies (Gao et al., 2012; Gao, Podlog, & Huang, 2013; Gao, Zhang, & Podlog, 2013; Gao, Zhang, & Stodden, 2013; Sun, 2012). Taken together, it is recommended that health professionals employ AVG interventions as a viable option to promote individuals' PA and health, as AVGs are more attractive and enjoyable for players in comparison with traditional PA (Figure 9.9). That is, AVGs can be used as an excellent addition to, but not a replacement for, traditional intensive PA or sports in individuals' daily lives (Gao, Zhang, & Stodden, 2013).

Regarding the implementation of AVG interventions, the findings suggest that AVG interventions in field-based settings should be developed based upon study characteristics which appear to have the greatest effect (i.e., intervention length). A meta-analysis demonstrated that children/adolescents benefit more from AVG interventions when the interventions are longer (Gao et al., 2015). This finding is consistent with the previous PA intervention studies (Gao, Hannan, Xiang, et al., 2013; Maloney et al., 2008; Sun, 2012). The involvement of greater muscle mass during AVG play should also be considered. Currently, only AVGs that mainly involved whole body movements and lower body movements (primarily DDR) have been implemented in field-based studies. Gao et al.

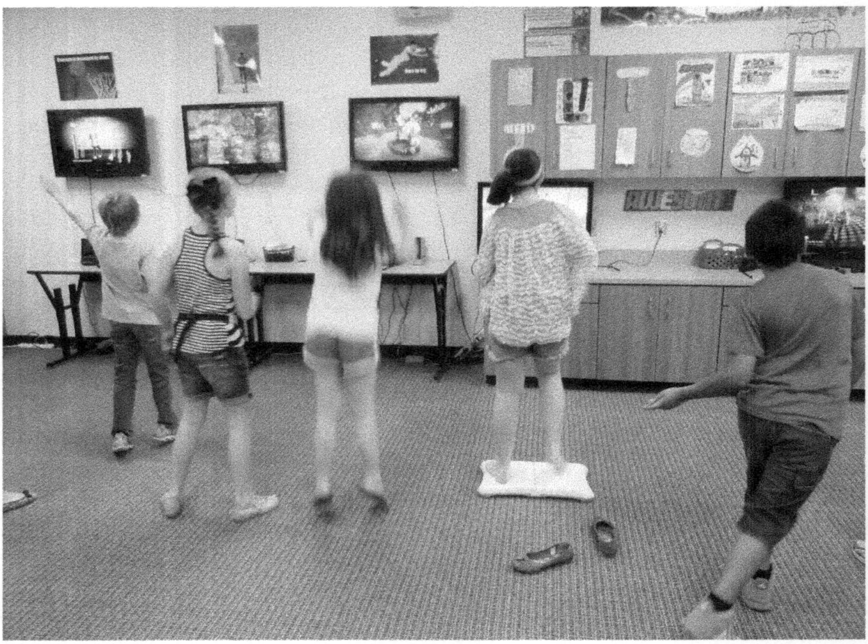

Figure 9.9 Kids playing active video games.

Source: Photo by Zan Gao.

(2015) suggested that these two types of AVGs generated similar health benefits, partially supporting findings by Peng et al. (2011). The finding further confirms that AVGs requiring large muscle group movement (lower body or whole body) are most effective in promoting PA (Biddiss & Irwin, 2010). Lastly, PA assessment methods did not moderate the relationship between PA interventions and health outcomes. Given the limited sample for assessing PA, future studies examining this moderator with larger samples are warranted.

Clinic-based context

Given the fact that increased PA has been shown to be a viable approach to prevent or lessen the risk of chronic diseases among a variety of populations, AVGs may represent an alternative means in prompting PA participation and improving the quality of life and life satisfaction (Baranowski, Maddison, Maloney, Medina, & Simons, 2014; Gao & Chen, 2014; Liang & Lau, 2014; Lu, Kharrazi, Gharghabi, & Thompson, 2013). As mentioned in the previous section of this chapter, the positive effects of AVGs on health-related outcomes have been reported among healthy populations (Gao et al., 2015; Peng et al., 2011). More recently, however, AVGs have received considerable attention from healthcare professionals and scholars alike as a rehabilitative tool in clinical settings to promote physical, psychological, and cognitive functioning among various populations (Gioftsidou et al., 2013; Hung et al., 2014). The reader is referred to the next section of this chapter to gain a better understanding of the application of AVG in the healthcare field.

Application of active video games in the healthcare field

As a result of the unique and enjoyable experience of game-based rehabilitation, AVGs may have the potential to increase motivation and adherence to physical and cognitive therapy at a low cost compared to traditional forms of treatment (Lange, Flynn, & Rizzo, 2009). Below we present the effects of AVG-based rehabilitation on various outcomes in different populations, the implications of AVG-based rehabilitation in healthcare field, as well as the limitations and recommendations for future research.

Effects of AVG-based rehabilitation on different populations

This section of the chapter will address the current literature with regard to the effectiveness of AVG-based rehabilitation on health and cognitive outcomes among various populations, namely, youth/young adults (5–25 years old) (Figures 9.10 and 9.11), middle-aged adults (40–65 years old), and older adults (≥65 years old).

AVG-based balance rehabilitation, specifically Wii Fit programs, have demonstrated a positive effect among youth and young adults with Down Syndrome (Rahman, 2010) or with a history of lower limb injury (Sims, Cosby,

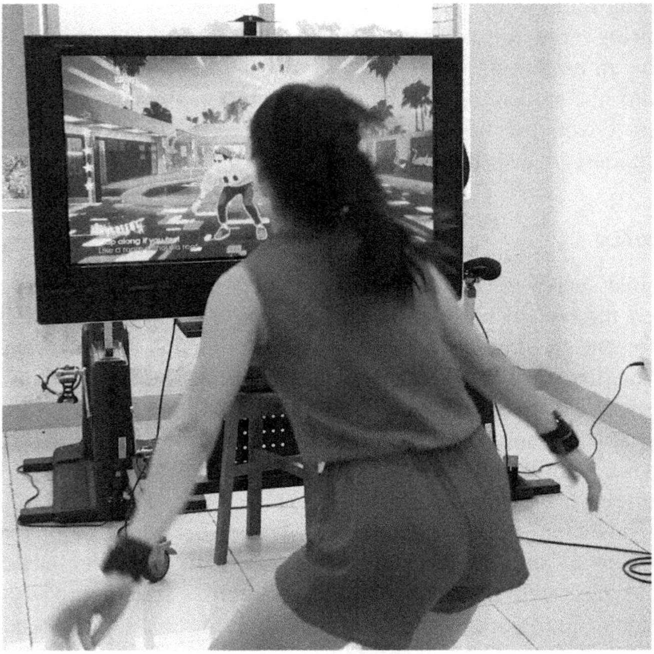

Figure 9.10 Young adults playing active video games.

Source: Photo by Zan Gao.

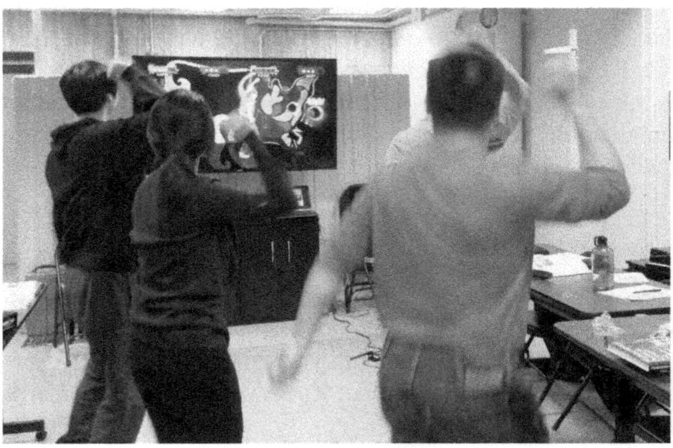

Figure 9.11 Young adults playing active video games.

Source: Photo by Zan Gao.

Saliba, Hertel, & Saliba, 2013) compared to control conditions which included traditional therapy-based strength exercises to improve balance using standard care procedures. In middle-aged adults, the vast majority of AVG-based rehabilitation used the Wii (Gil-Gómez, Lloréns, Alcañiz, Colomer, 2011; Kim, Kang, Park, & Jung, 2012; Kramer, Dettmers, & Gruber, 2014; Nilsagard, Forsberg, & von Koch, 2013; Robinson, Dixon, Macsween, van Schaik, & Martin, 2015) with one rehabilitation program among stroke patients using the Sony PlayStation Eye Toy (Yavuzer, Senel, Atay, & Stam, 2008). Specifically, AVGs were used for physical functioning and/or balance rehabilitation among patients with multiple sclerosis (Kramer et al., 2014; Nilsagard et al., 2013; Robinson et al., 2015), acquired brain injuries (Gil-Gomez et al., 2011) and stroke (Kim et al., 2012; Yavuzer et al., 2008). Generally, AVG-based rehabilitation had little effect on patients' physical functioning versus control conditions in middle-aged adults. However, AVG-based rehabilitation demonstrated positive effects on balance over control and comparison conditions.

The gaming systems used for rehabilitation in older adults included the Nintendo Wii (Daniel, 2012; Franco et al., 2012; Pluchino, Lee, Asfour, Roos, & Signorile, 2012), researcher-developed gaming platforms (Chen et al., 2012; Szturm, Betker, Moussavi, Desai, & Goodman, 2011), or the Microsoft Xbox Kinect (Sato, Kuroki, Saiki, & Nagatomi, 2015). Among older adults, AVG-based rehabilitation was used to improve physical functioning, balance, and falls efficacy for lower limb rehabilitation in frail elderly at risk of falls (Chen et al., 2012), pre-frail elderly at risk of falls (Daniel, 2012; Franco et al., 2012; Pluchino et al., 2012; Sato et al., 2015), or balance/mobility in impaired elderly (Szturm et al., 2011). Compared with control or comparison conditions, AVG-based physical functioning rehabilitation yielded similar effects in older adults. However, AVG-based balance rehabilitation had a small, marginally positive effect as compared to control conditions. Also, AVGs had a positive effect on falls efficacy versus control among older adults.

Effect of AVG-based rehabilitation on health and cognitive outcomes

Physiological and physical effects of AVGs

A number of AVG studies investigated a wide range of physiological and physical outcomes in patients, with the majority of the studies focusing on whether AVG-based rehabilitation has a positive effect on balance. Indeed, a number of studies examined the use of AVGs on static and dynamic balance ability, with most indicating AVG-based rehabilitation could improve balance performance. Among them, three experimental studies found positive results on balance (Esculier, Vaudrin, Bériault, Gagnon, & Tremblay, 2012; Pompeu et al., 2012; van den Berg et al., 2016) as compared to control/comparison groups after AVG-based rehabilitation. Yet, Bainbridge et al. (2011) failed to find balance change after an AVG-based rehabilitation program.

Many studies examined other components of physical functioning besides balance. Among them, seven studies comparing AVG-based rehabilitation with other treatment protocols observed comparable or equal improvements for several outcomes. In detail, one control trial found significant improvements for the Sit to Stand Test, the ten-meter Walk Test and Tinetti's Performance Oriented Mobility Assessment for the AVG group (Esculier et al., 2012). Further, four of six randomized controlled trials observed significant changes in the 2-minute Walk Test (Imam, Miller, Finlayson, Eng, & Jarus, 2015); the Unified Parkinson's disease rating scale (Pompeu et al., 2012); the Functional Independence Measure (Yavuzer et al., 2008); and the Senior Fitness Test, Late Life Function and Disability Index (Daniel, 2012) as compared to the control/comparison groups. Notably, two other randomized controlled trials indicated no significant differences in the Active Range of Knee Motion, the 2-minute Walk Test, the Lower Extremity Functional Scale (Fung, Ho, Shaffer, Chung, & Gomez, 2012) and the Nursing Home Physical Performance Test (Hsu, Thibodeau, Wong, Zukiwsky, Cecile, & Walton, 2011) between AVG-based rehabilitation and conventional therapy—providing evidence that the use of the AVGs might best be used as an adjunctive therapy to standard treatment.

Psychological effects of AVGs

Studies investigating psychological rehabilitative outcomes included enjoyment, quality of life, and depression. Specifically, three studies investigated enjoyment in relation to AVG-based rehabilitation with two randomized controlled trials indicating a positive effect on enjoyment (Hsu et al., 2011; van den Berg et al., 2016) for the AVG groups, compared to the comparison groups. Interestingly, two non-experimental studies seem to suggest AVGs could be an effective rehabilitative tool in improving quality of life but not to a degree sufficient to trigger changes in mood (Herz, Mehta, Sethi, Jackson, Hall, & Morgan, 2013; Mhatre et al., 2013). Conversely, one randomized controlled trial stated no significant change was found for the Wii group in quality of life despite a slight upward trend indicating improvement after AVG-based treatment (van den Berg et al., 2016).

Cognitive effects of AVGs

A number of studies examined patients' cognitive functions, with most concerned with balance confidence. Generally, the findings are equivocal for balance confidence, with one randomized controlled trial (Daniel, 2012) indicating improvements while one control trial (Esculier et al., 2012) and two other randomized controlled trials (Fung et al., 2012; van den Berg et al., 2016) observing no changes following AVG-based rehabilitation as compared to control/comparison groups. Other cognitive rehabilitative outcomes included falls efficacy, pain intensity, and cognitive performance. Specifically, falls efficacy was examined exclusively in older adults (Chen et al., 2012; Pluchino et al., 2012) with AVGs demonstrating a positive effect over control/comparison groups. With regard to pain intensity, one randomized controlled trial demonstrated that AVGs were not effective for upper extremity pain management after an AVG intervention (Hsu et al., 2011) while another randomized controlled trial revealed no significant difference in lower extremity pain between an AVG group and physiotherapy group (Fung et al., 2012). Finally, one control trial demonstrated significantly improved cognitive performance for Wii groups for attention and decision-making (dos Santos Mendes et al., 2012) while one randomized controlled trial indicated significant improvements in executive function versus a comparison group (Pompeu et al., 2012).

Implications of AVG-based rehabilitation in the healthcare field

The findings indicate that AVG-based balance rehabilitation was most common across all age groups. The vast majority of findings favored AVG-based balance rehabilitation over control conditions among youth and young adults. While findings regarding AVG-based balance rehabilitation among middle-aged adults still favored AVGs in comparison with control conditions, the magnitude of effect decreased. The same was true when using AVG-based balance rehabilitation versus control conditions among older adults. Notably, previous experience with AVG may be a factor limiting the effectiveness of AVG-based balance rehabilitation among older populations in comparison to youth and young adults. Given this situation, AVGs may demonstrate greater effectiveness for balance rehabilitation among youth/young adults, as less time is required to learn how to play the game(s) and more time can be spent engaging in rehabilitation-oriented gameplay.

AVG-based physical functioning rehabilitation was observed only among middle-aged and older adult populations but not youth/young adults. This is logical given the fact that functional limitations among middle-aged and older adults are more common compared to youth and young adults (Holmes, Powell-Griner, Lethbridge-Cejku, & Heyman, 2009). Notably, although the majority of randomized controlled trials reported favorable results for AVGs with regard to physical functioning, a limited number of publications and the use of different instruments measuring dissimilar physical outcomes made it challenging to compare each study and draw a definite conclusion on the effectiveness of AVG-based rehabilitation. Additionally, as some randomized controlled trials (Daniel, 2012; Imam, Miller, Finlayson, Eng, & Jarus, 2015) were designed as feasibility trials, with the primary goal of assessing the feasibility of AVG-based rehabilitation as opposed to drawing conclusions regarding the efficacy of this treatment modality, the results cannot readily be interpreted to suggest AVG-based interventions are more effective than usual care. Moreover, the discrepancies between study findings might be attributable to the fact that some studies did not isolate the AVG intervention from traditional rehabilitation exercises. Not isolating the AVG-based physical functioning rehabilitation may have reduced the effects of AVGs. Finally, a generalized conclusion must be regarded with caution as the aforementioned studies had a wide range of sample sizes and relatively short intervention durations, which may limit the generalizability and practical implications of the findings. Consequently, the decision on the effectiveness of AVGs on non-balance physical functioning among patients is still inconclusive. Given the current aging population, continued investigation regarding how to promote balance and physical functioning among patients via AVGs is paramount in improving the ability to engage in activities of daily living and reducing later life disability.

One advantage of AVG-based rehabilitation over traditional physical therapy is that AVGs not only provide physical benefits, but also act as a form of entertainment. The most appealing aspect of AVGs lies in its motivating feature—meaning AVGs offer players a much higher level of engagement, which can significantly reduce players' level of perceived exertion (Gao, Gerling, Mandryk, & Stanley, 2014). As such, motivation to stick with AVGs is higher than with traditional rehabilitation. In this way, players may experience increased enjoyment during AVG gameplay, leading to improved quality of life over time and, more importantly, sustained participation in AVG-based rehabilitation activities. That said, research evidence regarding the effectiveness of AVGs on psychological rehabilitative outcomes is mixed, with some studies indicating positive effects while a small portion of studies reporting no effect. Taken together, the findings were not in line with previous studies indicating positive psychological effects of AVGs on enjoyment among healthy youth and adults (Li, Theng, & Foo, 2016; Verhoeven, Abeele, Gers, & Seghers, 2015). Notably, extrinsic factors in the included studies may have affected the results due to the high proportion of patients with preexisting depression (Mhatre et al., 2013). Additionally, it is plausible that the intensity and length of AVG-based rehabilitation were not high enough to elicit changes in mood. It is also possible that health professionals did not provide a variety of AVGs to the patients during the intervention periods—potentially increasing the monotony of the program and reducing enjoyment. Meanwhile, as modern technology is not part of daily life for many seniors, with many unfamiliar with technology, the motivation to learn how to use AVGs is rather weak, as the learning process may be frustrating for many older adults—particularly among older patients already burdened enough by treatments related to their diseases or impairments. Therefore, findings concerning the psychological rehabilitative effects of AVGs on older patients are inconclusive and, at times, contradictory.

At this point, it is unclear whether AVGs are a viable rehabilitative tool to improve cognitive outcomes in older patients. First, as previously stated, despite findings demonstrating improved balance confidence post-intervention, studies did not indicate whether these improvements were statistically significant (Broadbent, Crowley-McHattan, & Zhou, 2014; Clark & Kraemer, 2009; Daniel, 2012). Without providing inferential statistics, we cannot conclude that AVG-based rehabilitation is effective for balance confidence. Second, most current studies have been examining the acute effects of AVG-based rehabilitation without follow-up to assess the sustainability of intervention adaptations, which might cause researchers to under- or over-rate the potential of AVGs and result in inaccurate conclusions regarding the effectiveness of AVGs on patients' cognitive outcomes. Additionally, as individuals with higher education levels or socioeconomic status may possess greater cognitive ability than individuals of lower education levels or socioeconomic status, some factors such as education, occupation, and even personality could have affected individuals' cognitive performance within those studies. Finally, the nature of AVGs could also be a confounding factor influencing intervention results as some types of AVGs (e.g., games that require more executive functions) may have stronger cognitive demands than others. In this regard, patients may receive varying stimulation intensities from different AVG-based treatments leading to different results in cognitive rehabilitative outcomes.

Falls efficacy was another common cognitive outcomes between studies within any age group and was seen exclusively in older adults (Chen et al., 2012; Pluchino et al., 2012). Findings that revealed AVG-based rehabilitation to improve falls efficacy favored AVGs compared to control conditions. This finding is promising due to the following reasons. First, falls are prevalent among older adults. Second, older adults may not be able to commute to a clinic for rehabilitation to reduce fall risk and increase falls efficacy due to functional disabilities (Levasseur et al., 2015). AVG-based rehabilitative programs are likely to be better adhered to and can be implemented at home without the need of constant supervision by a physical therapist/nurse or patient travel, AVGs might represent an attractive and effective alternative in promoting greater falls efficacy and possible reduction in fall prevalence. Further, healthcare professionals may monitor the progress of patients engaging in AVG-based rehabilitation by having patients upload AVG data to an online portal. Healthcare professionals could then monitor the data and provide relevant feedback to increase the effectiveness of the rehabilitation program.

Limitations and recommendations

This section has synthesized the available evidence regarding the effectiveness of AVG-based rehabilitation in the therapeutic treatment of physiological/physical, psychological and cognitive ailments. The strength of this section lies in the provision of a comprehensive synthesis of the effects of AVG-based rehabilitation in the healthcare field in a systematic manner, yet some limitations should be noted. First, the heterogeneity of samples, outcomes, interventions, effects, measurement instruments, and research designs lessened the ability to detect significant differences and summarize overall significant findings. Second, the variety of AVGs limited the ability to investigate which specific games, and which aspects of those games, are most useful for the rehabilitation of specific diseases and/or impairments.

These findings have implications for healthcare professionals as AVG-based rehabilitation may be more easily adhered to, given the enjoyable nature of AVG play and the ability of this rehabilitation to be played within the comfort of the patients' home. Further, once trained in how to use AVGs as part of a rehabilitation program, patients can implement the program without assistance from health practitioners while health practitioners may be able to remotely monitor, via an online portal, the progress of the patient—potentially decreasing healthcare costs for both parties. To better understand and evaluate the effects of AVG-based rehabilitation on patients, future studies should continue to determine guidelines regarding the ideal dose of AVG gameplay among patients with specific diseases and/or impairments. This could be achieved through the use of more high-quality study designs and more follow-up testing with patients to discern the sustainability of the adaptations stimulated by certain durations and frequencies of AVG-based rehabilitation. Second, researchers may want to isolate AVG-based rehabilitation and standard therapy procedures during rehabilitation with patients. Isolating these treatments will permit better examination of the standalone benefits that AVG-based rehabilitation may have in comparison to standard therapy. Additionally, researchers may integrate newer technology and employ multiple types of AVGs to distinguish and surmise the effectiveness of specific AVGs on specific diseases and/or impairments. Lastly, larger samples and greater concentration on the cognitive rehabilitative outcomes resulting from AVG gameplay are warranted with a larger and more diverse number of variables assessed. Methodological improvements such as those outlined previously will ensure the development of AVG-based rehabilitation programs that are most effective and capable of treating a wider array of health-related outcomes.

Augmented reality games and active video games

Augmented reality games, such as Zombies, Run! and Pokémon Go, have successfully attracted the attention of youth and adults alike in recent years, with particular excitement noted after the release of Pokémon Go in July 7, 2016. Indeed, Pokémon Go generated lots of public interest, with an estimated 65 million users downloading the game within one week of its release, including thousands of young children (Baranowski, 2016) (Figure 9.12). While a full review of augmented reality games is beyond the scope of this book, we would like to briefly introduce these augmented reality games and their relationships with AVGs.

Augmented reality games are unique because they integrate the physical and virtual worlds into one interface using mobile devices applications (a.k.a., apps). Unlike the traditional sedentary video games that encourage solitary and sedentary activity, augmented reality games require players to walk around and explore their local surroundings such as parks, schools, gyms, and home neighborhoods, and hence offer potential physical, social, and emotional benefits to players (Serino, Cordrey, McLaughlin, & Milanaik, 2016). In this way, augmented reality games serve very similar functions to those of AVGs, and consequently can be considered a type of AVG that elicits PA. In fact, augmented reality games have been around since the early 1990s but little attention had been given to this technology in promoting PA and health. For instance, an early augmented reality game, Finding Yosh, attempted to elicit PA through a geocaching approach but failed to expand its use to a larger population. In 2002, a

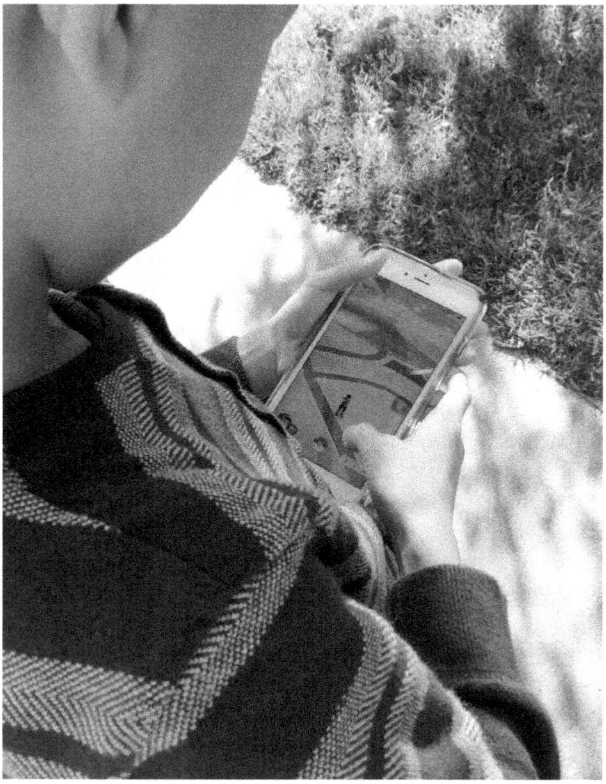

Figure 9.12 A kid playing Pokémon Go.
Source: Photo by Zan Gao.

then-pioneering game named Majestic made significant contributions to the field, followed by several attempts to advance this technology. As a result of the contributions made by Majestic, there are a number of available augmented reality games on the market presently, including but not limited to: Ingress, Zombies, Run!, Zombies Everywhere, The Walk, Superhero Workout, SpecTrek, Clandestine Anomaly, Temple Treasure Hunt Game, Geocaching, Real Strike, Night Terrors, and Pokémon Go, among others.

Clearly, this technology has been gaining momentum in the past decade, particularly with the advances in virtual reality and augmented-reality headsets. Prior to Pokémon Go's arrival, another augmented reality game entitled "Zombies, Run!" achieved some popularity. This immersive game motivates players up off their couch, and gets them fit with the help of zombies. Specifically, the game partially immerses players into a world full of zombies, requiring players to run or jog to survive zombie attacks while listening to the undead scream. Players also have to collect supplies and unlock daily missions too. Overall, this game provides an experience in which the players' real world blends into a virtual one on the screen of their mobile device while simultaneously encouraging individuals to be physically active.

In 2012, Niantic Labs, the developers behind Pokémon Go, released a new augmented reality game: Ingress. Ingress encourages players to leave their houses and embrace the environment to gain game experience. Niantic later developed Pokémon Go, to an unprecedented level of fanfare given Pokémon's consistent and committed fan base—making it the most popular augmented reality game of all time. Pokémon Go is a free app available on iPhone and Android devices that is also a GPS-based augmented reality game. Users are encouraged to track and catch Pokémon that are virtually superimposed onto physical and real-world surroundings, such as local parks, schools, historical sites, and gyms. Contrary to the original Pokémon sedentary video game, Pokémon Go encourages its users be physically active through exploration of the physical environment while simultaneously engaging in the game's fantasy world. Similar to Zombies, Run!, Pokémon Go is also deemed an innovative AVG (Baranowski, 2016).

The newly available augmented reality games are promising in bringing potential health benefits to the users, particularly among children and adolescents. For instance, Pokémon Go encourages a physically active lifestyle and promotes active learning as well through the interaction with the local neighborhoods and historical sites. The game also enhances social interaction by playing against nearby players. Additionally, the game may exert a positive effect on mood and emotion (Serino et al., 2016). Despite the attractiveness and benefits of aforementioned augmented reality games, readers should be aware of the adverse consequences of these games. Based upon the media reports, it has been observed that physical harm may occur as a result of playing Pokémon Go while walking or driving. Playing the game also increases economic burden as a result of in-app purchasing and heavy data usage, and potentially leads the users to inappropriate or dangerous areas. The most concerning downside of playing Pokémon Go may be due to its geo-locating feature (i.e., the "lure" function) an interactive aspect of the game which can lead to crime. For example, criminals have taken advantage of the game and conducted a number of recent first-degree robberies and felonies. It is, therefore, imperative to be cautious and alert all the time while playing such augmented reality games (Serino et al., 2016).

Overall, augmented reality games can improve positive health behavior (i.e., PA behavior), socialization, and emotion. These games have the potential to promote PA and other aspects of health in the naturalist contexts. As the technology advances, the efficacy and effectiveness of emerging augmented reality games such as Pokémon Go deserve further investigation. Baranowski (2016) has proposed a series of future research questions and directions in the new field. It is expected that greater number of empirical studies will emerge in the next five years.

Practical implications

Although the increased frequency of publications in this field indicate AVGs' increased popularity, AVG research is still lagging behind, given the rapid development of the gaming industry and the volume of AVGs on the market. According to the preceding, extensive review, research design and other methodological issues of AVG studies need improvement—particularly as AVGs have more frequently been taken from laboratories and placed in field-based contexts, such as schools, community centers, homes, and health clinics. Research studies reviewed in this chapter have suggested that, in laboratory-based contexts, AVGs had a positive effect on healthy individuals' physiological and psychological outcomes compared to rest, with these effects similar to those of light-to-moderate-intensity PA. Studies have also supported some types of AVGs in field-based contexts which, when implemented with careful planning and guidance, are efficacious in providing physical, psychosocial, motor, and cognitive benefits (Figure 9.13). In this regard, AVGs offer more benefits than downsides with regard to the promotion of individuals' PA and health outcomes.

Notably, while PA as a result of AVG use can contribute toward daily recommendations of PA duration, solely depending on AVG as a PA promotion strategy among individuals is not realistic, as the light-to-moderate intensity of PA generated from AVG play is, at times, insufficient to help individuals meet the recommended PA intensity needed for the greatest health benefit. These findings have

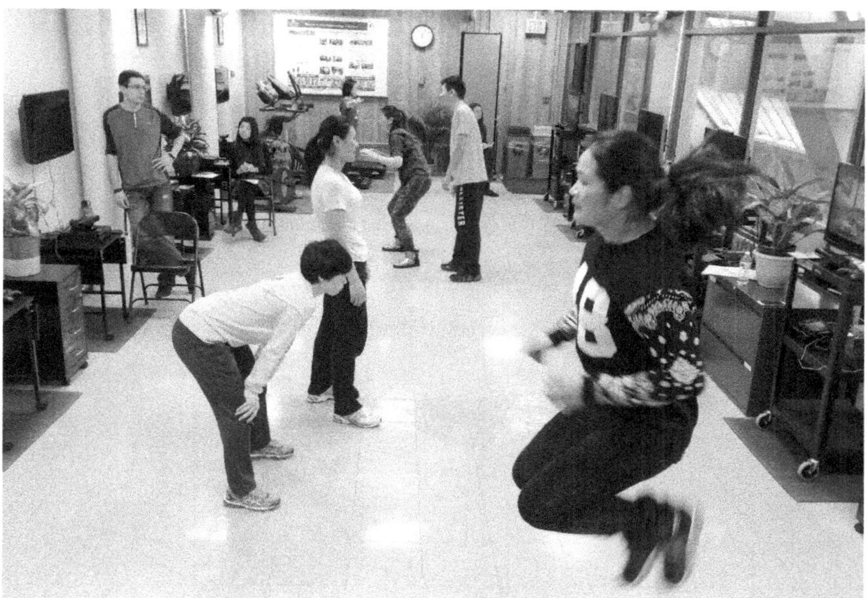

Figure 9.13 Elite athletes playing active video games.

Source: Photo by Zan Gao.

public health implications that can help inform healthcare stakeholders regarding AVG interventions. For example, health professionals may integrate AVGs in schools, community centers, and homes to help individuals develop a healthy lifestyle habits—striving only to replace sedentary behavior, but not the traditional PA and sports, with AVGs.

Meanwhile, the fun and/or boredom factors of AVGs should be taken into consideration during program implementation as well. In particular, AVGs need to be constantly upgraded or updated to hold children's interest and promote sustainability with regard to changes in health behaviors. However, given the fun component programmed into the games, AVGs are desirable as a promising addition to promote PA and health by replacing these sedentary behaviors. Additionally, when implementing AVGs, health professionals should provide systematic instructions on AVG use and provide PA opportunities for players. The ultimate goal of this instruction is to take advantage of the enthusiastic nature of AVGs, and achieve long-term success in making AVG play part of individuals' daily workout routine. Finally, it also needs to be recognized that the potential of AVGs in field-based contexts might have been underestimated due to a variety of limitations inherent in many published studies. Future research and practice should take into account these limitations to unravel and exploit the maximal effectiveness of AVGs. Simply stated, high quality and well-designed research is warranted to investigate how various AVGs may affect individuals' health-related outcomes from a longitudinal perspective (Figures 9.14, Figure 9.15).

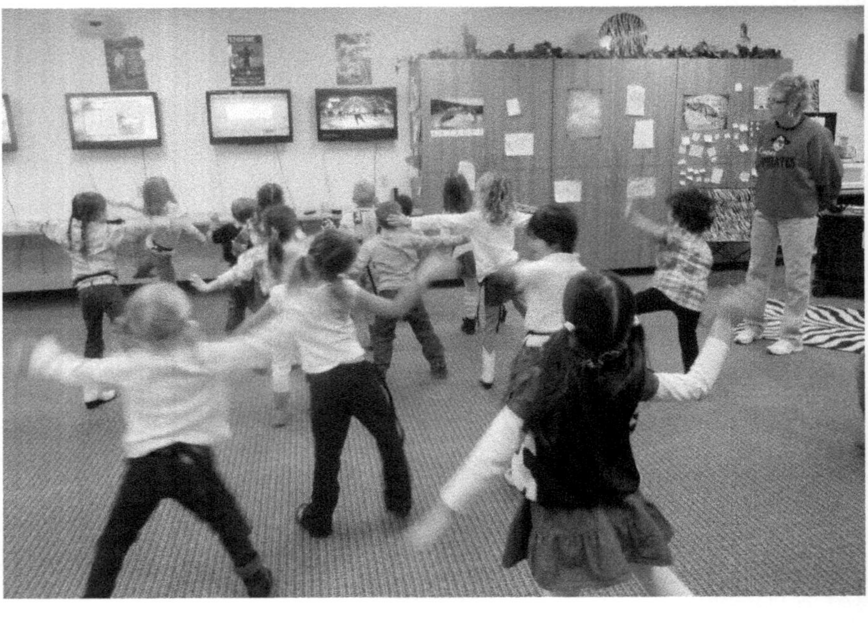

Figure 9.14 Kids playing active video games.

Source: Photo by Zan Gao.

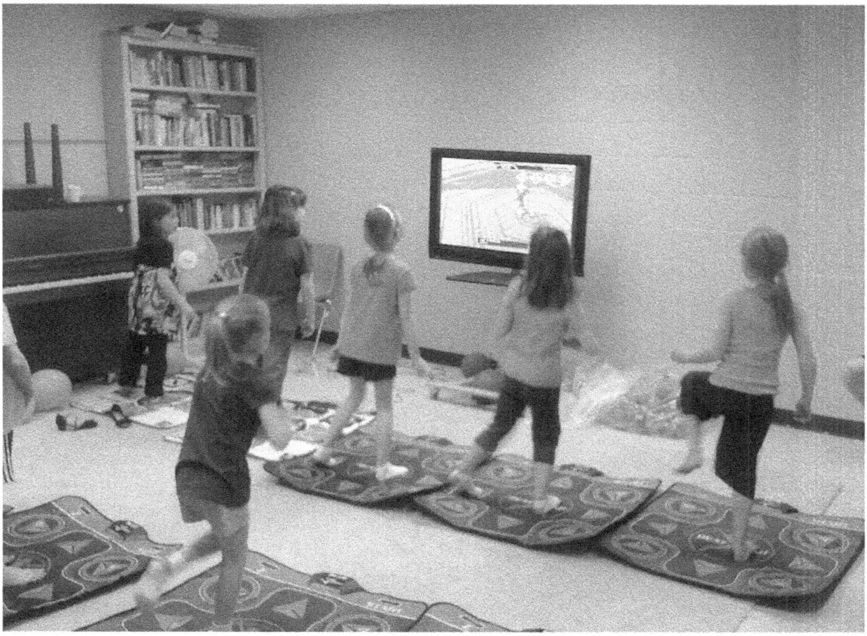

Figure 9.15 Kids playing active video games.
Source: Photo by Zan Gao.

This chapter provides an overview and synthesis of the health benefits of AVGs in healthy and clinical populations. Given the limitations inherent in the empirical studies reviewed, researchers and practitioners have a number of research questions to answer prior to being able to conclude if AVGs can effectively promote healthy individuals' moderate-to-vigorous PA in fun and innovative ways. Gao (2017) has offered some recommendations for future research in different contexts among various populations, including but not limited to: (1) examine the long-term efficacy of AVG use in non-structured home settings for PA promotion using high-quality randomized controlled trials, and the potential benefits of family/group play and potential barriers in such settings; (2) determine whether children/adolescents with access to AVGs actually replace their screen time with AVGs as opposed to traditional sports or PA; (3) conduct process evaluation for AVGs to ensure the intervention fidelity; (4) examine the efficacy and effectiveness of augmented reality games such as Pokémon Go on individuals' PA behavior and health outcomes, particularly youth and young adults; (5) investigate other gaming consoles such as the Xbox and Play Station on rehabilitation; and (6) examine the effectiveness of home-based, patient-implemented AVG-based rehabilitation as compared with clinic-based rehabilitation research. More details can be found in Gao (2017).

Acknowledgments

Please note that a small portion of statements and sentences are abstracted from Gao and Chen (2014) and Gao et al. (2015). Copyright permission has been secured from *Obesity Reviews.*

References

Adamo, K. B., Rutherford, J. A., & Goldfield, G. S. (2010). Effects of interactive video game cycling on overweight and obese adolescent health. *Applied Physiology, Nutrition, and Metabolism, 35*(6), 805–815.

Bailey, B. W., & McInnis, K. (2011). Energy cost of exergaming: A comparison of the energy cost of 6 forms of exergaming. *Archives of Pediatrics & Adolescent Medicine, 165*(7), 597–602. http://doi.org/10.1001/archpediatrics.2011.15.

Bainbridge, E., Bevans, S., Keeley, B., & Oriel, K. (2011). The effects of the Nintendo Wii Fit on community-dwelling older adults with perceived balance deficits: A pilot study. *Physical & Occupational Therapy in Geriatrics, 29*(2), 126–135.

Baranowski, T. (2013). Games and childhood obesity. *Games for Health Journal, 2*(3), 113–115. http://doi.org/10.1089/g4h.2013.1502.

Baranowski, T. (2016). Pokémon Go, go, go, gone? *Games for Health Journal, 5*(5), g4h.2016.01055.tbp. http://doi.org/10.1089/g4h.2016.01055.tbp.

Baranowski, T., Abdelsamad, D., Baranowski, J., O'Connor, T. M., Thompson, D., Barnett, A., … Chen, T.-A. (2012). Impact of an active video game on healthy children's physical activity. *Pediatrics, 129*(3), e636–e642. http://doi.org/10.1542/peds.2011-2050.

Baranowski, T., Maddison, R., Maloney, A., Medina, E., & Simons, M. (2014). Building a better mousetrap (exergame) to increase youth physical activity. *Games for Health Journal, 3*(2), 72–78. http://doi.org/10.1089/g4h.2014.0018.

Barnett, A., Cerin, E., & Baranowski, T. (2011). Active video games for youth: A systematic review. *Journal of Physical Activity & Health, 8*(5), 724–37.

Barnett, L. M., Hinkley, T., Okely, A. D., Hesketh, K., & Salmon, J. (2012). Use of electronic games by young children and fundamental movement skills? *Perceptual & Motor Skills, 114*(3), 1023–1034.

Barnett, L. M., Ridgers, N. D., Hanna, L., & Salmon, J. (2014). Parents' and children's views on whether active video games are a substitute for the "real thing." *Qualitative Research in Sport, Exercise and Health, 6*(3), 366–381.

Barnett, L. M., Ridgers, N. D., Reynolds, J., Hanna, L., & Salmon, J. (2015). Playing active video games may not develop movement skills: An intervention trial. *Preventive Medicine Reports, 2*, 673–678.

Bateni, H. (2012). Changes in balance in older adults based on use of physical therapy vs the Wii Fit gaming system: A preliminary study. *Physiotherapy, 98*(3), 211–216.

Bethea, T. C., Berry, D., Maloney, A. E., & Sikich, L. (2012). Pilot study of an active screen time gamecorrelates with improved physical fitness in minority elementary school youth. *Games for Health Journal, 1*(1), 29–36. http://doi.org/10.1089/g4h.2011.0005.

Biddiss, E., & Irwin, J. (2010). Active video games to promote physical activity in children and youth: A systematic review. *Archives of Pediatrics & Adolescent Medicine, 164*(7), 664–672. http//:doi: 10.1001/archpediatrics.2010.104.

Broadbent, S., Crowley-McHattan, Z., Zhou, S., & Shaw, B. S. (2014). The effect of the Nintendo Wii Fit on exercise capacity and gait in an elderly woman with CREST syndrome. *International Journal of Therapy and Rehabilitation, 21*(11), 539–546.

Chaput, J. P., Genin, P. M., Le Moel, B., Pereira, B., Boirie, Y., Duclos, M., & Thivel, D. (2015). Lean adolescents achieve higher intensities but not higher energy expenditure while playing active video games compared with obese ones. *Pediatric Obesity, 1*(11), 102–106.

Chen, P. Y., Wei, S. H., Hsieh, W. L., Cheen, J. R., Chen, L. K., & Kao, C. L. (2012). Lower limb power rehabilitation (LLPR) using interactive video game for improvement of balance function in older people. *Archives of Gerontology and Geriatrics, 55*(3), 677–682.

Christison, A., & Khan, H. A. (2012). Exergaming for health: A community-based pediatric weight management program using active video gaming. *Clinical Pediatrics, 51*(4), 382–388.

Clark, R., & Kraemer, T. (2009). Clinical use of Nintendo Wii™ bowling simulation to decrease fall risk in an elderly resident of a nursing home: A case report. *Journal of Geriatric Physical Therapy, 32*(4), 174–180.

Daley, A. J. (2009). Can exergaming contribute to improving physical activity levels and health outcomes in children? *Pediatrics, 124*(2), 763–771. http://doi.org/10.1542/peds.2008-2357.

Daniel, K. (2012). Wii-Hab for pre-frail older adults. *Rehabilitation Nursing, 37*(4), 195–201.

dos Santos Mendes, F. A., Pompeu, J. E., Lobo, A. M., da Silva, K. G., de Paula Oliveira, T., … Piemonte, M. E. P. (2012). Motor learning, retention and transfer after virtual-reality-based training in Parkinson's disease–effect of motor and cognitive demands of games: A longitudinal, controlled clinical study. *Physiotherapy, 98*(3), 217–223.

Duncan, M., & Staples, V. (2010). The impact of a school-based active video game play intervention on children's physical activity during recess. *Human Movement, 11*(1), 95–99. http://doi.org/10.2478/v10038-009-0023-1.

Errickson, S. P., Maloney, A. E., & Thorpe, D. (2012). "'Dance Dance Revolution'" used by 7- and 8-year-olds to boost physical activity: Is coaching necessary for adherence to an exercise prescription? *Games for Health Journal, 1*(1), 45–50. http://doi.org/10.1089/g4h.2011.0028.

Esculier, J. F., Vaudrin, J., Bériault, P., Gagnon, K., & Tremblay, L. E. (2012). Home-based balance training programme using Wii Fit with balance board for Parkinson's disease: A pilot study. *Journal of Rehabilitation Medicine, 44*(2), 144–150.

Fogel, V. a, Miltenberger, R. G., Graves, R., & Koehler, S. (2010). The effects of exergaming on physical activity among inactive children in a physical education classroom. *Journal of Applied Behavior Analysis, 43*(4), 591–600. http://doi.org/10.1901/jaba.2010.43-591.

Foley, L., & Maddison, R. (2010). Use of active video games to increase physical activity in children: A (virtual) reality. *Pediatric Exercise Science, 22*, 7–20.

Franco, J. R., Jacobs, K., Inzerillo, C., & Kluzik, J. (2012). The effect of the Nintendo Wii Fit and exercise in improving balance and quality of life in community dwelling elders. *Technology and Health Care, 20*(2), 95–115.

Fung, V., Ho, A., Shaffer, J., Chung, E., & Gomez, M. (2012). Use of Nintendo Wii Fit™ in the rehabilitation of outpatients following total knee replacement: A preliminary randomized controlled trial. *Physiotherapy, 98*(3), 183–188.

Gallahue, D. L., Ozmun, J. C., & Goodway, J. (2012). *Understanding motor development: Infants, children, adolescents, adults* (7th ed.). Boston, MA: McGraw-Hill.

Gao, Y., Gerling, K. M., Mandryk, R. L., & Stanley, K. G. (2014, October). Decreasing sedentary behaviours in pre-adolescents using casual exergames at school. In *Proceedings of the first ACM SIGCHI annual symposium on computer-human interaction in play* (pp. 97–106). ACM.

Gao, Z. (2012). Motivated but not active: The dilemmas of incorporating interactive dance into gym class. *Journal of Physical Activity & Health, 9*(6), 794–800.

Gao, Z. (2017). Fight fire with fire: Promoting physical activity and health through active video games. *Journal of Sport and Health Science*.

Gao, Z., & Chen, S. (2014). Are field-based exergames useful in preventing childhood obesity? A systematic review. *Obesity Reviews, 5*, 1–16. http://doi.org/10.1111/obr.12164.

Gao, Z., Chen, S., Pasco, D., & Pope, Z. (2015). A meta-analysis of active video games on health outcomes among children and adolescents. *Obesity Reviews, 16*(9), 783–794. http://doi.org/10.1111/obr.12287.

Gao, Z., Hannan, P., Xiang, P., Stodden, D. F., & Valdez, V. E. (2013). Video game-based exercise, Latino children's physical health, and academic achievement. *American Journal of Preventive Medicine, 44*(3 Suppl 3), 240–246. http://doi.org/10.1016/j.amepre.2012.11.023.

Gao, Z., Hannon, J. C., Newton, M., & Huang, C. (2011). Effects of curricular activity on students' situational motivation and physical activity levels. *Research Quarterly for Exercise and Sport, 82*(3), 536–544.

Gao, Z., Huang, C., Liu, T., & Xiong, W. (2012). Impact of interactive dance games on urban children's physical activity correlates and behavior. *Journal of Exercise Science & Fitness, 10*(2), 107–112. http://doi.org/10.1016/j.jesf.2012.10.009.

Gao, Z., & Podlog, L. (2012). Urban Latino children's physical activity levels and performance in interactive dance video games: Effects of goal difficulty and goal specificity. *Archives of Pediatrics & Adolescent Medicine, 166*(10), 933–937. http://doi.org/10.1001/archpediatrics.2012.649.

Gao, Z., Podlog, L., & Huang, C. (2013). Associations among children's situational motivation, physical activity participation, and enjoyment in an active dance video game. *Journal of Sport and Health Science, 2*(2), 122–128. http://doi.org/10.1016/j.jshs.2012.07.001.

Gao, Z., & Xiang, P. (2014). Effects of exergaming based exercise on urban children's physical activity participation and body composition. *Journal of Physical Activity & Health, 11*(5), 992–998. http://doi.org/10.1123/jpah.2012-0228.

Gao, Z., Zhang, P., & Podlog, L. W. (2013). Examining elementary school children's level of enjoyment of traditional tag games vs. interactive dance games. *Psychology, Health & Medicine, 19*(5), 605–613. http://doi.org/10.1080/13548506.2013.845304.

Gao, Z., Zhang, T., & Stodden, D. (2013). Children's physical activity levels and psychological correlates in interactive dance versus aerobic dance. *Journal of Sport and Health Science, 2*(3), 146–151. http://doi.org/10.1016/j.jshs.2013.01.005.

Gil-Gómez, J. A., Lloréns, R., Alcañiz, M., & Colomer, C. (2011). Effectiveness of a Wii balance board-based system (eBaViR) for balance rehabilitation: A pilot randomized clinical trial in patients with acquired brain injury. *Journal of Neuroengineering and Rehabilitation, 8*(1), 1–9.

Gioftsidou, A., Vernadakis, N., Malliou, P., Batzios, S., Sofokleous, P., Antoniou, P., … & Godolias, G. (2013). Typical balance exercises or exergames for balance improvement. *Journal of Back and Musculoskeletal Rehabilitation, 26*(3), 299–305.

Goldfield, G. S., Adamo, K. B., Rutherford, J., & Murray, M. (2012). The effects of aerobic exercise on psychosocial functioning of adolescents who are overweight or obese. *Journal of Pediatric Psychology, 37*(11), 1136–1147.

Graves, L. E. F., Ridgers, N. D., & Stratton, G. (2008). The contribution of upper limb and total body movement to adolescents' energy expenditure whilst playing Nintendo

Wii. *European Journal of Applied Physiology, 104*(4), 617–623. http://doi.org/10.1007/s00421-008-0813-8.

Guy, S., Ratzki-Leewing, A., & Gwadry-Sridhar, F. (2011). Moving beyond the stigma: Systematic review of video games and their potential to combat obesity. *International Journal of Hypertension, 2011*, 1–13. http://doi.org/10.4061/2011/179124.

Hammond, J., Jones, V., Hill, E. L., Green, D., & Male, I. (2014). An investigation of the impact of regular use of the Wii Fit to improve motor and psychosocial outcomes in children with movement difficulties: A pilot study. *Child: Care, Health and Development, 40*(2), 165–175.

Herz, N. B., Mehta, S. H., Sethi, K. D., Jackson, P., Hall, P., & Morgan, J. C. (2013). Nintendo Wii rehabilitation ("Wii-hab") provides benefits in Parkinson's disease. *Parkinsonism & Related Disorders, 19*(11), 1039–1042.

Hilton, C. L., Cumpata, K., Klohr, C., Gaetke, S., Artner, A., Johnson, H., & Dobbs, S. (2014). Effects of exergaming on executive function and motor skills in children with autism spectrum disorder: A pilot study. *American Journal of Occupational Therapy, 68*(1), 57–65.

Holmes, J., Powell-Griner, E., Lethbridge-Cejku, M., & Heyman, K. (2009). Aging differently: Physical limitations among adults aged 50 years and over: United States, 2001–2007. *NCHS Data Brief, 20*(1). Retrieved from http://origin.glb.cdc.gov/nchs/products/databriefs/db20.htm.

Hsu, J. K., Thibodeau, R., Wong, S. J., Zukiwsky, D., Cecile, S., & Walton, D. M. (2011). A "Wii" bit of fun: The effects of adding Nintendo Wii® Bowling to a standard exercise regimen for residents of long-term care with upper extremity dysfunction. *Physiotherapy Theory and Practice, 27*(3), 185–193.

Hung, J. W., Chou, C. X., Hsieh, Y. W., Wu, W. C., Yu, M. Y., Chen, P. C., … & Ding, S. E. (2014). Randomized comparison trial of balance training by using exergaming and conventional weight-shift therapy in patients with chronic stroke. *Archives of Physical Medicine and Rehabilitation, 95*(9), 1629–1637.

Imam, B., Miller, W. C., Finlayson, H., Eng, J. J., & Jarus, T. (2015). A randomized controlled trial to evaluate the feasibility of the Wii Fit for improving walking in older adults with lower limb amputation. *Clinical Rehabilitation, 31*(1), 82–92.

Jelsma, D., Geuze, R. H., Mombarg, R., & Smits-Engelsman, B. C. (2014). The impact of Wii Fit intervention on dynamic balance control in children with probable developmental coordination disorder and balance problems. *Human Movement Science, 33*, 404–418. http://dx.doi.org/10.1016/j.humov.2013.12.007.

Johnson, T. M., Ridgers, N. D., Hulteen, R. M., Mellecker, R. R., & Barnett, L. M. (2016). Does playing a sports active video game improve young children's ball skill competence? *Journal of Science and Medicine in Sport, 19*(5), 432–436. http://dx.doi.org/10.1016/j.jsams.2015.05.002.

Kim, E. K., Kang, J. H., Park, J. S., & Jung, B. H. (2012). Clinical feasibility of interactive commercial Nintendo gaming for chronic stroke rehabilitation. *Journal of Physical Therapy Science, 24*(9), 901–903.

Kramer, A., Dettmers, C., & Gruber, M. (2014). Exergaming with additional postural demands improves balance and gait in patients with multiple sclerosis as much as conventional balance training and leads to high adherence to home-based balance training. *Archives of Physical Medicine and Rehabilitation, 95*(10), 1803–1809.

Lange, B., Flynn, S. M., & Rizzo, A. A. (2009). Game-based telerehabilitation. *European Journal of Physical and Rehabilitation Medicine, 45*(1), 143–151.

LeBlanc, A. G., Chaput, J.-P., McFarlane, A., Colley, R. C., Thivel, D., Biddle, S. J. H., … Tremblay, M. S. (2013). Active video games and health indicators in children and youth: A systematic review. *PloS One, 8*(6), e65351. http://doi.org/10.1371/journal.pone.0065351.

Levasseur, M., Généreux, M., Bruneau, J. F., Vanasse, A., Chabot, É., Beaulac, C., & Bédard, M. M. (2015). Importance of proximity to resources, social support, transportation and neighborhood security for mobility and social participation in older adults: Results from a scoping study. *BMC Public Health, 15*(1), 1. http//doi: 10.1186/s12889-015-1824-0.

Li, J., Theng, Y. L., & Foo, S. (2016). Effect of exergames on depression: A systematic review and meta-analysis. *Cyberpsychology, Behavior, and Social Networking, 19*(1), 34–42.

Liang, Y., & Lau, P. W. C. (2014). Effects of active videogames on physical activity and related outcomes among healthy children: A systematic review. *Games for Health Journal, 3*(3), 122–144. http://doi.org/10.1089/g4h.2013.0070.

Lu, A. S., Kharrazi, H., Gharghabi, F., & Thompson, D. (2013). A systematic review of health videogames on childhood obesity prevention and intervention. *Games for Health Journal, 2*(3), 131–141. http://doi.org/10.1089/g4h.2013.0025.

Lwin, M. O., & Malik, S. (2014). Can exergames impart health messages? Game play, framing, and drivers of physical activity among children. *Journal of Health Communication, 19*(2), 136–151. http://doi.org/10.1080/10810730.2013.798372.

Maddison, R., Foley, L., Mhurchu, C. N., Jiang, Y., Jull, A., Prapavessis, H., … & Rodgers, A. (2011). Effects of active video games on body composition: A randomized controlled trial. *The American Journal of Clinical Nutrition, 94*(1), 156–163. http//doi: 10.3945/ajcn.110.009142.

Maddison, R., Mhurchu, C. N., Jull, A., Prapavessis, H., & Rodgers, A. (2007). Energy expended playing video console games: An opportunity to increase children's physical activity? *Pediatric Exercise Science, 19*, 334–343.

Madsen, K. A., Yen, S., Wlasiuk, L., Newman, T. B., & Lustig, R. (2007). Feasibility of a dance videogame to promote weight loss among overweight children and adolescents. *Archives of Pediatrics & Adolescent Medicine, 161*(1), 105–107. http//doi: 10.1001/archpedi.161.1.105-c.

Maloney, A. E., Bethea, T. C., Kelsey, K. S., Marks, J. T., Paez, S., Rosenberg, A. M., … Sikich, L. (2008). A pilot of a video game (DDR) to promote physical activity and decrease sedentary screen time. *Obesity, 16*(9), 2074–2080.

Maloney, A. E., Stempel, A., Wood, M. E., Patraitis, C., & Beaudoin, C. (2012). Can dance exergames boost physical activity as a school-based intervention? *Games for Health Journal, 1*(6), 416–421. http://doi.org/10.1089/g4h.2011.0010.

Marti, A. C., Alvarez-Pitti, J. C., Provinciale, J. C., Lison, J. F., & Rivera, R. B. (2015). Alternative options for prescribing physical activity among obese children and adolescents: Brisk walking supported by an exergaming platform, *Nutrición Hospitalaria, 31*(2), 841–848.

McCarthy, H., Brazil, S. T., Greene, J. C., Rendell, S., & Rohr, L. E. (2013). The impact of Wii Fit yoga training on flexibility and heart rate. *International SportMed Journal, 14*(2), 67–76.

McManus, A. M., & Mellecker, R. R. (2012). Physical activity and obese children. *Journal of Sport and Health Science, 1*(3), 141–148. http://doi.org/10.1016/j.jshs.2012.09.004.

Mears, D., & Hansen, L. (2009). Active gaming: Definitions, options and implementation. *Strategies, 23*(2), 26–29.

Mhatre, P. V., Vilares, I., Stibb, S. M., Albert, M. V., Pickering, L., Marciniak, C. M., … & Toledo, S. (2013). Wii Fit balance board playing improves balance and gait in Parkinson disease. *PM&R, 5*(9), 769–777.

Miller, T. A., Vaux-Bjerke, A., McDonnell, K. A., & DiPietro, L. (2013). Can E-Gaming be useful for achieving recommended levels of moderate- to vigorous-intensity physical activity in inner-city children? *Games for Health Journal, 2*(2), 96–102. http://doi.org/10.1089/g4h.2012.0058.

Murphy, E. C.-S., Carson, L., Neal, W., Baylis, C., Donley, D., & Yeater, R. (2009). Effects of an exercise intervention using Dance Dance Revolution on endothelial function and other risk factors in overweight children. *International Journal of Pediatric Obesity, 4*(4), 205–214. http://doi.org/10.3109/17477160902846187.

Ni Mhurchu, C., Maddison, R., Jiang, Y., Jull, A., Prapavessis, H., & Rodgers, A. (2008). Couch potatoes to jumping beans: A pilot study of the effect of active video games on physical activity in children. *The International Journal of Behavioral Nutrition and Physical Activity, 5*(1), 1. http://doi.org/10.1186/1479-5868-5-8.

Nilsagard, Y. E., Forsberg, A. S., & von Koch, L. (2013). Balance exercise for persons with multiple sclerosis using Wii games: A randomised, controlled multi-centre study. *Multiple Sclerosis Journal, 19*(2), 209–216.

Orsega-Smith, E., Davis, J., Slavish, K., & Gimbutas, L. (2012). Wii Fit balance intervention in community-dwelling older adults. *Games for Health: Research, Development, and Clinical Applications, 1*(6), 431–435.

Pate, R. R. (2008). Physically active video gaming: An effective strategy for obesity prevention. *Archives of Pediatrics & Adolescent Medicine, 162*(9), 895–896. http//doi: 10.1001/archpedi.161.1.105.

Paw, M. J. C. A., Jacobs, W. M., Vaessen, E. P., Titze, S., & van Mechelen, W. (2008). The motivation of children to play an active video game. *Journal of Science and Medicine in Sport, 11*(2), 163–166.

Peng, W., Lin, J. H., & Crouse, J. (2011). Is playing exergames really exercising? A meta-analysis of energy expenditure in active video games. *Cyberpsychology, Behavior and Social Networking, 14*(11), 681–688. http://doi.org/10.1089/cyber.2010.0578.

Penko, A. L., & Barkley, J. E. (2010). Motivation and physiologic responses of playing a physically interactive video game relative to a sedentary alternative in children. *Annals of Behavioral Medicine, 39*(2), 162–169.

Pluchino, A., Lee, S. Y., Asfour, S., Roos, B. A., & Signorile, J. F. (2012). Pilot study comparing changes in postural control after training using a video game balance board program and 2 standard activity-based balance intervention programs. *Archives of Physical Medicine and Rehabilitation, 93*(7), 1138–1146.

Pompeu, J. E., dos Santos Mendes, F. A., da Silva, K. G., Lobo, A. M., de Paula Oliveira, T., Zomignani, A. P., & Piemonte, M. E. P. (2012). Effect of Nintendo Wii™ based motor and cognitive training on activities of daily living in patients with Parkinson's disease: A randomised clinical trial. *Physiotherapy, 98*(3), 196–204.

Pope, Z., Lee, J., Li, X., & Gao, Z. (2016). Effects of exergaming on college students' energy expenditure, physical activity and enjoyment. *Medicine and Science in Sports and Exercise, 48*(5), S594.

Primack, B. a, Carroll, M. V, McNamara, M., Klem, M. Lou, King, B., Rich, M., … Nayak, S. (2012). Role of video games in improving health-related outcomes: A systematic review. *American Journal of Preventive Medicine, 42*(6), 630–638. http://doi.org/10.1016/j.amepre.2012.02.023.

Rahman, S. A. (2010). Efficacy of virtual reality-based therapy on balance in children with Down syndrome. *World Applied Sciences Journal, 10*(3), 254–261.

Rendon, A. A., Lohman, E. B., Thorpe, D., Johnson, E. G., Medina, E., & Bradley, B. (2012). The effect of virtual reality gaming on dynamic balance in older adults. *Age and Ageing, 41*(4), 549–552.

Robinson, J., Dixon, J., Macsween, A., van Schaik, P., & Martin, D. (2015). The effects of exergaming on balance, gait, technology acceptance and flow experience in people with multiple sclerosis: A randomized controlled trial. *BMC Sports Science, Medicine and Rehabilitation, 7*(1), 1. http//doi:10.1186/s13102-015-0001-1.
Salem, Y., Gropack, S. J., Coffin, D., & Godwin, E. M. (2012). Effectiveness of a low-cost virtual reality system for children with developmental delay: A preliminary randomised single-blind controlled trial. *Physiotherapy, 98*(3), 189–195.
Sato, K., Kuroki, K., Saiki, S., & Nagatomi, R. (2015). Improving walking, muscle strength, and balance in the elderly with an exergame using Kinect: A randomized controlled trial. *Games for Health Journal, 4*(3), 161–167. http//doi: 10.1089/g4h.2014.0057.
Serino, M., Cordrey, K., McLaughlin, L., & Milanaik, R. L. (2016). Pokémon Go and augmented virtual reality games: A cautionary commentary for parents and pediatricians. *Current Opinion in Pediatrics, 28*(5), 673–677. http//doi: 10.1097/MOP.0000000000000409.
Sheehan, D. P., & Katz, L. (2012). The impact of a 6-week exergaming curriculum on balance with grade three school children using the Wii Fit. *International Journal of Computer Science in Sport, 11*(3), 5–22.
Sheehan, D. P., & Katz, L. (2013). The effects of a daily, 6-week exergaming curriculum on balance in fourth grade children. *Journal of Sport and Health Science, 2*(3), 131–137. http://doi.org/10.1016/j.jshs.2013.02.002.
Sims, J., Cosby, N., Saliba, E. N., Hertel, J., & Saliba, S. A. (2013). Exergaming and static postural control in individuals with a history of lower limb injury. *Journal of Athletic Training, 48*(3), 314–325.
Staiano, A. E., Abraham, A. A., & Calvert, S. L. (2013). Adolescent exergame play for weight loss and psychosocial improvement: A controlled physical activity intervention. *Obesity, 21*(3), 598–601. http//doi:10.1002/oby.20282.
Staiano, A. E., Marker, A. M., Beyl, R. A., Hsia, D. S., Katzmarzyk, P. T., and Newton, R. L. (2016) A randomized controlled trial of dance exergaming for exercise training in overweight and obese adolescent girls. *Pediatric Obesity*, http//doi: 10.1111/ijpo.12117.
Sun, H. (2012). Exergaming impact on physical activity and interest in elementary school children. *Research Quarterly for Exercise and Sport, 83*(2), 212–220.
Sun, H. (2013). Impact of exergames on physical activity and motivation in elementary school students: A follow-up study. *Journal of Sport and Health Science, 2*(3), 138–145. http://doi.org/10.1016/j.jshs.2013.02.003.
Szturm, T., Betker, A. L., Moussavi, Z., Desai, A., & Goodman, V. (2011). Effects of an interactive computer game exercise regimen on balance impairment in frail community-dwelling older adults: A randomized controlled trial. *Physical Therapy, 91*(10), 1449–1462.
Toulotte, C., Toursel, C., & Olivier, N. (2012). Wii Fit® training vs. adapted physical activities: Which one is the most appropriate to improve the balance of independent senior subjects? A randomized controlled study. *Clinical Rehabilitation, 26*(9), 827–835.
Trost, S. G., Sundal, D., Foster, G. D., Lent, M. R., & Vojta, D. (2014). Effects of a pediatric weight management program with and without active video games: A randomized trial. *JAMA Pediatrics, 168*(5), 407–413. http//doi: 10.1001/jamapediatrics.2013.3436.
Van Biljon, A., & Longhurst, G. K. (2012). The influence of exergaming on the functional fitness in overweight and obese children: Physical activity, health and wellness.

African Journal for Physical Health Education, Recreation and Dance, 18(42), 984–991.

van den Berg, M., Sherrington, C., Killington, M., Smith, S., Bongers, B., Hassett, L., & Crotty, M. (2016). Video and computer-based interactive exercises are safe and improve task-specific balance in geriatric and neurological rehabilitation: A randomised trial. *Journal of Physiotherapy, 62*(1), 20–28.

Van Diest, M., Lamoth, C. J., Stegenga, J., Verkerke, G. J., & Postema, K. (2013). Exergaming for balance training of elderly: State of the art and future developments. *Journal of Neuroengineering and Rehabilitation, 10*(1), 1.

Verhoeven, K., Abeele, V. V., Gers, B., & Seghers, J. (2015). Energy expenditure during Xbox Kinect play in early adolescents: The relationship with player mode and game enjoyment. *Games for Health Journal, 4*(6), 444–451. http//doi: 10.1089/g4h.2014.0106.

Vernadakis, N., Gioftsidou, A., Antoniou, P., Ioannidis, D., & Giannousi, M. (2012). The impact of Nintendo Wii to physical education students' balance compared to the traditional approaches. *Computers & Education, 59*(2), 196–205.

Vernadakis, N., Papastergiou, M., Zetou, E., & Antoniou, P. (2015). The impact of an exergame-based intervention on children's fundamental motor skills. *Computers & Education, 83*, 90–102.

Wagener, T. L., Fedele, D. A., Mignogna, M. R., Hester, C. N., & Gillaspy, S. R. (2012). Psychological effects of dance-based group exergaming in obese adolescents. *Pediatric Obesity, 7*(5), e68-e74. http//doi: 10.1111/j.2047-6310.2012.00065.x.

Welk, G., & Blair, S. (2000). Physical activity protects against the health risks of obesity. *Research Digest, 3*, 1–8.

Whittman, G. (2010). Video gaming increases physical activity. *Journal of Extension, 48*(2), 1–4.

Yavuzer, G., Senel, A., Atay, M. B., & Stam, H. J. (2008). "Playstation Eyetoy games" improve upper extremity-related motor functioning in subacute stroke: A randomized controlled clinical trial. *European Journal of Physical and Rehabilitation Medicine, 44*(3), 237–244.

Zeng, N., Lee, J., Pope, Z., Li, X., & Gao, Z. (2016). College students' situational motivation, energy expenditure, and blood pressure in exergaming and treadmill walking. *Medicine and Science in Sports and Exercise, 48*(5), S717.

10 Virtual reality in physical activity promotion

Nan Zeng and Zan Gao

Among emerging technologies poised to aid in the assessment and promotion of physical activity (PA) and health, virtual reality and augmented reality (a.k.a., simulation technology) are arguably the most exciting and technologically advanced. Virtual reality is a digital technology that replicates a real or imagined environment, and simulates a user's physical presence in this environment allowing for user interaction (Isaac, 2016). Two types of virtual reality exist. The first is immersive virtual reality which frequently uses head-mounted displays, body-motion sensors, real-time graphics, and advanced interface devices (e.g., specialized helmets) in the simulation of an environment for the user. Conversely, non-immersive virtual reality uses interfaces such as flat-screen televisions/computer screens with associated keyboards, game pads, and joysticks—not simulating an environment to as deep a degree as immersive virtual reality. Simply stated, virtual reality creates an environment in which visual, auditory, and other perceptual stimuli are incorporated in a sequence of manipulated events to which a person is expected to react (Pasco, 2013). That is, virtual reality replaces the real world with a simulated world.

The latest commercially available virtual reality headsets, such as the Oculus Rift, PlayStation VR, Samsung Gear VR, or HTC Vive artificially generate sensory experiences, which may include visual, auditory, touch and scent stimuli, while allowing a user to manipulate objects within the virtual environment (Isaac, 2016). Notably, virtual reality environments are split into two categories. Simple virtual reality environments consist of a two-dimensional (2-D) viewing environment, whereas a complex virtual reality environment can include three-dimensional (3-D) digital objects and user-controlled avatars displayed in real-time (i.e., without any time delay in movement between the users' and avatars' actions). Since a 3-D environment provides a condition where individuals are immersed in close-to-reality situations while interacting with digital objects and other avatars, virtual reality interaction concepts within these environments have been widely used to help understand virtual reality applications and their features—immersion, interaction, and presence—in PA and health promotion (Pasco, 2013).

By contrast, augmented reality is a direct or indirect live view of a physical, real-world environment whose elements are supplemented by computer-generated sensory input such as sound, video, graphics or GPS data (Graham, Zook, & Boulton, 2013). Augmented virtual reality games, like Pokémon Go and Zombies, Run!, are unique in that they overlay aspects from the physical and virtual worlds into one cohesive experience. In fact, virtual reality and augmented reality are the inverse of one another as virtual reality offers a digital recreation of a real-life setting, while augmented reality delivers virtual elements as an overlay onto the real world (Augment, 2015) (Figure 10.1). Investigation and understanding of virtual reality and augmented reality interaction concepts are of paramount importance when applied to the PA and health promotion fields as it increases the likelihood of effective interventions.

To date, virtual reality is extensively used in many health domains, with most virtual reality systems designed to facilitate cognitive learning, motor function,

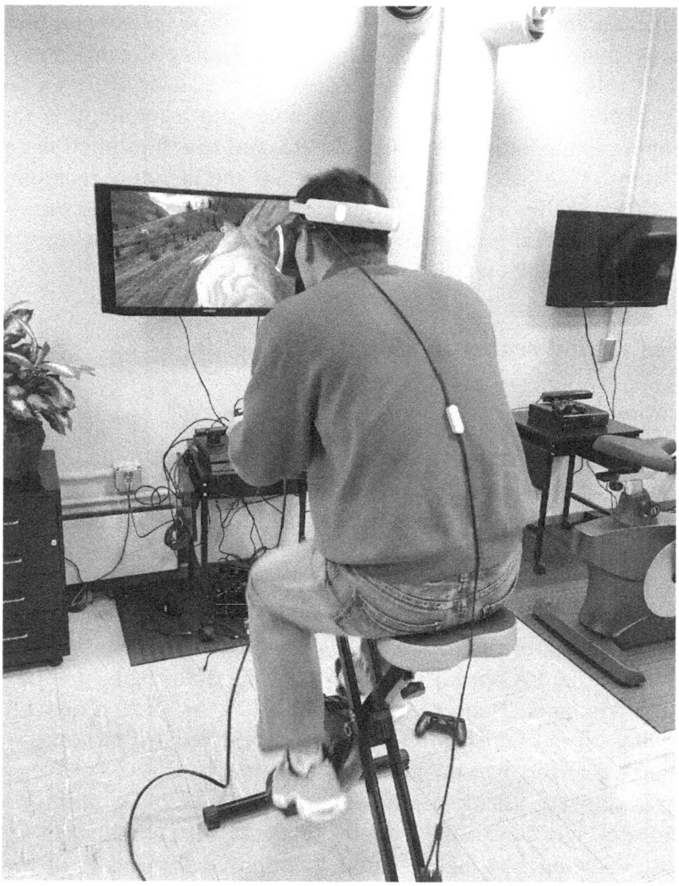

Figure 10.1 An adult playing a virtual reality active game.

Source: Photo by Nan Zeng.

and psychological well-being. Additionally, virtual reality is also considered a cutting-edge technology possessing great potential in PA and health promotion. Specifically, virtual reality systems present opportunities for the implementation of interventions aimed at increasing PA and promoting health in environments including, but not limited to, school-based physical education classes, community-based fitness programs, or home-based rehabilitation, among others. To this end, virtual reality has received considerable attention in the promotion of PA participation in healthy individuals in addition to being used for rehabilitation purposes in patients (Miller et al., 2014). Indeed, in an attempt to provide diverse workout experiences, some researchers and health professionals have even integrated traditional PA equipment with virtual reality technology. For example, combining virtual reality with standard gym-based exercise equipment, such as a stationary exercise bike, may serve to enhance the psychological benefits of exercise (Mestre, Dagonneau, & Mercier, 2011). These psychological benefits may increase the chances of long-term adherence to an exercise program through the provision of a sense of challenge and regulated competition, and result in a more enjoyable exercise experiences (Plante, Aldridge, Bogden, & Haneli, 2003). Therefore, virtual reality as an emerging technology is rapidly becoming a popular intervention technique for PA and health promotion among various populations. This chapter will mainly review the literature regarding the application of virtual reality in PA and health promotion in various settings (i.e., physical education, sports, and rehabilitation) and populations (i.e., young, middle-aged, and older adults with/without disabilities).

Application of virtual reality in different PA settings

Physical education

Due to support from organizations such as SHAPE America, in addition to the increasing presence of modern technology in healthcare, virtual reality is becoming widely accepted by physical educators for use in promoting children's PA (Hansen & Sanders, 2012). Physical educators nationwide have been integrating immersive and non-immersive forms of virtual reality systems into their curricula through provision of virtual reality exercise bikes, rhythmic dance machines, sporting games, martial arts simulators, balance boards, and other similar products—thereby increasing PA appeal and motivation in youth engaged in physical education/fitness programs (Hansen & Sanders, 2012). As such, a new area of research regarding virtual reality's ability to be integrated within the physical education setting has arisen over the last several years.

While the traditional physical education teaching methodology still predominates within most current physical education curricula, virtual reality in school-based physical education has the potential to improve students' self-training awareness, prevent injuries, and overcome gym space limitations, among other benefits (Liao, 2015) (Figure 10.2). In fact, some K-12 schools have begun using such devices in their physical education classes. For example, students in the San

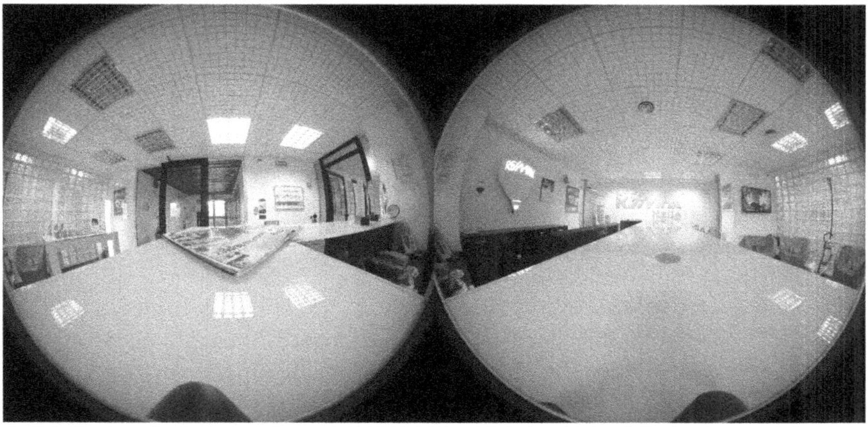

Figure 10.2 From the lens of a virtual reality game.
Source: pixabay.com.

Francisco Unified School District and Florida's Polk County Public Schools are among the first to use Nearpod VR virtual reality lesson plans. Using branded Google Cardboards, teachers can send classes on over 25 virtual field trip lessons across many curricular areas from math to science and from foreign language to health and physical education. Unfortunately, there is a paucity of experimental research on using virtual reality as an intervention tool in the K-12 physical education setting. As such, the effects of virtual reality in physical education classes are unclear. Despite initially positive results, the development and utilization of virtual reality within school-based physical education continue to be limited by many schools' reluctance to allocate gym/classroom space and funds to physical education (Liao, 2015)—explaining the relatively few virtual reality studies seen in physical education settings. Therefore, researchers and practitioners should address the following questions: (1) given the high cost of implementing school-based virtual reality programs, how do physical educators make school administration understand the potential effectiveness of virtual reality to improve PA and health outcomes among children in physical education?; (2) once implemented in physical education, how can virtual reality be used as a teaching medium capable of strengthening and improving teaching methods and optimizing teaching content?; and (3) using virtual reality-based teaching methodology and content provision, how effectively does virtual reality aid physical educators in helping youth meet national physical education standards (e.g., developing physical literacy and providing the knowledge and skills necessary to be "lifelong movers") (SHAPE America, 2013).

Sports

Biofeedback (e.g., heart rate, breathing mechanics, etc.) was previously the main technology used to provide information regarding athlete performance (Lieberman & Breazeal, 2007). Other previous technologies focused on transferring sports-related skills from a video game training context to performance of the sports-related skill on the actual field of play (Rosser et al., 2007). However, advances in virtual reality technology have offered new possibilities for sports performance training (Bailenson et al., 2008). Specifically, improvements in visualization, motion capture, and computing power have paved the way for the development of virtual reality simulations capable of training sensorimotor components of sports (Bideau et al., 2010). Indeed, virtual reality has been demonstrated to be useful for enhancing athletic performance when aiming to improve an existing skill (Bergamasco, Bardy, & Gopher, 2012; Bideau et al., 2010). Coaches and athletes find virtual reality training useful as this technology allows for a systematically controlled environment—likely reducing injury risk—and can be used to manipulate factors (e.g., creating simulated adverse weather conditions) that affect athletes' performance on the actual field of play. For example, a feasibility study by Stinson and Bowman (2014) used virtual reality to aid in improving soccer athletes' performance during high-pressure situations. To conduct this study, researchers developed an immersive virtual reality soccer goalkeeping environment in which users defended against simulated penalty kicks using their bodies. Findings indicated that a virtual reality sport-oriented system can induce increased anxiety (as assessed by physiological and subjective measures) compared to a baseline condition. These findings suggest that inducing anxiety (i.e., adverse conditions) using virtual reality systems is possible and may be used to train athletes in psychologically taxing situations that they might face on the actual field of play. Further research, however, is needed to determine if simulated virtual reality sporting environments can lead to improvement in sports psychology variables aside from anxiety. Nonetheless, through systematically manipulating these factors and analyzing the instant feedback generated during virtual reality training sessions which simulated these adverse conditions, coaches and athletes can then develop better training programs on the actual field of play that allow for improved performance despite the adverse conditions the athletes might face (Hoffmann, Filippeschi, Ruffaldi, & Bardy, 2014).

Aside from simulating potentially adverse conditions on the field of play, virtual reality has been used as a training aid in many sports (e.g., golf, rowing, skiing, cycling, etc.) to help evaluate athletic performance and analyze technique. For example, 3-D virtual reality systems can pinpoint certain aspects of an athlete's unique biomechanics and technique which need to be modified. In recent years, studies using virtual reality as a training tool have become more common. For instance, Hoffmann and colleagues (2014) investigated the use of virtual reality with novice rowers as a means to learn about energy management. Fifteen participants were assigned to an avatar group ($n=7$) asked to track a boat on the screen, whose speed was set individually to follow the appropriate to-be-learned speed profile. The control group ($n=8$) followed a traditional indoor training program. Findings demonstrated decreased racing times among rowing participants within the avatar group, whereas the control group did not obtain the same improvements—suggesting virtual reality may be an effective means of learning energy management and enhancing performance. In fact, virtual reality training has been widely recognized by some professional sports teams and The National Collegiate Athletic Association (NCAA) Division I institutions. Recently, the Minnesota Vikings announced that they had incorporated virtual reality into their quarterback training, joining the New York Jets, Dallas Cowboys, San Francisco 49ers, and Arizona Cardinals in the virtual realm. At the NCAA level, the Stanford, Auburn, Clemson, Vanderbilt, Dartmouth, Rice, and the University of Arkansas football programs are also using the system provided by STRIVR Labs (focusing on using virtual reality to improve the performance of athletes). Although there is a paucity of research on this topic, with the technology still in its infancy, virtual reality shows promise for a wide range of athlete training.

What is clear from the preceding literature review regarding the use of virtual reality in various PA settings is the fact that virtual reality technologies show initial potential in physical education and sports settings to promote PA and athletic performance. Nevertheless, few large-scale, methodologically rigorous studies have been conducted in the literature, with no study completed in physical education classes. While improvements to virtual reality technology have been significant in recent years, the technology is still young. Therefore, more research is warranted to prove the effectiveness of virtual reality technologies prior to adoption by physical educators and coaches for promoting PA and athletic performance, respectively.

Application of virtual reality technology in rehabilitation

Physical rehabilitation

Physical rehabilitation strives to aid patients with disabilities in the acquisition of lost motor skills that may have come about due to injury or illness—with the main goal being to ensure these individuals can perform activities of daily living (Weiss, Keshner, & Levin, 2014). Virtual reality-based physical rehabilitation technology shares the preceding objectives, with the improvement of functional capacity paramount, while also offering an easier-to-implement physical rehabilitation option to a diverse array of populations, such as adults suffering from stroke and Parkinson's disease and children/adolescents with developmental disabilities (Weiss, Keshner, & Levin, 2014).

To date, approximately 15 million people annually have a new or recurrent stroke worldwide, and nearly two-thirds of stroke survivors have motor deficits associated with diminished quality of life (Feigin et al., 2016; Krishnamurthi et al., 2015). As a result of motor deficits, most patients are unable to perform independent actions, tasks, and activities needed for self-care, home management, employment, and social activities. Conventional stroke rehabilitation techniques, such as motor relearning, neurodevelopmental therapy, or proprioceptive neuromuscular facilitation, are similarly effective in improving motor function (Saposnik, 2016). However, traditional physical rehabilitation can be resource-intensive and costly—often requiring specialized facilities not always widely available (Jutai & Teasell, 2003). Resulting from the limitations of traditional physical rehabilitation, virtual reality is now seen as a novel rehabilitation strategy and is regarded as an enjoyable alternative to promote motor recovery. Indeed, promising evidence from previous research has shown the effectiveness of virtual reality for improving motor function after stroke.

In a recent randomized controlled trial, Saposnik and colleagues (2016) found a non-immersive virtual reality group using the Nintendo Wii gaming system (VRWii) improved upper extremity motor performance time from baseline and posttest. Yet, there was no significant difference between the virtual reality and control group playing recreational activities (e.g., cards, ball games, Jenga). The study suggests that innovative non-immersive virtual reality technologies might be as effective as recreational activities in enhancing upper extremity motor function among stroke patients. Similarly, Subramanian et al. (2013) revealed that endpoint speed, overall performance on a reach-to-grasp task, and activity levels increased in both virtual reality environment and physical environment groups. However, only participants in the virtual reality environment group improved shoulder horizontal adduction and flexion at post-test. As such, virtual reality training might be a suitable alternative for stroke patients to promote upper-limb recovery.

Additionally, the effects of virtual reality-based physical rehabilitation on lower extremity function (e.g., to improve balance and reduce risk of falls) among stroke populations has also been proved. For example, McEwen and colleagues (2014) investigated whether a 3-week adjunct virtual reality therapy improves balance, mobility, and gait in stroke rehabilitation inpatients. The treatment group ($n=30$) received a standard stroke rehabilitation therapy plus virtual reality exercises that challenged balance (e.g., soccer goaltending and snowboarding) performed while standing. The control group ($n=29$) received identical treatment but did not challenge balance and, instead, performed treatments while sitting. Findings indicated the treatment group had reduced impairment in the lower extremity compared to the control group. Further, Cho, Lee, and Song (2012) conducted a 6-week randomized controlled trial to examine the effects of virtual reality training on the balance of chronic stroke patients. Although there was no increase in static balance for either group, greater improvements for dynamic balance in the virtual reality training group were observed, indicating virtual reality balance training is feasible and suitable for chronic stroke patients with balance deficit in clinical settings.

Virtual reality-based physical rehabilitation has also been used among patients with Parkinson's disease. For example, Yang et al. (2016) examined whether a 6-week home-based virtual reality balance training program was more effective than conventional home balance training for improving balance and walking in patients with Parkinson's disease. Although no significant differences were seen between these two groups, researchers found both groups to demonstrate improved balance after training. The study suggests the two training approaches were equally effective in improving balance and walking among community-dwelling Parkinson's disease patients. In a randomized controlled study by Robles-García and colleagues (2016), the impact of 4 weeks of imitation-therapy on movement hypometria in Parkinson's disease was assessed. While the experimental group imitated full-amplitude repetitive finger-tapping movements presented by the virtual reality avatar at three different tapping rates, the control group performed a protocol matching the same features presented to the experimental group, but without imitation. Findings indicated significantly increased movement amplitude after the therapy in the experimental group for the trained and untrained hands, suggesting that virtual reality-based therapy has the potential to enhance the effect of motor functioning in patients with Parkinson's disease.

With regard to children and adolescents with developmental disabilities, the positive effects of virtual reality-based physical rehabilitation in these populations have been presented. In a recent study, increased upper-limb motor skills on the affected side and bilateral coordination ability were observed by Do and associates (2016), following virtual reality-based bilateral arm training. This study concluded that bilateral arm training based using virtual reality can be an effective intervention method for enhancing motor function in children with hemiplegic cerebral palsy. Ashkenazi et al. (2013) explored the feasibility of using a low-cost, off-the-shelf virtual reality game to treat young children with developmental coordination disorder. Following the intervention, significant changes were observed in fine and gross motor skills, including hand writing, manual dexterity, aiming, catching, balance, and walking. Furthermore, the children seemed to be motivated and to enjoy the interaction with the virtual reality environment. Similarly, Gonsalves and colleagues (2015) examined the effect of virtual reality on movement quality in children with developmental coordination disorder. Researchers found children with developmental coordination disorder display a slower hand path speed, greater wrist extension, and greater elbow flexion compared with children with typical development when engaging in virtual reality. The study suggests virtual reality is favorable for facilitating desired motor learning outcomes.

As seen, of the reviewed high-quality literature regarding the use of virtual reality in physical rehabilitation among a diverse array of populations, results are promising in relation to the effectiveness of virtual reality-based rehabilitation. It appears that virtual reality rehabilitation is favorable or of equal quality as compared to conventional rehabilitation in part because of the ability to provide the intensive repetition of meaningful task-related activities. That is, virtual reality is beneficial in improving individual motor functioning. Nevertheless, the virtual reality interventions are different due to divergent virtual reality instruments. Future research should compare the effects between dissimilar virtual reality treatments.

Psychological rehabilitation

Over the past two decades, virtual reality-based psychological rehabilitation has experienced increasing application in treating individuals with anxiety disorders, with particular emphasis on specific phobias (Morina, Ijntema, Meyerbröker, & Emmelkamp, 2015). In detail, this type of virtual reality-based psychological rehabilitation incorporates computer graphics, visual displays, and sensory inputs to create an immersive virtual environment capable of approximating the feeling of being in the real world (McCann et al., 2014). After immersing a patient in this virtual world, therapists can then introduce the anxiety-eliciting stimuli into the environment. The advantage of using virtual reality-based psychological rehabilitation is the therapists' ability to control the quality, intensity, duration, and frequency of exposure to the anxiety-eliciting stimuli (Emmelkamp, 2005). For instance, in a 12-month randomized controlled trial by Anderson and colleagues (2013), the effects of virtual reality exposure therapy on 97 participants' social anxiety disorder was evaluated. These researchers found that patients who were exposed in the virtual world reported less peak anxiety and spoke longer at the post-treatment speech, indicating virtual reality exposure therapy might be effective for treating social fears. Michaliszyn et al. (2010) assessed the efficacy of virtual reality in virtuo exposure and in vivo exposure on spider phobia. These two treatment conditions were compared to a wait-list condition. Researchers found participants in both the in virtuo and in vivo exposure therapies demonstrated significant improvements on objective and subjective measures of fear after eight 90-minute treatment sessions. That is, both in vivo and in virtuo exposure are efficient methods of treating spider phobia. Notably, a slight advantage of in vivo exposure over in virtuo exposure was found, as revealed by significant and continued improvement regarding catastrophic beliefs about spiders after posttest in the in vivo group. Further, Gaggioli and colleagues (2014) conducted a 5-week randomized controlled trial involving 121 teachers and nurses (i.e., all highly exposed to stress) to evaluate the effects of virtual reality for the management and prevention of psychological stress. These researchers found the virtual reality group to report significant reductions in chronic "trait" anxiety and a significantly increased coping and emotional support skills when compared to the wait-list group. Findings lead the authors to conclude that virtual reality protocol yields better effects than the traditionally accepted gold standard for psychological stress treatment (i.e., cognitive behavioral therapy).

In fact, previous meta-analyses have shown the effectiveness of virtual reality-based psychological rehabilitation on various mental disorders. For example, Powers and Emmelkamp (2008) conducted a meta-analytic review investigating the impact of virtual reality-based psychological rehabilitation on mental illnesses, with nine studies on specific phobias, two studies on social phobia, one study on panic disorder, and one study on post-traumatic stress disorder. Researchers found that virtual reality-based psychological rehabilitation is highly effective in treating phobias in comparison to traditional psychological rehabilitation (e.g., relaxation and bibliotherapy) or wait-list control conditions. Additionally, Opris and colleagues (2012) included 23 studies in a meta-analysis comparing virtual reality-based psychological rehabilitation for anxiety disorders as compared to standard rehabilitation procedures. The majority of the included studies were on specific phobias ($n = 12$), with the remaining studies investigating the use of virtual reality-based psychological rehabilitation on social phobia ($n = 5$), panic disorder with or without agoraphobia ($n = 5$), and post-traumatic stress disorder ($n = 1$). Similar to the aforementioned meta-analytic review, high effect sizes in favor of virtual reality-based psychological rehabilitation were observed when this novel rehabilitation methodology was compared to wait-list control conditions. As a result, the researchers concluded that virtual reality-based psychological rehabilitation is efficacious in treating anxiety disorders, in addition to demonstrating a powerful real-life impact and good stability of results over time. In the most recent meta-analysis conducted to date, Morina et al. (2015) included 14 studies regarding the effectiveness of virtual reality-based psychological rehabilitation in the treatment of arachnophobia (i.e., fear of spiders) and acrophobia (i.e., fear of heights). Findings revealed that patients undergoing virtual reality-based psychological rehabilitation for specific phobias (e.g., fear of flying, fear of spiders, etc.) resulted in significantly better behavioral assessments than patients undergoing standard rehabilitation or serving as wait-list controls.

As reviewed, present evidence indicates that virtual reality-based psychological rehabilitation has the potential to promote psychological well-being and can be a valuable tool in treating various mental disorders. It is also clear that virtual reality-based psychological rehabilitation shows considerable utility in allowing patients to engage in novel, highly interactive, and effective simulations of active face-to-face conditions (Figure 10.3). Nevertheless, most research regarding virtual reality and psychological rehabilitation has been conducted among adults or older adults. More studies, therefore, are warranted in determining the effects of virtual reality on mental health among children and adolescents.

Cognitive rehabilitation

Cognitive impairment is a considerable health concern worldwide, with a number of people unable to live independently due to these impairments (Seelye, Schmitter-Edgecombe, Das, & Cook, 2012). Virtual reality-based cognitive rehabilitation has experienced increasingly widespread use for the treatment of cognitive impairments. This emerging technology offers new rehabilitation options which can be tailored to suit specific clinical or research purposes (Rizzo et al., 2001; Tarnanas et al., 2013). Specifically, the engaging nature of virtual reality tasks makes this technology ideal for a wide range of applications including cognitive screening and evaluation (Zygouris et al., 2015). In fact, the potential of virtual reality-based cognitive rehabilitation is currently being investigated, with a focus on the treatment of cognitive processes, such as attention, working memory, verbal and visual memory, and general cognitive functioning (Gamito et al., 2011; Kim,

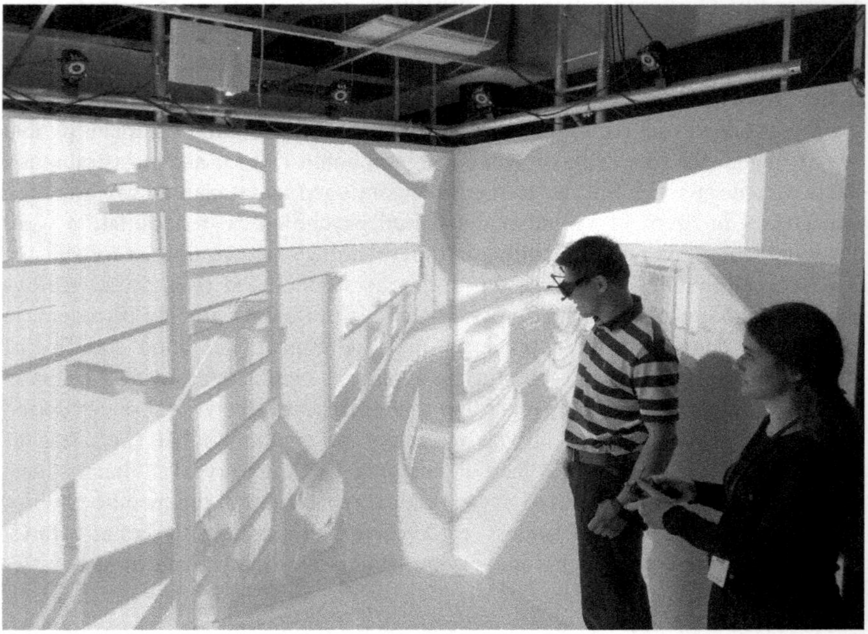

Figure 10.3 Experiencing virtual reality in CAVE.
Source: Photo by Denis Pasco.

Chun, Kim, & Park, 2011; Man, Chung, & Lee, 2012; Manzoni et al., 2016; Optale et al., 2010, Sorita et al., 2013; Yip & Man, 2013; Zygouris et al., 2015). For example, Optale and colleagues (2010) compared a 6-month virtual reality memory training to music therapy in the treatment of cognitive decline for 36 older adults, with the objective being to improve memory. These researchers found participants who underwent virtual reality memory training showed significant improvements in memory tests—particularly with regard to long-term recall, while the control group demonstrated continued cognitive decline. The beneficial effects observed in cognitive functions support the efficacy of using virtual reality in elderly adults and suggest that the virtual reality memory training protocol can be a valid and integral part of a rehabilitative strategy aimed at encouraging memory recovery. Similarly, in a 5-week randomized controlled study by Man et al. (2012), 44 older adults in the early stages of dementia were recruited to investigate the effectiveness of virtual reality-based memory training. At study's end, both the virtual reality-based cognitive rehabilitation group and traditional rehabilitation group demonstrated positive training effects, with the virtual reality group showing greater improvement in objective memory performance and the non-virtual reality group displaying better subjective memory tests, indicating the use of virtual reality is acceptable for treating older adults with dementia. Finally, Kim and colleagues (2011) evaluated the effectiveness of additional fully immersive virtual reality in the promotion of greater cognitive functioning. An intervention group comprised of 15 cognitive impairment patients underwent virtual reality-based cognitive rehabilitation and computer-based cognitive rehabilitation while 13 patients in a control group received only computer-based cognitive rehabilitation over four weeks. Researchers observed both groups to have improved neuropsychological outcomes following treatment. However, compared to the controls, the intervention group demonstrated improvements on a visual continuous performance test and on a backward visual span test—both positive findings in relation to visual attention and memory, leading the authors to conclude that virtual reality training combined with computer-based cognitive rehabilitation may be of additional benefit for treating patients with cognitive impairment.

Given the positive results reviewed above, the use of virtual reality-based cognitive rehabilitation promises to continue to be a research area of interest. Virtual reality-based cognitive rehabilitation offers great benefit as the immersive nature of the simulated environment capable of being created allows clinicians to approximate real-life situations in a well-controlled manner which reduces the risk of adverse patient outcomes (Rizzo et al., 2001). Further, as a result of being able to highly control the environment, clinicians can enhance the transfer of skills learned in the simulated environment of virtual reality to real-world conditions (Rose, Attree, Brooks, & Andrews, 2001). As such, future research using virtual reality-based cognitive rehabilitation should continue to increase the number of different applications of this technology in the field of cognitive rehabilitation.

Practical implications

Traditional informational approaches for promoting PA and health are to disseminate information through printed materials and mass media. However, technology sprawl has challenged this tradition, and advanced health promotion professionals are integrating email, text messaging, web sites, and online support groups into their repository (Tomnay, 2005). A less familiar, yet attractive, platform for PA and health promotion specialists is virtual reality. Nowadays, virtual reality is widely used in PA and health promotion settings among various populations (Figure 10.4). An appealing feature of virtual reality is to allow participants to see, hear, use, and modify simulated objects in a computer-created world (Tomnay, 2005). Specifically, the potential of virtual reality in PA and health promotion has been explored, with improved motor function and patients' rehabilitative outcomes have been observed among various settings. Nevertheless, the use virtual reality technology to promote PA and health is still in its infancy (Liu, 2011; Mohnsen, 2003; Pasco, 2013). Therefore, researchers and practitioners should continue to explore the benefits of virtual reality and harness its potential in the promotion of PA and health among a variety of populations in a trustworthy manner.

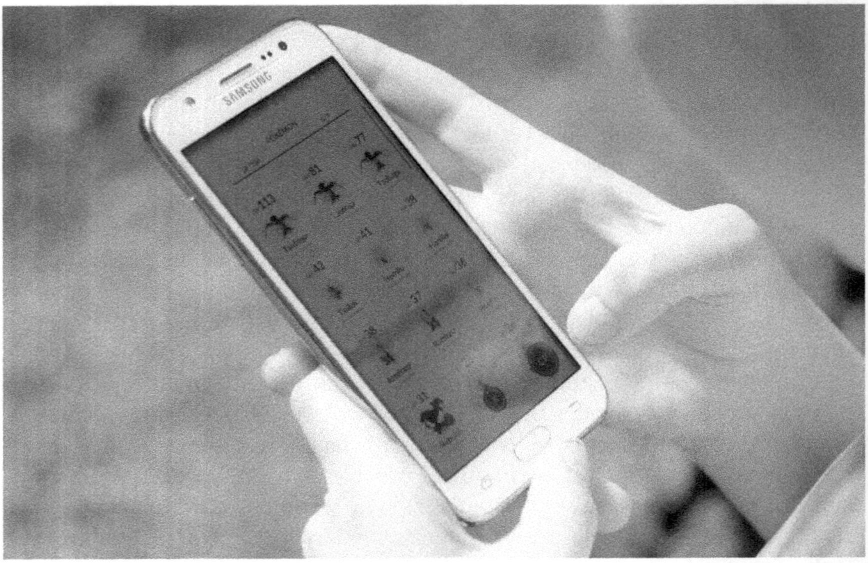

Figure 10.4 Playing an augmented reality game—Pokémon Go.

Source: pixabay.com.

References

Anderson, P. L., Price, M., Edwards, S. M., Obasaju, M. A., Schmertz, S. K., Zimand, E., & Calamaras, M. R. (2013). Virtual reality exposure therapy for social anxiety disorder: A randomized controlled trial. *Journal of Consulting and Clinical Psychology, 81*(5), 751–760.

Ashkenazi, T., Weiss, P. L., Orian, D., & Laufer, Y. (2013). Low-cost virtual reality intervention program for children with developmental coordination disorder: A pilot feasibility study. *Pediatric Physical Therapy, 25*(4), 467–473.

Augment (2015, October 6). *Virtual Reality vs. Augmented Reality*. Retrieved from www.augment.com/blog/virtual-reality-vs-augmented-reality/.

Bailenson, J., Patel, K., Nielsen, A., Bajscy, R., Jung, S. H., & Kurillo, G. (2008). The effect of interactivity on learning physical actions in virtual reality. *Media Psychology, 11*(3), 354–376.

Bergamasco, M., Bardy, B., & Gopher, D. (Eds.). (2012). *Skill training in multimodal virtual environments*. Boca Raton, FL: CRC Press/

Bideau, B., Kulpa, R., Vignais, N., Brault, S., Multon, F., & Craig, C. (2010). Using virtual reality to analyze sports performance. *IEEE Computer Graphics and Applications, 30*(2), 14–21.

Cho, K. H., Lee, K. J., & Song, C. H. (2012). Virtual-reality balance training with a video-game system improves dynamic balance in chronic stroke patients. *The Tohoku Journal of Experimental Medicine, 228*(1), 69–74.

Do, J. H., Yoo, E. Y., Jung, M. Y., & Park, H. Y. (2016). The effects of virtual reality based bilateral arm training on hemiplegic children's upper limb motor skills. *NeuroRehabilitation*, (Preprint), 1–12.

Emmelkamp, P. M. (2005). Technological innovations in clinical assessment and psychotherapy. *Psychother Psychosom*, *74*(6), 336–343.

Feigin, V. L., Roth, G. A., Naghavi, M., Parmar, P., Krishnamurthi, R., Chugh, S., ... & Estep, K. (2016). Global burden of stroke and risk factors in 188 countries, during 1990–2013: A systematic analysis for the Global Burden of Disease Study 2013. *The Lancet Neurology*, *15*(9), 913–924.

Gaggioli, A., Pallavicini, F., Morganti, L., Serino, S., Scaratti, C., Briguglio, M., ... & Tartarisco, G. (2014). Experiential virtual scenarios with real-time monitoring (interreality) for the management of psychological stress: A block randomized controlled trial. *Journal of Medical Internet Research*, *16*(7), e167.

Gamito, P., Oliveira, J., Pacheco, J., Morais, D., Saraiva, T., Lacerda, R., ... & Rosa, P. (2011). Traumatic Brain Injury memory training: A Virtual Reality online solution. *International Journal on Disability and Human Development*, *10*(4), 309–312.

Gonsalves, L., Campbell, A., Jensen, L., & Straker, L. (2015). Children with developmental coordination disorder play active virtual reality games differently than children with typical development. *Physical Therapy*, *95*(3), 360–368.

Graham, M., Zook, M., & Boulton, A. (2013). Augmented reality in urban places: Contested content and the duplicity of code. *Transactions of the Institute of British Geographers*, *38*(3), 464–479.

Hansen, L., & Sanders, S. W. (2012). Active Gaming: Is "virtual" reality right for your physical education program? *Strategies*, *25*(6), 24–27.

Hoffmann, C. P., Filippeschi, A., Ruffaldi, E., & Bardy, B. G. (2014). Energy management using virtual reality improves 2000-m rowing performance. *Journal of Sports Sciences*, *32*(6), 501–509.

Isaac, J. (2016). *Step into a new world – Virtual Reality (VR)*. Retrieved from www.completegate.com/2016070154/blog/virtual-reality-explained#vrdef.

Jutai, J. W., & Teasell, R. W. (2003). The necessity and limitations of evidence-based practice in stroke rehabilitation. *Topics in Stroke Rehabilitation*, *10*(1), 71–78.

Kim, B. R., Chun, M. H., Kim, L. S., & Park, J. Y. (2011). Effect of virtual reality on cognition in stroke patients. *Annals of Rehabilitation Medicine*, *35*(4), 450–459.

Krishnamurthi, R. V., Moran, A. E., Feigin, V. L., Barker-Collo, S., Norrving, B., Mensah, G. A., ... & Johnson, C. O. (2015). Stroke prevalence, mortality and disability-adjusted life years in adults aged 20–64 years in 1990–2013: Data from the global burden of disease 2013 study. *Neuroepidemiology*, *45*(3), 190–202.

Liao, T. (2015, August). Application of virtual reality technology to sports. In *2015 AASRI International Conference on Circuits and Systems*. Atlantis Press.

Lieberman, J., & Breazeal, C. (2007). TIKL: Development of a wearable vibrotactile feedback suit for improved human motor learning. *IEEE Transactions on Robotics*, *23*(5), 919–926.

Liu, J. K. (2011). The study on physical education method based on virtual reality. *Advanced Materials Research*, *271–273*, 1164–1167.

Man, D. W., Chung, J. C., & Lee, G. Y. (2012). Evaluation of a virtual reality-based memory training programme for Hong Kong Chinese older adults with questionable dementia: A pilot study. *International Journal of Geriatric Psychiatry*, *27*(5), 513–520.

Manzoni, G. M., Cesa, G. L., Bacchetta, M., Castelnuovo, G., Conti, S., Gaggioli, A., ... & Riva, G. (2016). Virtual reality-enhanced cognitive-behavioral therapy for morbid obesity: A randomized controlled study with 1 year follow-up. *Cyberpsychology, Behavior, and Social Networking, 19*(2), 134–140.

McCann, R. A., Armstrong, C. M., Skopp, N. A., Edwards-Stewart, A., Smolenski, D. J., June, J. D., … & Reger, G. M. (2014). Virtual reality exposure therapy for the treatment of anxiety disorders: An evaluation of research quality. *Journal of Anxiety Disorders, 28*(6), 625–631.

McEwen, D., Taillon-Hobson, A., Bilodeau, M., Sveistrup, H., & Finestone, H. (2014). Virtual reality exercise improves mobility after stroke an inpatient randomized controlled trial. *Stroke, 45*(6), 1853–1855.

Mestre, D. R., Dagonneau, V., & Mercier, C. S. (2011). Does virtual reality enhance exercise performance, enjoyment, and dissociation? An exploratory study on a stationary bike apparatus. *Presence, 20*(1), 1–14.

Michaliszyn, D., Marchand, A., Bouchard, S., Martel, M. O., & Poirier-Bisson, J. (2010). A randomized, controlled clinical trial of in virtuo and in vivo exposure for spider phobia. *Cyberpsychology, Behavior, and Social Networking, 13*(6), 689–695.

Miller, K. J., Adair, B. S., Pearce, A. J., Said, C. M., Ozanne, E., & Morris, M. M. (2014). Effectiveness and feasibility of virtual reality and gaming system use at home by older adults for enabling physical activity to improve health-related domains: A systematic review. *Age and Ageing, 43*(2), 188–195.

Mohnsen, B. (2003). Virtual reality applications in physical education. *Journal of Physical Education, Recreation and Dance, 74*(9), 13–15.

Morina, N., Ijntema, H., Meyerbröker, K., & Emmelkamp, P. M. (2015). Can virtual reality exposure therapy gains be generalized to real-life? A meta-analysis of studies applying behavioral assessments. *Behaviour Research and Therapy, 74*, 18–24.

Opriş, D., Pintea, S., García-Palacios, A., Botella, C., Szamosközi, Ş., & David, D. (2012). Virtual reality exposure therapy in anxiety disorders: A quantitative meta-analysis. *Depression and Anxiety, 29*(2), 85–93.

Optale, G., Urgesi, C., Busato, V., Marin, S., Piron, L., Priftis, K., … & Bordin, A. (2010). Controlling memory impairment in elderly adults using virtual reality memory training: A randomized controlled pilot study. *Neurorehabilitation and Neural Repair, 24*(4), 348–357.

Pasco, D. (2013). The potential of using virtual reality technology in physical activity settings. *Quest, 65*(4), 429–441.

Plante, T. G., Aldridge, A., Bogden, R., & Haneli, C. (2003). Might virtual reality promote the mood benefits of exercise? *Computers in Human Behavior, 19*(4), 495–509.

Powers, M. B., & Emmelkamp, P. M. (2008). Virtual reality exposure therapy for anxiety disorders: A meta-analysis. *Journal of Anxiety Disorders, 22*(3), 561–569.

Rizzo, A. A., Buckwalter, J. G., McGee, J. S., Bowerly, T., Van Der Zaag, C., Neumann, U., … & Chua, C. (2001). Virtual environments for assessing and rehabilitating cognitive/functional performance a review of projects at the usc integrated media systems center. *Presence: Teleoperators and Virtual Environments, 10*(4), 359–374.

Robles-García, V., Corral-Bergantiños, Y., Espinosa, N., García-Sancho, C., Sanmartín, G., Flores, J., … & Arias, P. (2016). Effects of movement imitation training in Parkinson's disease: A virtual reality pilot study. *Parkinsonism & Related Disorders, 26*, 17–23.

Rose, F. D., Attree, E. A., Brooks, B. M., & Andrews, T. K. (2001). Learning and memory in virtual environments: A role in neurorehabilitation? Questions (and occasional answers) from the University of East London. *Presence: Teleoperators and Virtual Environments, 10*(4), 345–358.

Rosser, J. C., Lynch, P. J., Cuddihy, L., Gentile, D. A., Klonsky, J., & Merrell, R. (2007). The impact of video games on training surgeons in the 21st century. *Archives of Surgery, 142*(2), 181–186.

Saposnik, G. (2016). Efficacy and safety of virtual reality in stroke rehabilitation: A multicenter randomized trial (EVREST Multicenter). *Lancet Neurology*, published Online June 27, 2016.

Saposnik, G., Cohen, L. G., Mamdani, M., Pooyania, S., Ploughman, M., Cheung, D., ... & Nilanont, Y. (2016). Efficacy and safety of non-immersive virtual reality exercising in stroke rehabilitation (EVREST): A randomised, multicentre, single-blind, controlled trial. *The Lancet Neurology, 15*(10), 1019–1027.

Seelye, A. M., Schmitter-Edgecombe, M., Das, B., & Cook, D. J. (2012). Application of cognitive rehabilitation theory to the development of smart prompting technologies. *IEEE Reviews in Biomedical Engineering, 5*, 29–44.

SHAPE America. (2013). *Grade-level outcomesfor K-12 physical education.* Reston, VA: Author.

Sorita, E., N'Kaoua, B., Larrue, F., Criquillon, J., Simion, A., Sauzéon, H., ... & Mazaux, J. M. (2013). Do patients with traumatic brain injury learn a route in the same way in real and virtual environments? *Disability and Rehabilitation, 35*(16), 1371–1379.

Stinson, C., & Bowman, D. A. (2014). Feasibility of training athletes for high-pressure situations using virtual reality. *IEEE Transactions on Visualization and Computer Graphics, 20*(4), 606–615.

St-Jacques, J., Bouchard, S., & Bélanger, C. (2010). Is virtual reality effective to motivate and raise interest in phobic children toward therapy? A clinical trial study of in vivo with in virtuo versus in vivo only treatment exposure. *The Journal of Clinical Psychiatry, 71*(7), 924–931.

Subramanian, S. K., Lourenço, C. B., Chilingaryan, G., Sveistrup, H., & Levin, M. F. (2013). Arm motor recovery using a virtual reality intervention in chronic stroke randomized control trial. *Neurorehabilitation and Neural Repair, 27*(1), 13–23.

Tarnanas, I., Schlee, W., Tsolaki, M., Müri, R., Mosimann, U., & Nef, T. (2013). Ecological validity of virtual reality daily living activities screening for early dementia: Longitudinal study. *Journal of Medical Internet Research Serious Games, 1*(1), e1.

Tomnay, J. E. (2005). New technology and partner notification – why aren't we using them? *American Journal of Health Promotion, 16*(1), 19–22.

Weiss, P. L., Keshner, E. A., & Levin, M. F. (2014). *Virtual reality for physical and motor rehabilitation.* New York, NY: Springer.

Yang, W. C., Wang, H. K., Wu, R. M., Lo, C. S., & Lin, K. H. (2016). Home-based virtual reality balance training and conventional balance training in Parkinson's disease: A randomized controlled trial. *Journal of the Formosan Medical Association, 115*(9), 734–743.

Yip, B. C., & Man, D. W. (2013). Virtual reality-based prospective memory training program for people with acquired brain injury. *Neurorehabilitation, 32*(1), 103–115.

Zygouris, S., Giakoumis, D., Votis, K., Doumpoulakis, S., Ntovas, K., Segkouli, S., ... & Tsolaki, M. (2015). Can a virtual reality cognitive training application fulfill a dual role? Using the virtual supermarket cognitive training application as a screening tool for mild cognitive impairment. *Journal of Alzheimer's Disease, 44*(4), 1333–1347.

Part III

Applications for physical activity and health promotion

11 Negative aspects of emerging technologies in physical activity promotion

Zachary Pope and Zan Gao

Throughout this book, the reader has been presented with a number of emerging technologies used in promoting physical activity (PA) and health. From active video games to wearable technology and mobile device apps to social media and state-of-the-art GPS/GIS systems as well as virtual reality, the current generation of technology is redefining how individuals improve their health and well-being and prevent or attenuate diseases and conditions precipitated by poor health behaviors (e.g., physical inactivity, smoking, poor diet). Despite the promise many of these technologies hold for PA promotion, negative aspects, limitations, and challenges for researchers and clinicians are still present and need to be considered before further effective integration of emerging technology into the field of PA and health can take place. Notably, the negative aspects, limitations, and challenges reviewed below do not constitute an exhaustive list. The content is, however, representative of the major obstacles currently facing emerging technology in the promotion of PA for improved health and well-being.

Negative aspects and limitations of emerging technologies

Privacy

Perhaps the greatest negative aspect of emerging technologies for use in PA promotion is the privacy of health information when using these novel technologies (Lobelo et al., 2016; Richardson & Ancker, 2015). For example, if a clinician is having a patient use a free, commercially available smartphone app to track their steps per day, the app is likely not subject to the confidentiality and security regulations stipulated in the Health Insurance Portability and Accountability Act (HIPAA), to which apps specifically developed by physicians for healthcare purposes are required to adhere (Lobelo et al., 2016). This lack of regulation exposes the patient to unlawful use and sharing of private health information. As a result, questions regarding the security and privacy of personal health information assessed and provided to health professionals via different forms of emerging technology are a limiting factor with regard to client/patient use of emerging technology for health promotion—as is the fact that many applications require log-in information which further exposes the user to identity theft. Therefore, it is up to researchers to find ways in which to develop technology which protects a user's health information while still being able to acquire enough information from users to inform personal health practices (Figure 11.1).

Validity and reliability of PA and physiological data

The validity and reliability of PA and physiological data (e.g., METs, calories, steps) provided by emerging technologies such as mobile device health apps (i.e., mHealth apps) are, at times, questionable (Lobelo et al., 2016)—a term that might also be used to describe the PA and physiological data provided during active video game play or during health wearable use. For instance, in a recent study by Bai et al. (2016), consumer health wearables used to track PA (e.g., Fitbit Flex, JU24, etc.) had error values of 15%–20% for energy expenditure when compared to energy expenditure values provided by a portable metabolic analyzer—errors which have major implications for health professionals using these devices to develop PA and dietary plans to improve client/patient health. Further, with numerous technologies currently being released with the intention to promote health and well-being in ways that are more fashionable (e.g., necklaces, belts, and upscale smartwatches capable of capturing physiological data; see Charara, 2016), more research will be needed to discern whether or not these newer technologies are addressing some of the measurement errors present in past technologies of the same type. Bottom line, any health professional who

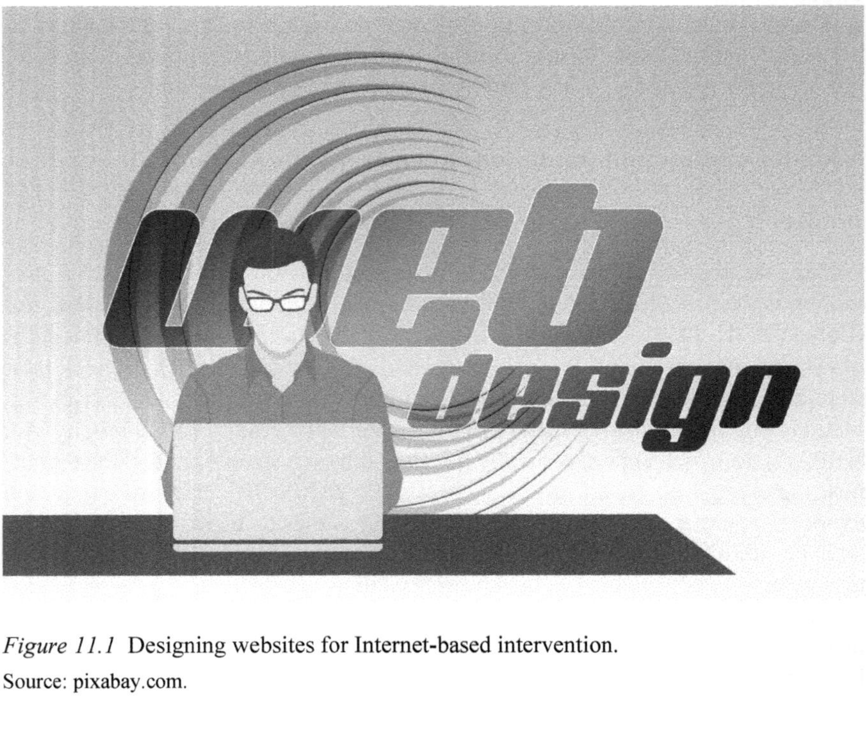

Figure 11.1 Designing websites for Internet-based intervention.

Source: pixabay.com.

wants to use emerging technology for health promotion purposes needs to keep in mind the error rates for heart rate, calories, and other physiological variables related to the type of technology being implemented. Indeed, not taking into account physiological data error rates for specific technologies might produce unwanted outcomes among patients—particularly patient populations where outcomes such as weight loss is of utmost importance or in populations where baseline fitness is poor.

Stigma

Stigma is also a barrier. For example, reviews on active video games have pointed out that while active video games are changing the perception that all video games contribute to poor health—as opposed to just sedentary video games contributing to poor health—continued work needs to be done to prove the effectiveness of this PA modality in the promotion of improved health (Guy, Ratzki-Leewing, & Gwadry-Sridhar, 2011). Fortunately, more recent meta-analytic reviews have statistically proven the effectiveness of active video games in PA and health promotion across numerous studies among children and adolescents (Gao, Chen, Pasco, & Pope, 2015)—results of which can be used to further decrease the stigma some individuals hold regarding the use of active video games to improve health. Within the context of active video games, King, Glanz, and Patrick (2015) have posited that health professionals need to "frame" this PA modality in terms of health, rather than just defining the games as a way to have fun. Extrapolating this "health framing" idea to other emerging technologies currently being used for PA promotion may improve the perception of these technologies' ability to improve health, while also decreasing the stigma or resistance of key stakeholders (e.g., school and hospital administrators) to adopting these technologies.

Integration framework and compensation for personnel

Lobelo et al. (2016) makes the point that if we are to more successfully integrate technology into healthcare treatments—of which PA is often a component—a framework through which to integrate this technology is needed. A proper integration framework is important for at least three reasons. First, this framework may allow us to discern the best ways by which to protect patient/client health information when placed within electronic medical records. Second, we will be able to increase the effectiveness of interventions using certain types of novel technology (e.g., health wearables, mHealth apps, etc.) for PA promotion. Finally, a proper integration framework will pemit new policies regarding the compensation of healthcare providers for time spent providing care via technological mediums such as mHealth apps. Indeed, as West (2012) indicated, most established mHealth programs do not compensate physicians and other healthcare professionals (e.g., physicians assistants, physical/occupational therapists) for the time they spend providing care to patients via a mHealth app—increasing resistance among this cohort to integrate this technology into practice. While more reasons could be listed regarding the importance of an established integration framework, one thing is clear: if the adoption of emerging technology into healthcare is to become more mainstream and greatly impact and revolutionize the manner by which health professionals provide care, an integration framework will be vital.

Lack of studies using an established theoretical framework or intervention fidelity

While some emerging technology fields, such as active video gaming, have numerous intervention literature which has properly integrated established theory and ensured proper intervention fidelity measures (e.g., putting methodology in place to assess, monitor, and correct any threats to the reliability and internal validity of an intervention; see Borrelli, 2011), other newer fields of emerging technology research have not been as successful in this task. Establishing theory allows researchers to develop and implement interventions with greater effectiveness due to the indirect effects theory has on the intervention's main objective (Brug, Oenema, & Ferreira, 2005). Further, theory allows for a more accurate interpretation of the phenomena seen as a result of the intervention's implementation (Patten, 2014). Finally, more studies using emerging technology to promote PA and improve health need to implement intervention fidelity measures to ensure the reliability and internal validity of the study. Intervention fidelity measures include the proper selection of intervention design and the implementation of provider/research team training, in addition to the ongoing assessment of intervention delivery (i.e., how will providers deliver the intervention systematically and consistently among all participants?), intervention receipt (i.e., do the participants understand the different components of the intervention?), and intervention enactment (i.e., does the participant enact the behavior changes taught during the intervention in a "real-world" setting?). Importantly, interventions with sound theoretical backing may still not be effective if the proper intervention fidelity measures were not set in place. The reader is directed to Chapter 6 and the authors' detailed discussion of intervention theory and fidelity within the context of mHealth app-based PA interventions.

Internet gaming disorder

In the 5th edition of their *Diagnostic and Statistical Manual of Mental Disorders* (DSM-5), the American Psychiatric Association included, for the first time, the diagnosis of Internet Gaming Disorder (IGD; American Psychiatric Association, 2013). According to the DSM-5, IGD has nine distinct criteria and, of these nine criteria, five must be present for greater than 12 months for a diagnosis with IGD. These criteria include: (1) gaming preoccupation; (2) foregoing other hobbies or activities to play games; (3) continued gameplay despite other life problems; (4) using gaming to cope with poor moods; (5) lying about the amount of time spent gaming; (6) reluctance to curtail or discontinue gaming habits; (7) experiencing withdrawal when unable to game; (8) becoming tolerant to an unusually high amount of gaming play; and (9) placing oneself in jeopardy of losing relationships, jobs, or education as a result of gaming (Figure 11.2). Depending upon the population studied, the prevalence of IGD can be as low as 0.2% (Festl, Scharkow, & Quandt, 2013) to nearly 9% (Choo et al., 2010). Recently, work has been completed to validate the Internet Gaming Disorder Questionnaire in multiple populations so health professionals can better assess and treat this disorder (Jeromin, Rief, & Barke, 2016). Nonetheless, health professionals using gaming technology to promote PA need to be aware of the signs of IGD in order to properly intervene if and when these signs start to appear in participants. That said, health professionals implementing game-based interventions (e.g., active video games and augmented/virtual reality games) need to make clear to participants that the games are only to be used to supplement a well-rounded PA plan.

Technology-related accidents, unlawful behavior, and safety

Emerging technology in the promotion of PA and health has many benefits which do, in general, outweigh the potential negative aspects of using these technologies. That said, use of these technologies does have downsides. For example, Pokémon Go, a hugely popular augmented reality game played using a smartphone,

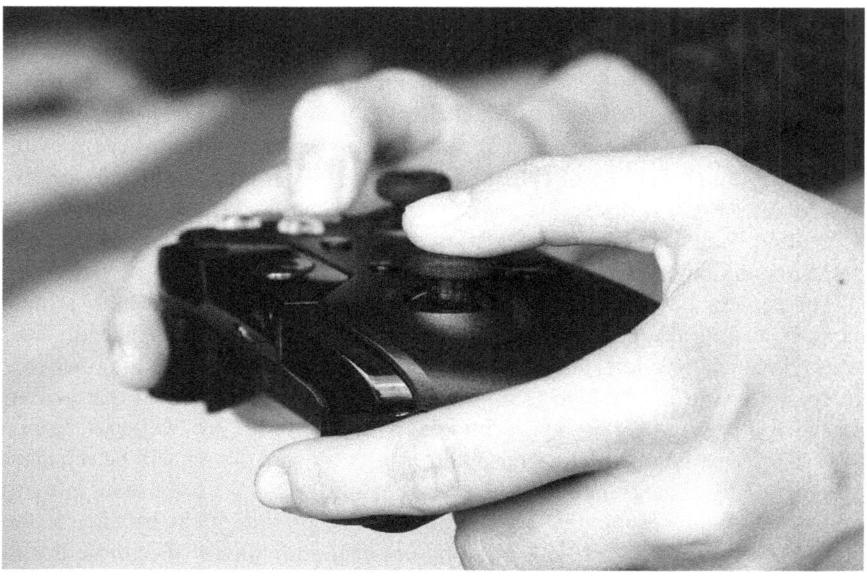

Figure 11.2 Playing video games.

Source: pixabay.com.

has facilitated increased PA among players. Unfortunately, as Serino and colleagues (2016) state, Pokémon Go has resulted in accidents due to players not paying attention while walking, riding a bike, or even driving a car to catch Pokémon, as well as increasing trespassing activity on private properties by players with an extreme desire to catch their next Pokémon. Moreover, as a result of using this game's "lure" function, criminals have used this game to attract other players to their location after which these criminals rob players who were simply looking for the nearest Pokémon character (Serino, Cordrey, McLaughlin, & Milanaik, 2016). While other emerging technologies such as GPS-based geocaching might also result in unlawful acts (e.g., trespassing on private property), Pokémon Go is a superb example of how the misuse of potentially health-benefiting technology can result in negative outcomes. Given these potentially negative outcomes, health professionals need to clearly outline to participants the need to remain attentive to their environment and engage in law-abiding actions. Finally, more research will also be needed regarding the safety of emerging technology when used to promote PA and health. Indeed, innovative new tech such as skateboard helmets which light up during activity have been developed (see Exertion Games Lab, 2016a), yet no empirical research has been conducted to ensure that technologies akin to this form of wearable technology are as safe as their traditional counterparts.

Challenges for researchers and clinicians

Now that several negative aspects/limitations associated with the implementation of emerging technology in PA promotion and, more broadly, health promotion, have been reviewed, it is worthwhile briefly discussing what challenges will face researchers and clinicians within this field over the next decade. While one could think of an endless list of challenges, many can fit into five broad categories: (1) stakeholder buy-in; (2) reduction of health disparities; (3) proving the validity and reliability of emerging technology in promotion of health behaviors such as PA; (4) dissemination of technology observed to be efficacious in promoting health; and (5) incorporation of Big Data analysis to improve health at the population level.

Stakeholder buy-in is likely the most pressing challenge for health professionals seeking to promote health via emerging technology. Indeed, until researchers and/or clinicians can develop proper security measures to protect the electronic health information (e.g., the amount of PA an individual engages in) provided by some emerging technologies for analysis by wellness teams/physicians, institutions such as hospitals or primary care clinics will be reluctant to integrate technology into their healthcare practices. As we have seen, integration of emerging technology has the potential to provide great benefits to the patient/client (see West, 2012), meaning ensuring individuals' electronic health information security is vital before administrators would consider fully adopting emerging technology as a means of treatment delivery (Figure 11.3). Schools, institutions which have great ability to use emerging technology to promote

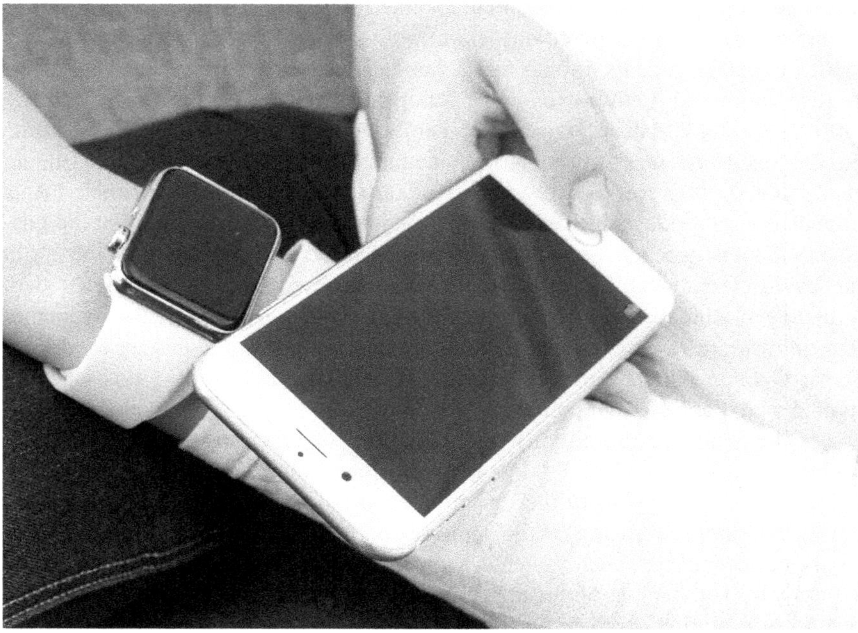

Figure 11.3 Application of a smart watch in health promotion.
Source: pixabay.com.

health among the large percentage of youth who attend, also need stakeholder buy-in. Particularly, school administrations and teachers need to see data on the effectiveness of emerging technology, such as mHealth apps and active video games, in the promotion of health within physical education and the classroom. This will go a long way in challenging the stigma associated with technology and technology's perceived negative relationship with youth health—providing opportunities for PA and health interventions to be implemented in novel and impactful ways within the school setting.

Second, a challenge for health professionals will be to decrease the health disparities present in society due, in part, to lack of access to healthcare. As Lobelo et al. (2016) noted, due to the greater access that individuals with higher socioeconomic status have compared to individuals of lower socioeconomic status, health professionals need to be careful that the use of emerging technology to improve health does not widen the health disparities between the two aforementioned populations. Frameworks for integrating emerging technology into healthcare need to be aware of this potential to increase the health disparity between populations of high and low socioeconomic status and concentrate efforts on underserved populations by creating avenues by which emerging technology is available to them. Fortunately, in recent years, researchers have been working on emerging technology which can be used by individuals in high- and low-income populations. For example, Gao and associates (2013) used active video games to promote health and improved academic performance in low-income Latino elementary school students finding that a Dance Dance Revolution-based PA intervention improved math scores and cardiorespiratory endurance versus control. Further, the tablet-based "Discovery Tool" has been used among low-income populations to document barriers in these individuals' PA environment (Buman et al., 2013). The users simply take a picture of a location where their PA is impeded (e.g., a sidewalk that is broken or ends abruptly) at which point the Discovery Tool geocaches the picture—providing direct coordinates to the object in the environment which is limiting PA. This information can then be used to influence modifications in the built environment to better facilitate PA. Nonetheless, until more research teams focus their attention on not widening the health disparities gap with the implementation of emerging technology, this gap will remain a challenge to overcome.

Greater study of the validity and reliability of emerging technology when assessing variables such as PA intensity/type, heart rates and energy expenditure needs to be conducted to further improve upon the accuracy of devices used for these assessment purposes. While some research has been completed to validate emerging technology, such as health wearables (Bai et al., 2016), only a paucity of literature is available on testing these devices in the provision of physiology-related information. Further, health wearables (e.g., Fitbits, and Jawbones) are not the only devices being used to provide information on PA intensity/type and energy expenditure. As other devices, such as smartphones, are more frequently being used to provide the aforementioned type of data to health professionals by way of mHealth apps, more research also needs to be devoted to the validation of these devices in the tracking of physiological outcomes (i.e., heart rate, calories, etc.) as well as the ability of patients/clients to accurately report PA and related health information via mHealth apps (Figure 11.4). While examples within the context of other emerging technologies could be provided, the need for greater study of the validity and reliability of emerging technology in the provision of health information is vital. Indeed, if health professionals do not prove the data provided by emerging technology for healthcare purposes to be valid and reliable, stakeholder buy-in will always remain elusive—particularly within primary care settings where provision of accurate information via these technologies is of paramount importance.

Finally, dissemination of technology that has been proved efficacious in the promotion of PA and health, in addition to the integration of Big Data analysis in technology-based interventions, represent two grand challenges to researchers in the future. Dissemination of efficacious technology is often troublesome in health technology research. While some laboratories investigating the use of technology to improve health and well-being are working hard with industrial collaborators to put these technologies onto the market (see Exertion Games Lab, 2016b), most laboratories lack the resources, reputation, or desire to commercialize their health technology. In order to reverse this trend, more emphasis needs to be placed on

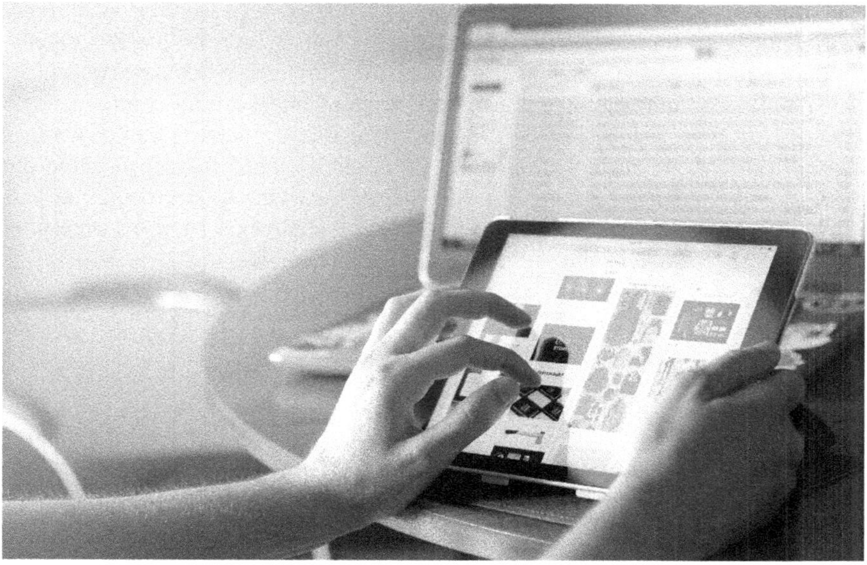

Figure 11.4 Combination of a mobile device and a computer.
Source: pixabay.com.

rewarding researchers for placing their health technology onto the public market, in the form of research grant monies which stipulate researchers shuld have a detailed plan for technology dissemination at the conclusion of the study.

As a final and potentially related challenge, integration of emerging technology needs to place emphasis on Big Data analysis. In the simplest terms, Big Data analysis refers to our ability to used advanced techniques to capture, store, and analyze the rapidly accumulating information present in numerous formats (e.g., text, audio, and video) in our technologically advanced society (TechAmerica Foundation's Federal Big Data Commission, 2012). In brief, the ability to analyze large volumes of health data produced by emerging technologies like the Fitbit might have major implications for healthcare. Specifically, examination of the individual-environment relationship using these large volumes of data could be used in the healthcare system to inform health behavior decisions while also facilitating the development of novel innovations which improve our ability to prevent, treat, and manage diseases. One thing is clear, however. Specifically, the general population needs to decide upon the trade-off between the privacy they wish when using emerging technology (e.g., health wearables) to track health indices as opposed to the amount of personal health information that could potentially be shared by these devices—information which could ultimately be evaluated using Big Data analysis techniques and used by health professionals to improve population-level health and well-being (Kvedar, 2015).

Despite the challenges which face numerous areas of emerging technology in the promotion of health and well-being, one thing remains certain: technology will continue to transform how health professionals treat/train patients/clients. Emerging technology has the power to improve intervention outcomes and facilitate quicker communication and feedback between interventionists and patients/clients. However, just as with any worthwhile endeavor, barriers and challenges are still present. As such, future health professionals need to keep in mind the barriers and challenges outlined in this chapter—striving to overcome the barriers which will subsequently make meeting the challenges of using emerging technology in PA and health promotion more manageable.

References

American Psychiatric Association. (2013). *Diagnostic and statistical manual of mental disorders* (5th ed.). Arlington, VA: American Psychiatric Association.

Bai, Y., Welk, G., Nam, Y., Lee, J., Lee, J.-M., Kim, Y., … Dixon, P. (2016). Comparison of consumer and research monitors under semistructured settings. *Medicine and Science in Sport and Exercise, 48*(1), 151–158.

Borrelli, B. (2011). The assessment, monitoring, and enhancement of treatment fidelity in public health clinical trials. *Journal of Public Health Dentistry, 71*, S52–S63.

Brug, J., Oenema, A., & Ferreira, I. (2005). Theory, evidence, and intervention mapping to improve behavior, nutrition, and physical activity interventions *International Journal of Behavioral Nutrition and Physical Activity, 22*(2), 1–7.

Buman, M., Winter, S., Sheats, J., Hekler, E., Otten, J., Grieco, L., & King, A. (2013). The Standford healthy neighborhood discovery tool: A computerized tool to assess active living environments. *American Journal of Preventive Medicine, 44*(4), e41–e47.

Charara, S. (2016). *Fashion tech: 20 wearables that are more chic than geek.* Retrieved from www.wareable.com/fashion/wearable-tech-fashion-style.

Choo, H., Gentile, D., Sim, T., Li, D., Khoo, A., & Liau, A. (2010). Pathological video-gaming among Singaporean youth. *Annals Academy of Medicine, 39*(11), 822–829.

Exertion Games Lab. (2016a). *LumaHelm-interactive helmet.* Retrieved from http://exertiongameslab.org/projects/lumahelm.

Exertion Games Lab. (2016b). *Projects.* Retrieved from http://exertiongameslab.org/projects.

Festl, R., Scharkow, M., & Quandt, T. (2013). Problematic computer game use among adolescents, younger and older adults. *Addiction, 108*, 592–599.

Gao, Z., Chen, S., Pasco, D., & Pope, Z. (2015). A meta-analysis of active video games on health outcomes among children and adolescents. *Obesity Reviews, 16*, 783–794.

Gao, Z., Hannan, P., Xiang, P., Stodden, D., & Valdez, V. (2013). Video game-based exercise, Latino children's physical health, and academic achievement. *American Journal of Preventive Medicine, 44*(3S3), S240–S246.

Guy, S., Ratzki-Leewing, A., & Gwadry-Sridhar, F. (2011). Moving beyond the stigma: systematic review of video games and their potential to combat obesity. *International Journal of Hypertension, 2011,* 1–13.

Jeromin, F., Rief, W., & Barke, A. (2016). Validation of the Internet Gaming Disorder Questionnaire in a sample of adult German-speaking Internet gamers. *Cyberpsychology, Behavior, and Social Networking, 19*(7), 453–459.

King, A., Glanz, K., & Patrick, K. (2015). Technologies to measure and modify physical activity and eating environments. *American Journal of Preventive Medicine, 48*(5), 630–638.

Kvedar, J. (2015). The privacy trade-offs. In *The internet of healthy things*. Boston, MA: Partners HealthCare Connected Health.

Lobelo, F., Kelli, H., Tejedor, S., Pratt, M., McConnell, M., Martin, S., & Welk, G. (2016). The wild wild west: A framework to integrate mHealth software applications and wearables to support physical activity assessment, counseling, and interventions for cardiovascular disease risk reduction. *Progress in Cardiovascular Diseases, 58*(6), 584–594.

Patten, M. (2014). The role of theory in research. In M. Patten (Ed.), *Understanding research methods: An overview of the essentials* (9th ed., pp. 27–29). Glendale, CA: Pyrczak Publishing.

Richardson, J., & Ancker, J. (2015). Public health perspectives of mobile phones' effects on healthcare quality and medical data security and privacy: A 2-year nationwide survey. Paper presented at the The American Medical Informatics Association Annual Conference Proceedings, 2015.

Serino, M., Cordrey, K., McLaughlin, L., & Milanaik, R. (2016). Pokémon Go and augmented virtual reality games: A cautionary commentary for parents and pediatricians. *Current Opinions in Pediatrics, 28*(5), 673–677.

TechAmerica Foundation's Federal Big Data Commission. (2012). *Demystifying big data: a practical guide to transforming the business of government*. Retrieved from www-304.ibm.com/industries/publicsector/fileserve?contentid=239170.

West, D. (2012). How mobile devices are transforming healthcare. *Issues in Technology Innovation, 18*(1), 1–11.

12 Emerging technologies in promoting physical activity and health

Zan Gao

Throughout this book, an illustration of how emerging technologies have changed and continue to change our lives has been provided. Indeed, emerging technologies have left no scientific field untouched, including the field of physical activity (PA) and health. As stated a number of times within this book, however, technology is like a double-edged sword when viewed through the lens of PA and health promotion. On one hand, technology contributes significantly to physical inactivity and sedentary behavior. On the other hand, researchers are striving to "fight fire with fire"—attempting to use emerging technology to promote PA participation. Notably, as a result of the work of intrepid researchers, emerging technologies have contributed tremendously to the understanding and promotion of PA behaviors—particularly over the past decade. This chapter will conclude the book with an overview of the most pressing issues and relevant considerations related to the implementation of emerging technologies in the promotion of PA and health.

Adoption of social and behavioral theories in promoting PA

To better understand and predict individuals' PA behaviors using emerging technologies, it is imperative to adopt appropriate social and behavioral theories for different target populations. In Chapter 3, we thoroughly elaborated three classifications for these theories: personal-level theories, behavior micro-environmental theories, and behavior macro-environmental theories (King, Stokols, Talen, Brassington, & Killingsworth, 2002). Although only seven out of the numerous social and behavioral theories available were discussed in this book, it is apparent that one personal-level theory (Transtheoretical Model) and one behavior micro-environmental theory (Social Cognitive Theory) have received the most attention in the literature. Undoubtedly, these two theories have greatly enhanced our understanding concerning key correlates and/or determinants of PA behavior. That said, researchers have reached a consensus that human behavior is not exclusively influenced by factors present only at the intrapersonal level or only at the interpersonal level. Rather, PA behavior change is a complex and multifaceted phenomenon influenced by a number of factors at multiple levels. Consequently, relying exclusively on certain intrapersonal or interpersonal level theories does not necessarily lead to successful behavior changes among target populations included in interventions. With the preceding fact in mind, researchers should consider embracing the Social Ecological Model of behavior change as this theory includes intrapersonal (i.e., self-efficacy) and interpersonal level variables (i.e., social support) as well as environmental and policy variables (Buchan, Ollis, Thomas, & Baker, 2012).

Notably, however, recent emerging technologies, including online social media, active video games, and health wearable devices and apps, have brought new challenges to the implementation of theory-based PA intervention strategies—providing a new area of potential exploration for future research. Nonetheless, the choice of assessment and intervention strategy will always be paramount, no matter what emerging technology is employed by researchers implementing PA interventions. In the next section, the reader will be treated to an overview of PA assessment and intervention using emerging technologies to promote PA at different levels (Figure 12.1). Specifically, technology-based PA assessment and intervention will be illustrated at the intrapersonal level (individual) first, followed by an overview of assessment and intervention at the interpersonal and ecological levels (groups and larger population segments and locales).

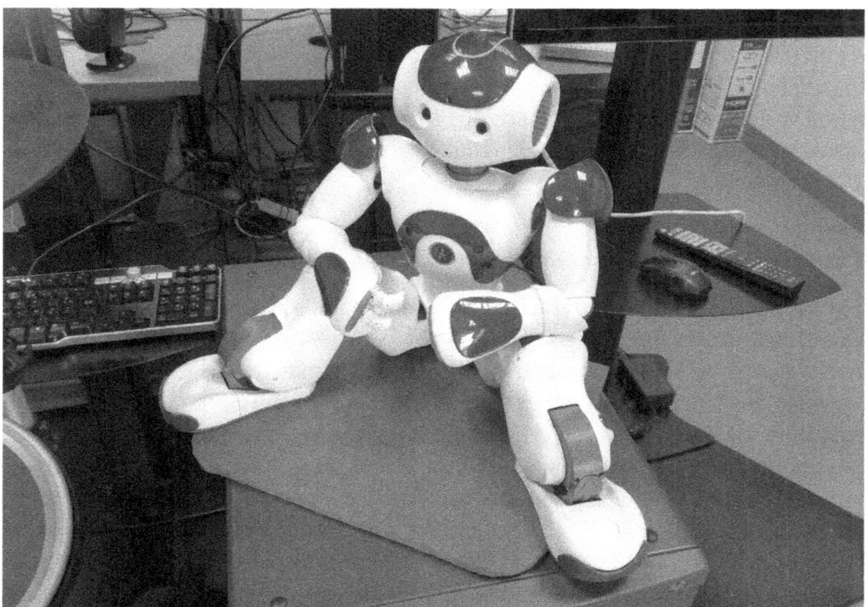

Figure 12.1 Robot, the future direction in technology in promoting health.

Source: Photo by Zan Gao.

Emerging technologies for PA assessment and intervention

Emerging technologies at the intrapersonal level

Use of emerging technologies at the intrapersonal level often include technology which captures an individual's personal PA data, beliefs, health status, and environments—typically in conjunction with proximal contextual information and real-time feedback (King, Glanz, & Patrick, 2015). Given the fact mobile devices are becoming smaller, faster, and less expensive as technology advances, the ubiquity of these devices is increasing daily. In fact, the prevalence of smartphones and other health wearable devices provides tremendous opportunities for assessing a variety of PA data, health outcomes, social interactions, and built environments at the intrapersonal level. For example, MapMyFitness, a popular smartphone exercise app, can track PA variables spatially through use of smartphones' embedded GPS in addition to other attractive functions.

In addition to assessing PA, some emerging technologies can provide platforms for using dynamic personal PA data in combination with local contextual information to provide real-time feedback and guidance for behavior change, thus making intervention programs possible. For instance, in a mobile device intervention study, subjects tracked their walking data, as well as personal and perceived environments (Hekler et al., 2012). Findings suggested that subjects walked, on average, approximately 20 minutes more during instances when they had direct access to a walking path. Further, when employing active video games, empirical studies have indicated that intervention children reported higher levels of self-efficacy and enjoyment and had similar PA levels as compared to control children—perhaps due to the built-in real-time feedback mechanisms of the games (Gao, Huang, Liu, & Xiong, 2012; Gao, Zhang, & Podlog, 2013) (Figure 12.2).

Emerging technologies at the interpersonal and ecological level

Emerging technologies at interpersonal and ecological levels can assess relevant data in the following ways: (1) use of web-based tools such as Google Earth, Google Streetview, and Walk Score to gain a more comprehensive view of individuals' built environments; (2) use of portable mobile or health wearable devices to collect PA data and travel information about larger groups and the environmental factors that might collectively influence individuals' health; (3) designing mobile device apps to facilitate capture of observational PA data (e.g., System for Observing Play and Recreation in Communities); (4) use of self-reported information paired with technological data and aggregate the data among large numbers of people with the goal of tracking PA behavior patterns and determinants for a large population; and (5) tracking a variety of PA data (e.g., duration, distance, frequency, location information, and daily patterns) through Facebook or Twitter or other similar programs (King et al., 2015).

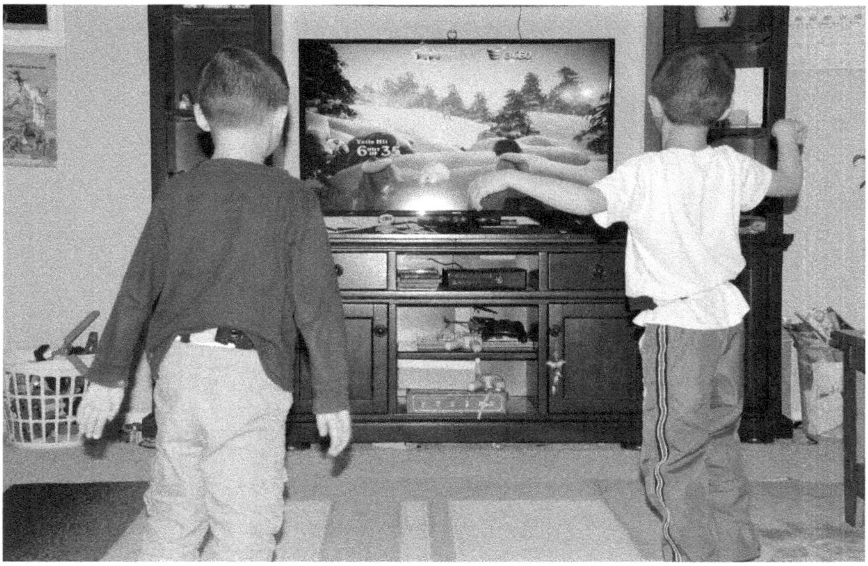

Figure 12.2 Young children playing active video games.
Source: Photo by Zan Gao.

PA interventions at interpersonal and ecological level usually employ online social networking, active video games (Figure 12.3), GPS/GIS, and web-based virtual worlds and community-oriented social networking games to gather data in the abovementioned manners. For example, iDance, an active video game, implemented within school physical education classes, is an example of a PA intervention at the interpersonal level. In detail, iDance allows up to 32 children to dance interactively with the game console, while providing instant scores and voice feedback to all players and stimulating competition among children. Regarding an example of an ecological level PA intervention, one might consider the newly released Pokémon Go app/game. Specifically, Pokémon Go allows users to explore community environments while also building social networks when outside competing with different people for the newest and best Pokémon characters. The preceding examples represent two of many different manners by which researchers and health professionals can intervene to promote PA at the interpersonal and ecological levels. That said, the target level of the PA intervention must always be kept in mind as some emerging technologies lend themselves better to intrapersonal level interventions (e.g., health wearables) while others are more effective at interpersonal or ecological level interventions (e.g., social media, augmented reality mobile device apps.such as Pokémon Go) (Figure 12.4).

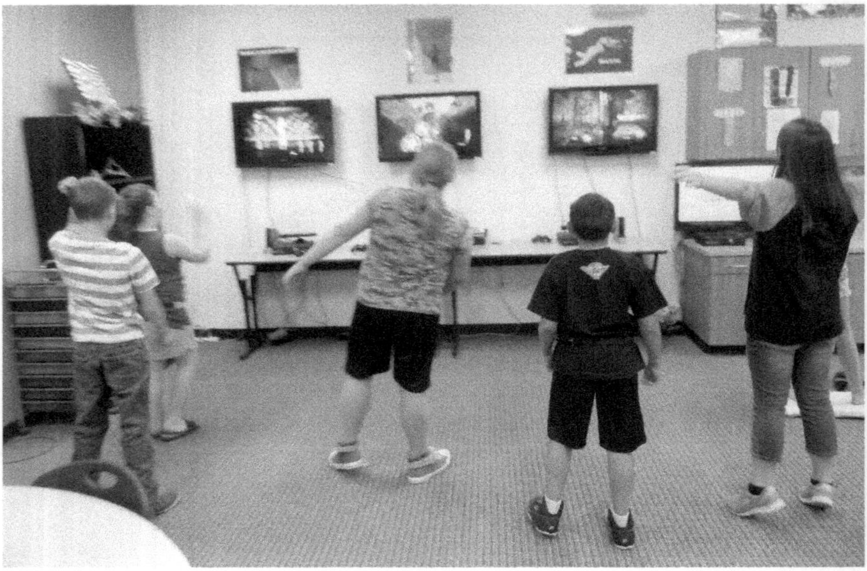

Figure 12.3 Young children playing active video games.

Source: Photo by Zan Gao.

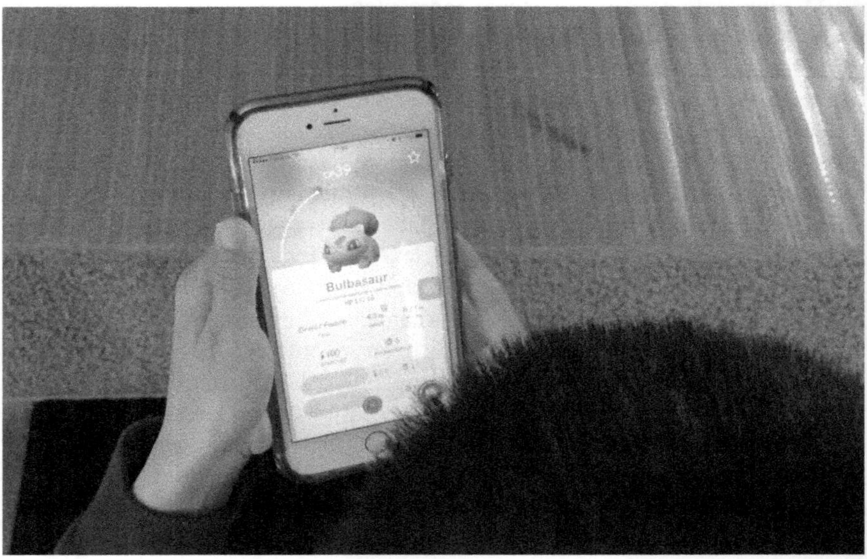

Figure 12.4 A kid playing Pokémon Go.

Source: Photo by Zan Gao.

The Internet of health things

A handful of emerging technologies, as well as the challenges and opportunities associated with these technologies' integration into PA and health promotion, have been elaborated throughout this book. During this review, the following questions might have been posed: What emerging technologies will we use 5 to 10 years from now to promote more healthful behaviors? Relatedly, what should we be doing currently to prepare for that future?

Fortunately, new smart mobile devices and other Internet-based emerging technologies make it possible for all parties (e.g., researchers, healthcare providers, technology companies) to work together in promoting PA and health in powerful and innovative ways that were previously unimaginable. Indeed, many of the cutting-edge studies reviewed in this book have demonstrated the power of smart mobile devices and Internet-based technologies in transforming PA assessment and intervention. Akin to the changing landscape of healthcare over the past decade from reactive to preventive forms of treatment, we can build our own Internet of Health Things with technology and PA to attenuate and prevent chronic diseases. For example, we can connect PA specialists with clients via smart devices such as health wearable devices, smartphones, and wireless weight scales, among other technologies, which these clients possess. Specifically, we would have the potential to provide clients with access to their own real-time health data (e.g., weight taken via a wireless scale, blood pressure taken with a wireless blood pressure cuff) via mobile device apps while using a health wearable device to monitor PA. The preceding data could then be uploaded daily to the Internet via a secure server to healthcare providers. On the basis of the PA specialists' review of a client's real-time health data, health professionals could then proactively develop well-designed, personalized exercise prescriptions to improve clients' health and well-being—offering external incentives to clients for staying physically active and adhering to exercise protocols.

It should be noted, however, that technological advances and the prevalence of chronic diseases are currently driving the development of thousands of apps, devices, sensors, wearables, and Internet-based tools. Despite the well-meaning reasons behind organizations and entities development of these products, research into the effectiveness of many of these emerging technologies is still in its infancy. For instance, little longitudinal data is available concerning how successful these emerging technologies are at enabling users to lose weight, get fit, or sleep better. Further, how emerging technologies empower clients to change health behaviors (e.g., participate in greater PA) and become healthier remains largely unexplored. Therefore, while pursuing this area of inquiry, it is important for researchers and health professionals to keep in mind that improved technology, data, and connectivity will not promote PA and health *per se*. Rather, emerging technologies and their applications have the potential to enable users to change behavior and/or work more effectively when health professionals take care to implement a PA and health intervention using sound theoretical backing and proper intervention fidelity measures.

Cross-technology issues

Advances in emerging technology also raise cross-technology issues. In some cases, health wearable or mobile devices incorporate several technologies, such as accelerometers, GPS, gyroscopes, cameras, light and sound sensors, and even physiological sensors for assessing electrocardiography and heart rate, to better understand correlates and determinants of PA behavior. Recently, platforms integrating multiple sensors have been developed in order to explain complex phenomena that fuse data simultaneously from one or more sensors and one or more behaviors (e.g., tracking both PA and diet data like MapMyFitness). For example, MapMyFitness, a GPS-enabled smartphone app, has been used to assess PA, dietary intake, and other health-related outcomes in a growing number of users. In fact, this type of app may provide detailed contextual information on PA environments on a sizable geographic scale (Hirsch et al., 2014). Indeed, the Personal Activity Location Measurement System, another fully integrated instrument, can provide estimated PA energy expenditure based upon data collected with accelerometers and heart rate monitors along with location data from GPS data loggers (Ellis et al., 2014). Therefore, it seems the next step in this area of inquiry is to more fully integrate data from motion sensors (e.g., accelerometer), contextual sensors (e.g., GPS), and physiological sensors while also including self-reported indicators of health as well (e.g., perceived PA environment, self-efficacy to adhere to an exercise program). As a result of this integration, researchers will be capable of providing a deeper understanding of the interactive effects of contextual and individual-level factors on PA behavior. That said, the following two issues need to be kept in mind when considering cross technology integration. First, smartphones typically run out battery quickly when GPS is utilized. The alternative options would be to use power banks, if possible, or use smartwatches or sports watches with associated app functionality. Second, few studies have employed crowdsourcing to evaluate and manage large datasets in an effort to promote PA and health. Yet, crowdsourcing data in PA and health is the newest and among the most powerful tools presently at researchers' disposal. It is warranted to take advantage of crowdsourcing data in promoting PA in the future. A brief review of crowdsourcing is provided in Chapter 7.

Promote and model digital citizenship

As alluded to above and mentioned throughout the book, it is challenging to assure present-day privacy and anonymity in an era when geo-coded data can be easily associated with behavioral and social data (Gutman & Stern, 2007). Further, although self-tracking and mobile device–based data have been increasingly used for PA promotion, few studies reported how subjects' privacy and confidentiality were handled. In fact, there are substantial concerns regarding how the new digital era is compromising anonymity. Although most people take actions to reduce identifying information associated with their online activities, re-identification of anonymous individuals in separate databases can be accomplished with advanced mathematical strategies (Pew Research Center, 2013). As a result, the expectations of anonymity in traditional PA and health research may be much more difficult to maintain when using present-day emerging technology. To resolve these issues, we must increase the use of technological safeguards such as robust passwords, encryption, and use of secure servers while improving industry vigilance in the prevention of misuse of information. Further, more rigorous consumer education regarding threats to privacy should be offered to facilitate users' expectations concerning data security and protection. According to King et al. (2015), many of the data theft and user identification problems might be alleviated if data security companies offer, at little to no cost, information technology services such as the installation of basic data protection programs to decrease data access vulnerabilities. That said, we advocate that legislative and policy action take place to speed this process.

Additionally, PA research using self-tracking mobile devices and other emerging technologies raises new issues regarding the need to get informed consent from participants. More specifically, if researchers collect PA data over a long period of time or re-use the data in successive experiments, questions arise regarding whether they still need to obtain consent from subjects. Traditionally, informed consent has generally been used for time-limited studies where assessments occurred infrequently. As such, protocols may need to be changed if researchers collect daily PA data from participants using emerging technology. Therefore, it is recommended to fully inform participants of the multiple uses of their data and ensure the participants that the data will be destroyed upon completion of a study. Notably, ethical issues pertinent to new forms of digital data have been investigated since the inception of Internet. Currently, however, Institutional Review Boards hold different perspectives concerning whether issues related to the collection of data via emerging technologies are unique, and thus there is a need to develop formal universal guidelines to address these issues (Buchanan, 2010).

As complex challenges and opportunities regarding the use of emerging technologies in PA and health interventions have been thoroughly discussed in Chapter 2, we wll not reiterate this information here; nor will we restate the directions for future research discussed in each emerging technology's individual chapter. Yet, it is important to note that careful consideration of these challenges, opportunities, and directions for future research set the stage for transformative approaches to scientific discovery and effective intervention implementation in the field of PA and health. Indeed, technology is continuously changing our lives, with the use of these technologies in the promotion of PA taking place most frequently over the last decade. As technology has become more advanced, however, these emerging technologies offer numerous exciting opportunities to assess and promote PA from an innovative paradigm when properly implemented to change individuals' PA behaviors. That said, to effectively assess and promote PA using emerging technology, we need to take into consideration the design, cost, and behavioral theories, as well as build partnerships with the technology industry, communities, interdisciplinary teams, and other relevant public sectors. In this manner, the promise of emerging technology in the facilitation of a more physically active and healthy global population can be more fully realized.

References

Buchan, D. S., Ollis, S., Thomas, N. E., & Baker, J. S. (2012). Physical activity behaviour: An overview of current and emergent theoretical practices. *Journal of Obesity, 2012*. http://doi.org/10.1155/2012/546459.

Buchanan, E. A. (2010). *Internet research ethics and IRBs.* Chicago IL: OHRP Research Forum.

Ellis, K., Godbole, S., Marshall, S., Lanckriet, G., Staudenmayer, J., & Kerr, J. (2014). Identifying active travel behaviors in challenging environments Using GPS, accelerometers, and machine learning algorithms. *Frontiers in Public Health, 2*(April), 36. http://doi.org/10.3389/fpubh.2014.00036.

Gao, Z., Huang, C., Liu, T., & Xiong, W. (2012). Impact of interactive dance games on urban children's physical activity correlates and behavior. *Journal of Exercise Science & Fitness, 10*(2), 107–112. http://doi.org/10.1016/j.jesf.2012.10.009.

Gao, Z., Zhang, P., & Podlog, L. W. (2014). Examining elementary school children's level of enjoyment of traditional tag games vs. interactive dance games. *Psychology, Health & Medicine, 19*(5), 1–9. http://doi.org/10.1080/13548506.2013.845304.

Gutman, M., & Stern, P. (2007). *Putting people on the map: Protecting confidentiality with linked social/spatial data.* Washington, DC: National Academies Press.

Hekler, E. B., Buman, M. P., Dunton, G. F., Atienza, A. A., & King, A. C. (2012). Are daily fluctuations in perceived environment associated with walking after controlling for implementation intentions? *Psychology & Health, 27*(9), 1009–1020.

Hirsch, J. A., James, P., Robinson, J. R. M., Eastman, K. M., Conley, K. D., Evenson, K. R., & Laden, F. (2014). Using MapMyFitness to place physical activity into neighborhood context. *Frontiers in Public Health, 2*, 1–9. http://doi.org/10.3389/fpubh.2014.00019.

King, A. C., Glanz, K., & Patrick, K. (2015). Technologies to measure and modify physical activity and eating environments. *American Journal of Preventive Medicine, 48*(5), 630–638. http://doi.org/10.1016/j.amepre.2014.10.005.

King, A. C., Stokols, D., Talen, E., Brassington, G. S., & Killingsworth, R. (2002). Theoretical approaches to the promotion of physical activity. *American Journal of Preventive Medicine, 23*(2), 15–25. http://doi.org/10.1016/S0749-3797(02)00470-1.

Pew Research Center (2013). *Anonymity, privacy, and security online*. Retrieved from www.pewinternet.org/Reports/2013/Anonymity-online.aspx.

Index

For Product Safety Concerns and Information please contact our EU representative GPSR@taylorandfrancis.com
Taylor & Francis Verlag GmbH, Kaufingerstraße 24, 80331 München, Germany

www.ingramcontent.com/pod-product-compliance
Ingram Content Group UK Ltd.
Pitfield, Milton Keynes, MK11 3LW, UK
UKHW020011200926
475702UK00014B/1825
* 9 7 8 0 3 6 7 3 7 4 4 9 5 *